Counseling across Cultures

Counseling
across
Cultures

THIRD EDITION

Edited by

Paul B. Pedersen
Juris G. Draguns
Walter J. Lonner
Joseph E. Trimble

University of Hawaii Press

Honolulu

94 93 92 91 90 89   5 4 3 2 1

Library of Congress Cataloging-in-Publication Data

Counseling across cultures / edited by Paul B. Pedersen . . . [et al.].
   —3rd ed.
     p.   cm.
   Includes bibliographies and index.
   ISBN 0-8248-1231-X
   1. Cross-cultural counseling.   2.   Psychiatry, Transcultural.
I. Pedersen, Paul, 1936–   .
   [DNLM: 1. Counseling. 2. Cross-Cultural Comparison.   WM 55 C853]
BF637.C6C63   1989
616.89'14—dc19
DNLM/DLC   88-39249
for Library of Congress   CIP

(∞)^TM   *The paper used in this publication meets the minimum requirements of American National Standard for Information Sciences—Per-
manence of paper for Printed Library Materials*
                                        ANSI Z39.48–1984

To our wives
Anne B. Pedersen
Marie Draguns
Marilyn S. Lonner
Molly E. Trimble

Contents

Preface

Counseling across Cultures is generally recognized as the earliest of a number of comprehensive books addressing the problems that are inevitably involved in multicultural counseling. The idea for the book originated from the 1973 meeting of the American Psychological Association in Montreal, at which a group of seven psychologists organized a symposium entitled "Counseling across Cultures." The symposium was well attended and positively received by its audience. The presenters were so enthusiastic about their shared interest that the papers were developed further, revised, and organized into a manuscript that, with the addition of several more chapters, was published in 1976 by the University Press of Hawaii as an East-West Culture Learning Institute monograph entitled *Counseling across Cultures*. The first edition went through five printings. The need to update certain chapters and add new ones resulted in a second edition, published in 1981. Now once again we have found it necessary to revise and augment the book. This third edition builds on the success of the previous editions to provide an updated review of the issues, alternative models, and applications of cultural data and information that are important to the process of counseling.

Mental health professionals generally agree that the cultural background of both the client and the counselor influences the way counseling is conducted and the way it is received. There are, however, few training opportunities for counselors who work with culturally different clients. Instead, mental health services tend to be delivered as though clients and counselors shared the same value assumptions, in spite of abundant evidence to the contrary. Additionally, there continue to be few mental health training programs available where mental health professionals can receive credentials in cross-cultural counseling or therapy. No validated tests, scales, or measures of intercultural counseling exist to gauge effectiveness. There are no review boards that can be used to appraise the readiness of a counselor for work in multicultural settings. Moreover, disproportionately few minority members are trained as mental health workers, even though minorities contribute a large share of clientele. Prominent professional journals in the mental health field still contain relatively few articles on cross-cultural counseling and therapy, although there seems to be a slight increase over the past decade. Professional mental health associations, likewise, continue to give scant attention to these issues at their annual meetings, despite the fact that some positive change can be discerned during the past few years. And until recently there was a dearth of textbooks attempting to present a comprehensive overview of cross-cultural counseling.

The same general belief that stimulated the initial publication of *Counseling across Cultures* in 1976 provides the impetus for this new edition—that cross-cultural counseling and therapy, because they are so frequently done either by referral, by circumstance, and sometimes by choice, require that their practitioners be acquainted with the central issues and problems affecting competent work in the area.

This edition of *Counseling across Cultures* contains thirteen chapters that are organized in four parts, with each part filling a separate function. The reader may want to read the book from start to finish, which proceeds from the general to the specific. Or the reader may elect to concentrate initially on particular chapters of special importance that complement other publications on multicultural counseling. The book is designed for people without an extensive background in either cross-cultural counseling or cross-cultural research. Moreover, the chapters do not presume an extensive clinical background. The book is essentially an introduction to the exciting and important field of counseling across cultures.

The first part is a basic introduction to the ideas, language, methods, and approaches that have been used in multicultural counseling. Draguns' chapter introduces the basic themes that cut across theories and methods of cross-cultural counseling. The chapter provides a framework for organizing the unique aspects of multicultural counseling with the more familiar aspects of what might be called "generic" counseling. Pedersen, Fukuyama, and Heath review the research literature on which counseling across cultures is based. The same basic themes of client, counselor, or environmental variables that are familiar to all counselors take on a special meaning when the research is focused on multicultural populations.

The second part deals with controversial issues likely to arise both within multicultural counseling and between those with a multicultural perspective and colleagues who do not share that perspective. Ridley's chapter identifies the elements of racism as they influence counseling and counselors. Although the emphasis in Ridley's chapter is on ethnic minority issues, the principles apply to the full range of relationships between minority and majority cultures. Wohl's chapter provides a more international and cross-disciplinary perspective to the wider field of cross-cultural counseling. LaFromboise and Foster provide the best review to date of ethical issues related to multicultural counseling. This important matter has been referred to most national counseling associations in the United States, and now LaFromboise and Foster provide the documentation for an informed discussion on multicultural ethics.

Part three considers some of the many alternative models of multicultural counseling. The selection presented here is not complete, but it does provide a sample of different approaches that contrast with a dominant culture description of counseling. Kitano reviews the ways in which a Japanese-American background influences the counseling process, combining both "Japanese" and "American" stereotyped aspects. Casas and Vasquez document the importance of bilingual and bicultural counseling approaches with special reference to Hispanic people. The rapid growth of Hispanics relative to other segments of the U.S. population indicates a considerable need to know more about models that work in a Hispanic setting. Trimble and Fleming review literature describing counseling the American Indian client. The great diversity within the American Indian population is often overlooked in stereotyped treatments. Thomas and Althen provide practical guidelines for counseling international students. This large and complex cadre of multivaried populations requires the special application of multicultural counseling skills. In her chapter, Lefley reviews the extensive literature on counseling refugees from a variety of different cultural backgrounds. The considerable differences among refugees has sometimes disguised the patterns of similarities across cultures for persons with refugee status.

Part four explores measurement and research applications. Tanaka-Matsumi and Higginbotham integrate the extensive literature on behavioral counseling and its use in multicultural settings. Identifying appropriate reinforcing events and interpreting culturally different behaviors accurately requires specialized knowledge. Lonner and Ibrahim review the problems and opportunities associated with the use of psychological tests and related data-gathering devices that may be useful in cross-cultural counseling. Sundberg and Sue examine the research process for colleagues doing dissertations or writing research proposals on multicultural issues. There are a great many research projects in multicultural issues waiting to be designed and carried out.

The composition of the United States population is changing. According to the 1980 census, 50 million (21%) of the 240 million Americans are black, Hispanic, or Asian. Demographic projections suggest that by the year 2000 one of every three Americans will be nonwhite. Between 1970 and 1980 Hispanics alone increased their share of the U.S. population by 61%, and numbers of Hispanics are estimated to have grown an additional 30% since 1980. Comparative growth rates for the period 1970–1980 are 6% for whites, and 18% for blacks, and 11% for the U.S. population as a whole. Projecting these current growth rates, Hispanics will outnumber blacks by the turn of the century and become the largest segment of the minority population. In addition to these internal data, there is also a high rate of immigration, including 544,000 legal and 3,500,000 illegal immigrants in 1984. Counselors and counseling must prepare for a multicultural clientele.

This book is inevitably oriented toward cross-cultural counseling in the United States. After all, the four editors are American, as are all the authors. However, many of the problems, issues, and principles raised here may, with minor adjustments, generalize to other pluralistic societies. Canadian mental health workers, for example, should benefit from most of the material in this book. The extent to which the ideas and principles contained here will generalize to other societies is an open question. However, it is our opinion that there will be many similarities in problems and issues encountered by those who engage in cross-cultural counseling wherever it may be practiced or attempted.

Counseling across Cultures is an attempt to help persons from all cultural backgrounds prepare to work more constructively with one another. We, the editors and contributors, have found the preparation of this book to be challenging and rewarding. We continue to be intrigued and excited about the complex phenomenon known as cross-cultural counseling, and we hope that you will share our enthusiasm.

> Paul B. Pedersen
> Juris G. Draguns
> Walter J. Lonner
> Joseph E. Trimble

PART ONE

Introduction and Overview

The chapters in this section introduce the problems, topics, language, and issues of multicultural counseling to guide the reader unfamiliar with counseling across cultures. The chapters will provide a useful framework for discussion of specific issues for readers more familiar with the multicultural counseling literature as well.

Juris B. Draguns' chapter on dilemmas and choices in cross-cultural counseling combines a perspective of universal issues that apply to all counseling with those aspects unique to specific cultural settings. This chapter seeks to define, or perhaps redefine, counseling in a cultural setting. There are certain assumptions that must be challenged, language that must be defined, and concepts that must be explained before the reader proceeds further into the literature on counseling across cultures.

Paul B. Pedersen, Mary Fukuyama, and Anne Heath build on the definition of counseling across culture to look at the abundance of research on client, counselor, and contextual variables in multicultural counseling. Multicultural counseling is not an exotic topic that applies to remote regions but is the heart and core of good counseling with any client. The considerable research documenting the importance of cultural variables is readily available and needs to be included in the study of counseling generally. This chapter seeks to guide the reader through that literature.

1

Dilemmas and Choices in Cross-Cultural Counseling: The Universal versus the Culturally Distinctive

JURIS G. DRAGUNS

The Present Status of Cross-Cultural Counseling

In the early 1970s there were no books on counseling and culture. Now there are many. This trend shows the increased professional awareness of cultural factors and of their relevance in counseling. In this chapter I propose to identify those factors, consider their importance, and, in general, provide a raison d'être for cross-cultural counseling. I also intend to articulate a number of major issues on which the practitioner of cross-cultural psychology must take a stand. In the process, I will try to disentangle the humanly universal and the culturally distinctive components of counseling.

Defining Culture

Counseling and culture refer to concepts that most of us intuitively understand. Yet, both of these terms have fuzzy boundaries; their outer limits are not easily determined. With Herskovits (1948, 17) we define culture as the "man-made part of the environment." But here we want to consider the less tangible aspects of culture, the socially shared aspects of experience and knowledge. This "culture in our heads" or, more formally, subjective culture (Triandis 1972) is part and parcel of our personal reality. It is not explicitly taught nor is it effortfully learned. Rather, it is absorbed in the process of socialization and strengthened and amplified in the course of lifelong incidental learning. The perceptions, expectations, and other cognitions that are culturally mediated are experienced as both unobtrusive and self-evident. In its unobtrusiveness, culture is like the air we breathe; only when we are deprived of it do we become aware of it. Typically, such a state occurs

3

when we are removed from our customary habitat. The confrontation with a different way of doing things brings into bold relief our relative and human-made—that is, cultural—assumptions, beliefs, and practices. We would be able to recognize strong cultural differences if we were to come into contact with the Inuit of the Canadian Arctic or the Pygmies of Central Africa. But the relative and conditional nature of our working assumptions about human beings and the world they live in is also evident in our interactions even with our immediate neighbors, who are quite possibly of different ethnic or racial backgrounds. Cultural differences impinge upon us not only around the globe but also around the block. In the pluralistic society of North America, and of many other places, cultural diversity is an inevitable part of day-to-day experience.

Defining Counseling

Not surprisingly then, cultural variety invades and challenges the operations of counseling. The scope of counseling is here broadly defined to encompass any and all professional techniques and activities that are undertaken to resolve human problems. That goal is usually accomplished by principally verbal techniques in the context of a client-counselor relationship in which the roles of the participants are sharply distinguished. The client brings to this task questions, conflicts, choices, often accompanied by personal distress; the counselor supposedly has the professional skills to facilitate the resolution of these problems. This objective is usually accomplished by marshalling the client's own, actual or potential, personal resources. Certain interventions are generally avoided in counseling, such as imposing an external solution by exhortation or persuasion, and disregarding the client's feelings, values, or inclinations in the process.

Counseling is thus a generic term for helpful interpersonal communication. At one extreme is guidance counseling, with its important component of providing information related to careers and schooling. At the other extreme is psychotherapy, which focuses on changing behavior and personality and promoting more adaptive functioning. The difference between counseling and psychotherapy is not sharp, and quite often the same professional practices both, under either or both titles. The objective of the counselor is usually to change a specific activity or behavior in an otherwise adequately functioning person; for example, getting a client to stop smoking. The goal of the psychotherapist is more global; it involves the change and reorganization of a person's adaptive resources, that is, his or her personality. We will use the term counseling to encompass the continuum from guidance to psychotherapy.

Counseling and Culture in Contact

Counseling is the product of twentieth-century Euroamerican civilization. In particular, its ethos is bound up with certain key features of American culture: individualism, egalitarianism, glorification of social mobility and social change. From the start counseling has been imbued with a strong sense of respect for self-determination. The counselor's task was conceived as helping the counselee chart his or her best course of action, and it was assumed that this could best be accomplished in the presence of a sympathetic but not meddlesome helper. For several generations, however, American counselors did not accord the same recognition to their clients' cultural diversity as they did to their individuality. No doubt many counselors implicitly and intuitively recognized and accommodated the importance of cultural components in their clients' lives. In many other cases, however, the experience of counseling floundered on the rocks of cultural misunderstandings, failures of communication, and clashes of expectations.

Specifically, practitioners of a generation ago found many of their culturally different clients unmotivated, resistant, and lacking in psychological mindedness. Undoubtedly, many of their clients thought their counseling sessions baffling, irrelevant, and generally unhelpful. We have only gradually come to realize that much counseling as it was then generally practiced did not fit the needs of a great many actual or potential counselees and that this lack of fit was the result of the diverging, or even clashing, expectations of counselees and counselors, both the products of different cultural backgrounds. The challenge to bridge this gap, which has been taken up in the past two decades, is expressed widely in the cross-cultural literature (Abel, Métraux, and Roll 1987; Atkinson, Morten, and Sue 1979; Henderson 1979; Marsella and Pedersen 1981; Pedersen 1985; Pedersen, Lonner, and Draguns 1976; Pedersen et al. 1981; Samuda and Wolfgang 1984; Pedersen, Sartorius, and Marsella 1984; Sue 1981; Vontress 1979; Walz and Benjamin 1978).

The Practical Challenge

Recognizing the need for cross-cultural counseling is a problem encountered by a great many practitioners. And the culturally different or atypical client may be bewildered and confused by the counseling services offered. Consequently, such a client does not benefit from counseling and frequently fails to return for any future appointments. Unfortunately, the responsibility for these failures has been often attributed to the client. The consensus among modern counselors is to accommodate culturally different clients instead of reject them. Three developments

are responsible for this shift. First and foremost, the growing assertiveness of minority and ethnic groups in the United States and elsewhere
has made it politically unrealistic to reject a large proportion of minority
or ethnic group counselees as unsuitable for counseling services. Second, the emerging subdiscipline of cross-cultural psychology (Triandis
et al. 1980; Brislin 1983; Segall 1986) has succeeded in demonstrating
the impact of culture upon all domains of behavior and experience,
including the counselor-client relationship. Third, a more sophisticated
conceptualization of psychotherapy as a "transaction" has superseded
the simplistic assignment of blame for any failures to either counselor or
counselee. Rather, conflicts are now more constructively understood in
light of their contexts and structures. And these contextual variables are
inevitably embedded in culture. Concurrent with these developments,
models have been proposed that incorporate cultural factors into counseling. Even when the counselor and counselee are of the same culture,
counseling (as well as psychotherapy) can be construed as a culture-
learning process (Draguns 1975). In that formulation culture is considered an invisible and silent participant in the counseling transactions of
the counselor and counselee. The role of culture is even more obvious
when clients and counselors of different cultural backgrounds encounter
one another. Expectations, meanings, and unspoken assumptions have
to be considered lest misunderstandings lead to disappointment, frustration, and failure. If the role of culture is overlooked, the flow of communication can become obstructed, and the development of a relationship may be aborted.

The Emerging Consensus

Most proponents of cross-cultural counseling agree on a few basic
points. First, the techniques or activities of counselors have to be modified as they are applied across a cultural gulf. Not everything about
counseling as it is practiced with typical middle-class North American
clients is immutable or sacrosanct. Second, complications in the counseling process are anticipated as the distance between the cultural backgrounds of the counselor and the counselee increases. The culturally
sensitive and competent counselor not only expects difficulties to occur
but is prepared to cope with them and to resolve them. Third, conceptions of counseling or, more broadly, of the helping process are cultural
as are approved modes of self-presentation and of the communication of
distress. Fourth, complaints and symptoms differ in their frequency of
occurrence in cultural groups (see Draguns 1973, 1980, 1985, 1987;
Leff 1981; Marsella 1979; Murphy 1982; Favazza and Oman 1978);
there may also be qualitative differences, that is certain symptoms may

be absent and others uniquely present in a group. This last point remains controversial and subject to debate (see Draguns 1980; Weidman and Sussex 1971; Yap 1969), and its relevance for the practical enterprise of counseling is open to question. Fifth, cultural norms and expectations may also vary. Thus, clients from different cultures have adjusted to different social realities. What the culturally perceptive counselor needs to know is how cultural characteristics translate into the subjective goals of clients.

Contexts of Application

When and where are cross-cultural considerations relevant? In the culturally diverse settings of the United States and Canada as well as of many other countries, these concerns apply first of all to minority groups, distinct from the majority or mainstream cultures and defined on the basis of racial characteristics, historical heritage, and language background. In the United States the minority groups officially recognized by the Department of Health and Human Services—Blacks, Hispanics, American Indians, several East and Southeast Asian groups, and Pacific Islanders—share the experience of institutionalized oppression; discrimination; and social, political, educational, and economic disadvantage. Added to these legally recognized minorities, there is a host of other ethnic groups, sometimes inexactly and casually subsumed under the label of "white ethnics," whose languages, customs, and, above all, identities are linked with their ancestral cultures in Europe and elsewhere. Included are Americans of Irish, Polish, Greek, German, Eastern European and Middle Eastern Jewish, Swedish, Lithuanian, and Italian descent. Some of these are first-generation immigrants; others may be four, five, or more generations removed from their ancestral roots. Some bonds to their culture of origin always remains, however, and in some cases they are pervasive and strong enough to require modifications in counseling. A standard reference work (Thernstrom 1980) lists and describes more than 110 distinct ethnic groups in the United States. Some of them include only a few hundred people, others several million. All of them constitute important, and in some cases central, reference groups for their members. It is impossible and unnecessary to adjust counseling techniques to each of these, and it is certainly inadvisable to do so just on the basis of a person's known descent or heritage. For some of the more frequently seen groups, Giordano and Giordano (1976, 1977) and McGoldrick, Pearce, and Giordano (1982) have provided practical hints that should be kept in mind—although not automatically applied—when counseling members of the group in question.

There are two additional categories of individuals included as potential candidates for cross-cultural counseling. A large number of temporary residents and "sojourners" (Church 1982) converge upon the educational institutions of their host countries. In contrast to other visitors, such as tourists or diplomats, the success of their stay in the host country is often predicated upon their ability to plunge into the new culture and to interact with its members. Often this process is stressful; it can also generate helplessness and distress. Counseling may enhance coping and alleviate distress in sojourners.

Outside of North America another prominent category of sojourners and potential users is that of guest workers. Attracted to the superior wage-earning opportunities in the developed and prosperous countries of Western Europe, they and their families have left their homes in the Mediterranean region to establish themselves in the very different cultural milieus of their host countries. Their stay is expected to be limited to the duration of a labor contract. For a variety of reasons, however, years often stretch into decades, and some of these sojourners never return to their own countries. A descriptive, clinical, and experimental literature has come into being on the psychological situation of guest workers and on their vulnerabilities and unmet needs (Deen 1985; Minsel and Herff 1985). One response to their situation has been the provision of counseling services (e.g., Martin and DeVolder 1983). In the United States there is no formal or official category of temporary residents admitted for employment reasons. But "internal" migrants similarly traverse an important cultural gulf. For example, the many Puerto Ricans who continually come and go between the continental United States and Puerto Rico (Prewitt-Diaz and Draguns 1987) cross no international frontier but are still faced with as different a cultural reality as that confronted by Algerians in Paris, Turks in Amsterdam, and Portuguese in Geneva. And, of course, the illegal or undocumented migrants in the United States, mainly from Latin America, share many experiences with the officially admitted guest workers of Western Europe. Added to the stresses of readaptation is the reality-based insecurity about being found out and deported. This ever-present fear stands in the way of initiating counseling services based on trust and the readiness to accept help from professionally qualified strangers.

Sojourners, whether students or guest workers, come voluntarily and, for the most part, individually or in small groups. Refugees typically leave their native lands under duress and are displaced suddenly and en masse. Their arrival in their countries of asylum is often preceded by traumatic and life-threatening experiences and is almost invariably associated with personal, social, and economic losses. At the same time, their sudden flight brings with it demands for rapid readaptation and integration into their host cultures, often leading to intense personal and occupational stresses. Counseling relationships can also help refugees.

The Outer Reaches of Cross-Cultural Counseling

The broad categories of individuals we have just discussed share the feature of being perceptibly and unambiguously different from the mainstream of the culture in which they find themselves. With many other groups of people, the relevance of cultural factors is a lot less easily detected. In pluralistic cultures, such as those of Canada and the United States, cross-cultural encounters are more of a rule then an exception. And as Pedersen (1981) has reminded us, differences in cultural backgrounds, even if subtle, are likely to come into play in the majority of counseling contacts in multicultural settings. Any two participants in a counseling transaction bring to it different combinations of socialization, heritage, expectations, and implicit theories of human nature and philosophies of life. Freedman (1985), a pioneer in the new field of clinical sociology, has provided numerous examples of cultural factors impinging upon a variety of clinical situations, including those affecting individuals in the cultural mainstream. Particularly prominent are the problems of traditionally religious clients, Orthodox Jews, Evangelical Protestants, Mormons, and others who often harbor distrust and skepticism toward mental health professionals and their allegedly antireligious orientation (Draguns and McLatchie 1986; Feinberg 1986; McLatchie and Draguns 1984). McLatchie and Draguns (1984) found that rural Evangelical Protestants, not usually considered a minority or culturally different group, were prepared to accept help from mental health professionals but were fearful of any attempts by secular therapists to alter their beliefs and values. The conceptions and practices of modern mental health intervention were found to fit poorly their needs and expectations. On the basis of these findings, however, treatment approaches have been designed to alleviate distrust and to augment the acceptance of psychotherapy by evangelical clients (Draguns and McLatchie 1986).

In other cases culture itself and its relationship to the individual have become the central issue in counseling (Giordano and Giordano 1976, 1977; McGoldrick et al. 1982). In a pluralistic society people have a number of options, from encapsulation within their own cultural reference group to a blanket rejection of their membership in it, behaviorally and psychologically (cf. Taft 1977). These choices often involve internal conflict associated with anxiety and distress. Giordano and Giordano (1977) have pioneered techniques to address issues of ethnic identity. I have observed with a small number of clinical cases that a serious psychological disturbance may disrupt the relationship with and even cause a violent rejection of the person's cultural group. This phenomenon is dramatically exemplified by a psychotic Jewish adolescent who was fascinated with Naziism and who even came to identify himself with it. On a less extreme and more commonly encountered level, counseling can often disentangle the nexus of ambivalent and complex feelings about a client's heritage and help the client define himself or herself in a socially complex and culturally pluralistic world.

Controversies and Misunderstandings

Cross-cultural counseling has generally provoked little controversy. The notion of accommodating the needs of culturally different clients and of modifying counseling techniques and practices to that end is widely, though not universally, accepted. Patterson (1978), for example, proceeding from an outspoken, universalist point of view, rejects the tenets and practices of cross-culturalism. The gist of his position is well expressed in the following quotation:

> The role of counseling and psychotherapy is to facilitate the development of self-actualization in clients. Cultures can be evaluated in terms of their contribution to the self-actualization of their members. The major conditions for the development of self-actualizing persons are known, and must be present in counseling and psychotherapy as practiced with any client regardless of culture. These conditions are not time-bound nor culture-bound. The problems of practicing counseling or psychotherapy in other cultures are viewed as problems of implementing these conditions. Certain characteristics of clients which present obstacles to the implementation of the conditions are associated with certain cultures. Until cultural changes lead to change in these characteristics, counseling or psychotherapy will be difficult and in some cases impossible with certain clients from certain cultures. Structuring and client education and training may change client expectations and make therapy possible. In any case, however, to accede to client expectations, abandoning methods which have been demonstrated to be related to self-actualization as an outcome of counseling or psychotherapy, is to abandon self-actualization as the goal, and to accept goals which are often inconsistent with self-actualization. (Patterson 1978, 133)

Patterson decries the efforts to modify counseling for application in other cultures. He finds the tenor of such proposals "negative, focusing upon the numerous problems and difficulties associated with cultural differences" (Patterson 1978, 120). The problems that are addressed, he maintains, are not unique to cross-cultural counseling but are inherent in counseling as a whole, which inevitably involves the counselor with clients different in age, gender, biographical experience, and social background. Patterson concedes the need to adjust counseling techniques to the expectation of the client, especially in his more recent writings (Patterson 1986). He disagrees, however, with some of the practitioners of cross-cultural counseling when they appear to advocate the development of different sets of skills, emphasis, and insights for use in each culture.

This critique rests on several misunderstandings of cross-cultural counseling in theory and in practice. Contrary to what Patterson asserts, cross-cultural counseling does not proceed from the assumption of radical cultural relativism, that is, the acceptance of the belief that each culture is unique and different and that all cultures are equal in value. Moreover, cross-cultural counselors do not view their clients' cultures as sacrosanct and immutable. Their attitude toward the cultural backgrounds of their counselees can be more accurately described as one of respect rather than of idealization or glorification. However, they recognize that their expertise and mandate is not to change the culture, but to enable change to take place in the counselee. As far as the counselee's relationship to his or her culture is concerned, it is a matter of the counselee's choice and decision. The basic premise of cultural extension and modification of the counseling enterprise is more modest. Cross-cultural counselors are only in agreement that cultural differences are relevant to counselor practices and that modifications in all aspects of counseling may be necessary for it to be effective with culturally different clients.

Cross-cultural counselors also reject the notion that whatever does not aim at self-actualization is not counseling. Counseling starts with distress that the counselee cannot alleviate or with a problem he or she cannot solve. In line with the ethos of counseling and psychotherapy as expressed by Rogers (1957), the goals of counseling are left up to the counselee. Self-actualization is an important and worthy but not a universal goal. If there is a pancultural feature in counseling, it involves redressing the balance between the individual and society, often toward self-actualization, but not infrequently toward the acceptance of greater social control (Draguns 1975). Moreover, in our empirical knowledge of the phenomenon of self-actualization we have not progressed much beyond Maslow's (1956) original descriptive accounts. Specifically, we know nothing about the manifestation and role of self-actualization in other cultures. That knowledge and, more generally, information on the characteristics of optimally functioning persons in other cultures would be extremely valuable to obtain (Draguns 1984).

Despite the misunderstandings in Patterson's critique, it constructively raises basic questions on the limits of cultural accommodation and on the universal versus the particular components of counseling services. Can its techniques and approaches be transformed without doing violence to counseling at its core? Patterson himself is not quite consistent in his attempts to answer that question. Originally, as we have seen, he allowed for the possibility that counseling may be impossible in some cultural settings. More recently, on the basis of his observation of counseling in Hong Kong, he offered a number of suggestions for modifying counselors' behavior and expectations as well as changing the interiors of counselors' offices. Patterson's suggestions are similar to recommendations in this volume and elsewhere for meeting the culturally different counselee halfway (e.g., Vontress 1981) that he had earlier castigated. The inconsistencies between his two positions illustrate the problem of delineating the degree to which counseling may change without compromising its basic nature.

The Evolution of Cross-Cultural Counseling: Dilemmas and Options

There are two main approaches to cross-cultural research. In the first approach an investigation may start with characteristics and constructs deemed to be universal, that is, applicable equally anywhere in the world. An investigator may, for example, assume that all human groups display aggressive behavior; then he might try to establish differences in aggression across cultures in manner and degree. This is the etic research strategy. (See Berry 1979; Malpass 1977; Price-Williams 1974.) The other approach begins with an indigenous characteristic or construct. An example is the Japanese concept of *amaeru*, translated "to presume upon another person's benevolence" (Doi 1973). This term is applied to a complex pattern of dependency and seeking gratification from others. An investigation of *amaeru* may try to reveal how it is inculcated in the course of socialization in Japan or how it accounts for a variety of normal and abnormal behaviors in adulthood. This is the emic strategy. Thus, the emic approach proceeds from within the culture; the etic approach is initiated from the outside on the basis of generic human dimensions, actual or alleged.

The same dichotomy applies to cross-cultural counseling. The counselor has the choice of starting with the different cultural reality of the client or with what the counselor and the counselee share with one another and with humanity. The two operations that come into play have been described by Stewart (1976, 1981) as of empathy and sympathy. In the former case the task of the counselor is to "tune into" a subjective reality different from his or her own; in the latter the counselor experiences sympathy, the recognition of commonality of emotions and experiences with another person.

Authorities on counseling—from Patterson (1978) to Wohl in this volume—have commented upon the difficulties of effectively offering helping services across a wide cultural gulf and have arrived at different conclusions on the likelihood and manner of crossing cultural barriers. At one end of the continuum, culturally perceptive counselors have been aware of the potential for misunderstandings and complications resulting from cultural differences, even when the language, residence, and many of the visible characteristics of the counseling dyad are the same. How can a white unicultural counselor understand the rage and fear of a black with a memory of lynchings in his family or the grief, guilt, and rage of some of the survivors of the Holocaust? There are few guidelines for blending the emic and the etic elements in the practice of counseling.

The major theories of counseling psychology—psychoanalytic, behavioral, cognitive, and existential—proceed from an etic point of departure. They have the potential, however, of coming to grips with and incorporating culturally characteristic elements, as demonstrated, for example, by Tanaka-Matsumi and Higginbotham in this volume. The principle of reinforcement is universal—in fact it is valid across the species—but effective reinforcers are determined culturally. Similarly, Abel, Métraux, and Roll (1987) have extended the psychoanalytic approach to culturally diverse groups and have demonstrated how cultural and personal influences are, for example, interwoven in transference or how the report and experience of dreams differ in several cultural groups. From the existential point of view, Vontress (1979) has proposed an outlook that is grounded in universals yet culturally sensitive.

The opposite route is taken by those whose counseling efforts are grounded in the culturally indigenous modes of helping, as exemplified by Jilek (1982) in incorporating Indian healing rituals and Indian healers' services in therapeutic programs in British Columbia. Another example is provided by Nishihara (1978) who incorporated the traditional Hawaiian technique of *ho'oponopono,* a communal approach to solving individual problems, in counseling Hawaiian clients. Such applications are as yet less frequent than the adaptations of Western therapies to culturally different clients. With the decline of Western ethnocentrism and the growing realization of the cultural origins of their own interventions among counselors and other helping professionals, their scope and impact can be expected to increase.

It is probably impossible to carry out counseling that is based purely on the etic or emic approach. The question remains as to what blend of these two ingredients to use. Counseling in exclusively the same, presumably universal, way reveals cultural insensitivity and is a prescription for failure. Yet, it is neither desirable nor practical to focus exclusively on cultural differences. To some degree all humans are cut of the same cloth, and this realization applies to their problems of living and their attempts at coping with them. The best approach is somewhere in between, even though we do not yet know exactly where.

Changing the Self versus Changing the Environment

In coping with the world, all humans respond either autoplastically, by modifying their behavior to accommodate external circumstances, or alloplastically, by imposing changes upon the world at large (cf. Vexliard 1968). This dichotomy is related to the balance between assimilation and accommodation that, as Piaget maintains, is present in all adaptation (Piaget 1950; Flavell 1963). Applied to counseling, the autoplastic-alloplastic distinction sparks the questions, How much should the counselee be helped to accept a situation as given and how much should he or she be encouraged to actively change it? We know that cultures differ in this variable. Latin Americans, for example, are traditionally socialized to accept the vicissitudes of life and to endure them gracefully; North Americans are taught throughout their lives to confront obstacles in their path and, if possible, to remove them (cf. Diaz-Guerrero 1967; Holtzman, Diaz-Guerrero, and Swartz 1975). To what extent are these two contrasting attitudes to be modified in counseling or, conversely, fostered and accommodated?

Historically, counseling and related services have been autoplastically slanted, whether they were applied within or across cultures. The mandate of the counselor, after all, is to reorganize and improve the skills and resources of the client rather than change the social structure within which he or she operates. But what should a counselor do when the attainment of clients' goals is blocked by societal oppression or discrimination? There are some leads in the cross-cultural literature that suggest that majority and minority counselors perceive this situation differently and advocate different courses of action. Berman (1979) found, in an analogue study, that white counselors explained their counselees' behavior on the basis of personal, internal factors. By contrast, black counselors in her study were more inclined to trace their clients' problems to social and external causes. Sue (1978) proposed a more elaborate typology based on the views held by the counselor and the counselee on the sources of responsibility and control in the counseling encounter. Anticipating the results by Berman, Sue cautioned counselors against imposing their own culturally bound notions of responsibility upon clients of different backgrounds. To sum up, cultures differ not only in their balance of autoplastic-alloplastic behavior, but also in their attribution of responsibility for such behaviors to self and others.

Correcting the traditionally autoplastic bias in counseling, especially with culturally different clients, is to be welcomed. There are serious problems to be expected, however, if the pendulum is allowed to swing too far in the opposite direction. Two issues in particular need to be resolved. One of these has to do with counselees' choices; the other involves the bases for counselors' actions. On the former issue Taft (1966) in Australia identified three options open to a person who lives and operates in two cultures: encapsulation in the community of one's compatriots, immersion into the social world of the host culture, or integration of elements from both cultures into a unique blend of personal experience. In addition, there is the residual category of individuals whose hold upon either culture is tenuous and fragile (see Berry and Kim 1988). Where the counselee stands on the issue of adaptation to the host or majority culture is an important and legitimate personal decision that may be facilitated or crystallized in counseling but that, in a tolerant, pluralistic society should not be externally imposed by anyone. If the counselee is conflict-torn on this issue, the goal of counseling should be to help him or her find the personally most satisfying solution on how to relate to the minority "in group" and majority "out group."

The other issue revolves around the alloplastic orientation of the counselor. What is the empirical justification for a social prescription for change? And what is the power of an individual counselor or counselee to implement these changes? Our knowledge as counselors is far greater about changing people than changing societies. Prescriptions for social change abound, but their justifications are grounded in ideologies, not facts. Our legitimate role as agents of social change is thus limited by our level of knowledge on the one hand and by the ethical imperative against imposing one's convictions and beliefs upon a counselee on the other.

In their hypothetical extremes the alloplastic bias degenerates into revolutionary rhetoric and bombast and the autoplastic bias into the scholasticism of the most rigid variants of the medical model misapplied to social problems. To elaborate, complex social problems are traced to the "mental illnesses" from which people expressing these problems are allegedly suffering. Steering clear of these two extremes, the counselor must help the counselee both to act upon people, objects, and situations and to be acted upon—to adapt to the environment. Combining these two modes realistically and sensitively, even creatively, is the goal of all counseling, a measure of its success, and a criterion of the counselor's skill and competence.

Relationships versus Techniques

A basic theme of this volume, and a hallmark of all cross-cultural counseling, is that the techniques of counseling are not immutable as they are applied across cultures. Even a skeptic such as Patterson (1978) recognizes that, albeit grudgingly. Culture enters the counseling process through the counselee's cognitions: their expectations, beliefs, and convictions based on their accumulated lifetime of experiences in what is proper, effective, and meaningful. Counseling techniques, then, must be plausible in order to be effective (see Goldstein 1962; Higginbotham 1977, 1984). In different milieus techniques may not be valued or accepted to the same extent.

These considerations suggest two things. First, as techniques of counseling are exported across cultural lines, they should be assessed for their fitness. Higginbotham (1984) has developed a culture accommodation scale to be applied to the delivery of mental health services. This instrument needs to be adapted to assess the cultural acceptability of various counselors' interventions. Second, an imperative of cross-cultural counseling is flexibility, the readiness to modify, adapt, and experiment during the counseling process.

Does nothing remain constant as counseling is modified through new adaptations? It would be hasty to answer this question in the affirmative. We just do not know enough to say what survives in the cultural transformation of the tangible and the intangible in counseling. It seems plausible, however, that any universals are more likely to be attitudinal rather than technical. We do not yet have a catalog of universal, culture-free elements of counseling.

In the absence of such a list, a précis addressed to the cross-cultural counselor might be as follows: Be prepared to adapt your techniques (e.g., general activity level, mode of verbal intervention, content of remarks, tone of voice) to the cultural background of the client; communicate acceptance of and respect for the client in terms that make sense within his or her cultural frame of reference; and be open to the possibility of more direct intervention in the life of the client than the traditional ethos of the counseling profession would dictate or permit. Parallel to well-known formulations in the literature of psychotherapy research (Strupp 1970, 1973), the non-specific attitudinal and relationship factors appear to be the most robust ingredient of the counseling experience regardless of site or context.

The Bilaterality of the Client-Counselor Relationship

If relationships are more enduring in the face of cultural transformation than are techniques, what demands does cross-cultural counseling place upon the counselor? There is general agreement that counseling across cultures is personally demanding and involving. Yet the counselor's reactions to these cross-cultural encounters have remained a neglected topic in the professional literature, which is understandably, if lopsidedly, focused on the counselee.

At various points in this book the silence on this subject has been broken. The conclusion is justified that, whatever the theoretical context of cross-cultural counseling, it is more experiential, "freewheeling," and bilateral than counseling in culturally uniform settings. Perhaps the cross-cultural counseling situation provokes a degree of culture shock, comparable to the experience of being plunged into an alien world in which accustomed behaviors and actions no longer work. Although the counselor is to some extent protected by the professional role and setting, feelings of inadequacy may be particularly painful in that they assail the counselor's competence as a professional. Li-Ripac (1980) documented some loss of accuracy in assessing clients outside of the therapist's cultural group, which may be related to the tendency to attribute more serious disturbances to clients outside of one's culture. "The clinician's prized tools, his empathy and sensitivity, may suffer impairment when carried across cultural lines" (Li-Ripac 1980, 339). But the resulting feelings of helplessness and inadequacy are not the only personal reactions experienced. The subjective reports that we do have, including those in this volume, indicate that cross-cultural counseling requires more effort and energy and that it may well produce more fatigue. Again, the parallel is obvious to cross-cultural adaptation; the counseling microcosm emerges as a replica of a cross-cultural encounter.

Research and the Clinical Experience

Research-based and clinical information about cross-cultural counseling has grown over the last two decades. (The yield of this accumulating evidence is summarized elsewhere in this volume.) Nonetheless, in a specific situation, the counselor is all too often left to his or her own devices. In general, the following are at the disposal of the cross-cultural counselor: (1) research-based findings on the cross-cultural counseling process; (2) published accounts of personal experiences by other cross-cultural counselors; (3) personally transmitted accounts; (4) the counselor's own experience with culturally different clients; and finally, (5) the counselor's professional, cultural, and personal sensitivity.

Each experience with a culturally different client becomes an adventure that takes both members of the dyad beyond what is currently known. The cross-cultural counselor must be prepared to act differently in each new situation and to learn from each new experience. Optimally, each new cross-cultural counseling session should become an experiment with an N of 1—meticulously observed, recorded and analyzed for its consequences. Practice informed by research and research sparked by practice will continue to develop the art of cross-cultural counseling.

References

Abel, T., Métraux, R., and Roll, S. 1987. *Psychotherapy and culture*. Albuquerque: University of New Mexico Press.

Atkinson, D. R., Morten, G., and Sue, D. W., eds. 1979. *Counseling American minorities: A cross-cultural perspective*. Dubuque, IA: William C. Brown.

Berman, J. 1979. Individual versus societal focus: Problem diagnoses of black and white male and female counselors. *Journal of Cross-Cultural Psychology* 10 (4): 497–507.

Berry, J. W. 1979. Research in multi-cultural societies: Implications of cross-cultural methods. *Journal of Cross-Cultural Psychology* 10:415–434.

Berry, J. W., and Kim, U. 1988. Acculturation and mental health. In P. R. Dasen, J. W. Berry, and N. Sartorius (eds.), *Health and cross-cultural psychology: Toward applications*, 207–236. Newbury Park, CA: Sage Publications.

Brislin, R. W. 1983. Cross-cultural research in psychology. *Annual Review of Psychology* 34:363–540.

Church, A. T. 1982. Sojourner adjustment. *Psychological Bulletin* 91:540–572.

Deen, N. 1985. Cross-cultural counseling from a West-European perspective. In P. B. Pedersen (ed.), *Handbook of cross-cultural counseling and therapy*, 45–54. Westport, CT: Greenwood Press.

Diaz-Guerrero, R. 1967. El sindrome activo y el passivo. *Revista Interamericana de Psicología* 1:263–272.

Doi, T. 1973. *The anatomy of dependence* (J. Bester, trans.). Tokyo: Kodansha.

Draguns, J. G. 1973. Comparisons of psychopathology across cultures: Issues, findings, directions. *Journal of Cross-Cultural Psychology* 4:9–47.

———. 1975. Resocialization into culture: The complexities of taking a worldwide view of psychotherapy. In R. W. Brislin, S. Bochner, and W. J. Lonner (eds.), *Cross-cultural perspectives on learning*, 273–289. Beverly Hills: Sage Publications.

———. 1980. Psychological disorders of clinical severity. In H. C. Triandis and J. G. Draguns (eds.), *Handbook of cross-cultural psychology*. Vol. 6, *Psychopathology*, 99–174. Boston: Allyn and Bacon.

———. 1984. Assessment of mental health and disorder. In P. B. Pedersen, N. Sartorius, and A. J. Marsella (eds.), *Mental health services: The cross-cultural context*, 31–58. Newbury Park, CA: Sage Publications.

———. 1985. Psychological disorders across cultures. In P. B. Pedersen (ed.), *Handbook of cross-cultural counseling and therapy*, 55–62. Westport, CT: Greenwood Press.

———. 1988. Personality and culture: Are they relevant for the enhancement of quality of mental life? In P. R. Dasen, J. W. Berry, and N. Sartorius (eds.), *Health and cross-cultural psychology: Toward applications*, 141–161. Newbury Park, CA: Sage Publications.

Draguns, J. G., and McLatchie, L. R. 1986. Psychotherapy with Evangelical Christians. Paper presented at the annual meeting of the American Psychiatric Association, Washington, DC.

Favazza, A. R., and Oman, M. 1978. Overview: Foundations of cultural psychiatry. *American Journal of Psychiatry* 135:293–303.

Feinberg, S. 1986. Psychotherapy with Orthodox Jewish patients. Paper presented at the annual meeting of the American Psychiatric Association, Washington, DC.

Flavell, J. H. 1963. *The developmental psychology of Jean Piaget.* New York: Van Nostrand.

Freedman, J. A. 1985. Clinical sociology. In P. B. Pedersen (ed.), *Handbook of cross-cultural counseling and therapy,* 117–124. Westport, CT: Greenwood Press.

Giordano, J., and Giordano, G. P. 1976. Ethnicity and community mental health. *Community Mental Health Review* 1 (3): 4–14, 15.

———. 1977. *The ethno-cultural factor in mental health: A literature review and bibliography.* New York Institute on Pluralism.

Goldstein, A. P. 1962. *Therapist-patient expectancies in psychotherapy.* New York: Pergamon Press.

Henderson, G., ed. 1979. *Understanding and counseling ethnic minorities.* Springfield, IL: Charles C. Thomas.

Herskovits, M. J. 1948. *Man and his works.* New York: Knopf.

Higginbotham, H. N. 1977. Culture and the role of client expectancy. In R. W. Brislin and M. P. Hammett (eds.), *Topics in culture learning* 5:107–124. Honolulu: East-West Center Press.

———. 1984. *Third World challenge to psychiatry.* Honolulu: University of Hawaii Press.

Holtzman, W. H., Diaz-Guerrero, R., and Swartz, J. D. 1975. *Personality: Development in two cultures.* Austin: University of Texas Press.

Jilek, W. 1982. *Indian healing: Shamanic ceremonialism in the Pacific Northwest today.* Surrey, B.C.: Hancock House Publishers.

Leff, J. 1981. *Psychiatry around the globe: A transcultural view.* New York: Marcel Dekker.

Li-Ripac, D. 1980. Cultural influences on clinical perception: A comparison of Caucasian and Chinese American therapists. *Journal of Cross-Cultural Psychology* 11:327–342.

McGoldrick, M., Pearce, J. K., and Giordano, J., eds. 1982. *Ethnicity and family therapy.* New York: Guilford Press.

McLatchie, L. R., and Draguns, J. G. 1984. Mental health concepts of Evangelical Protestants. *Journal of Psychology* 118:147–159.

Malpass, R. S. 1977. Theory and method in cross-cultural psychology. *American Psychologist* 32:1069–1079.

Marsella, A. J. 1979. Cross-cultural studies of mental disorders. In A. J. Marsella, R. Tharp, and T. Ciborowski (eds.), *Perspectives on cross-cultural psychology,* 233–262. New York: Academic Press.

Marsella, A. J., and Pedersen, P. B., eds. 1981. *Cross-cultural counseling and psychotherapy: Foundations, evaluation, and cultural considerations.* Elmsford, NY: Pergamon Press.

Martin, L., and DeVolder, J. 1983. Guidance and counseling services in the Federal Republic of Germany. *Personnel and Guidance Journal* 61:482–487.

Maslow, A. H. 1956. Self-actualizing people: A study of psychological growth. In C. E. Moustakas (ed.), *The self: Explorations in personal growth.* New York: Harper and Row.

Minsel, W. R., and Herff, W. 1984. Intercultural counseling: West German perspective. In R. J. Samuda and A. Wolfgang (eds.), *Intercultural counselling*, 97–108. Torpnto: Hogrefe.

Murphy, H. B. M. 1982. *Comparative psychiatry*. Berlin: Springer-Verlag.

Nishihara, D. P. 1978. Culture, counseling, and *ho'oponopono:* An ancient model in a modern context. *Personnel and Guidance Journal* 56:562–568.

Patterson, C. H. 1978. Cross-cultural or intercultural psychotherapy. *Hacettepe University Bulletin of Social Sciences* 1:119–134.

———. 1986. Culture and counseling in Hong Kong. *Chinese University Education Journal* 14 (2): 77–81.

Pedersen, P. B. 1981. The cultural inclusiveness of counseling. In P. B. Pedersen, J. G. Draguns, W. J. Lonner, and J. E. Trimble (eds.), *Counseling across cultures*, rev. ed., 22–58. Honolulu: University of Hawaii Press.

———, ed. 1985. *Handbook of cross-cultural counseling and therapy*. Westport, CT: Greenwood Press.

Pedersen, P. B., Draguns, J. G., Lonner, W. J., and Trimble, J. E., eds. 1981. *Counseling across cultures*. Rev. ed. Honolulu: University of Hawaii Press.

Pedersen, P. B., Lonner, W. J., and Draguns, J. G., eds. 1976. *Counseling across cultures*. Honolulu: University of Hawaii Press.

Pedersen, P. B., Sartorius, N., and Marsella, A. J., eds. 1984. *Mental health services: The cross-cultural context*. Beverly Hills: Sage Publications.

Piaget, J. 1950. *Psychology of intelligence*. New York: Harcourt Brace.

Pike, K. L. 1954. *Language in relation to a unified theory of a structure of human behavior*. Preliminary ed. Pt. 1. Glendale, CA: Summer Institute of Linguistics.

Prewitt-Diaz, J. O., and Draguns, J. G. 1987. Mental health of two-way migrants: From Puerto Rico to the United States and return. *Ciencias de la Conducta* 2:15–26.

Price-Williams, D. 1974. Psychological experiment and anthropology: The problem of categories. *Ethos* 2:95–114.

Prince, R. H. 1980. Variations in psychotherapeutic procedures. In H. C. Triandis and J. G. Draguns (eds.), *Handbook of cross-cultural psychology*. Vol. 6, *Psychopathology*. Boston: Allyn and Bacon.

Rogers, C. R. 1957. The necessary and sufficient conditions of therapeutic personality change. *Journal of Consulting Psychology* 21:95–103.

Samuda, R. J., and Wolfgang, A., eds. 1984. *Intercultural counselling*. Toronto: Hogrefe.

Segall, M. S. 1986. Culture and behavior: Psychology in global perspective. *Annual Review of Psychology* 37:523–564.

Stewart, E. C. 1976. Cultural sensitivities in counseling. In P. B. Pedersen, W. J. Lonner, and J. G. Draguns (eds.), *Counseling across cultures*. Honolulu: University of Hawaii Press.

———. 1981. Cultural sensitivities in counseling. In P. B. Pedersen, J. G. Draguns, W. J. Lonner, and J. E. Trimble (eds.), *Counseling across cultures*, rev. ed., 61–86. Honolulu: University of Hawaii Press.

Strupp, H. H. 1970. Specific or nonspecific factors in psychotherapy and the problem of control. *Archives of General Psychiatry* 23:393–401.

————. 1973. On the basic ingredients of psychotherapy. *Journal of Consulting and Clinical Psychology* 41:1–8.

Sue, D. W. 1978. World views and counseling. *Personnel and Guidance Journal* 56:458–463.

————. 1981. *Counseling the culturally different: Theory and practice.* New York: John Wiley and Sons.

Taft, R. 1966. *From stranger to citizen.* London: Tavistock.

————. 1977. Coping with unfamiliar environments. In N. Warren (ed.), *Studies of cross-cultural psychology.* Vol. 1. London: Academic Press.

Thernstrom, S., ed. 1980. *Harvard encyclopedia of American ethnic groups.* Cambridge, MA: Belknap Press.

Triandis, H. C. 1972. *Subjective culture.* New York: John Wiley and Sons.

Triandis, H. C., et al., eds. 1980. *Handbook of cross-cultural psychology.* Boston: Allyn and Bacon.

Vexliard, A. 1968. Tempérament et modalités d'adaptation. *Bulletin de Psychologie* 21:1–15.

Vontress, C. E. 1979. Cross-cultural counseling: An existential approach. *Personnel and Guidance Journal* 58:117–122.

————. 1981. Racial and ethnic barriers in counseling. In P. B. Pedersen, J. G. Draguns, W. J. Lonner, and J. E. Trimble (eds.), *Counseling across cultures,* rev. ed., 87–107. Honolulu: University of Hawaii Press.

Walz, G. R., and Benjamin, L., eds. 1978. *Transcultural counseling.* New York: Human Sciences Press.

Weidman, H. H., and Sussex, J. N. 1971. Culture values and ego functioning in relation to the culture-bound reactive syndromes. *International Journal of Social Psychiatry* 17:83–100.

Yap, P. M. 1969. The culture-bound reactive syndromes. In W. Caudill and T. Y. Lin (eds.), *Mental health research in Asia and the Pacific.* Honolulu: East-West Center Press.

2

Client, Counselor, and Contextual Variables in Multicultural Counseling

PAUL B. PEDERSEN
MARY FUKUYAMA
ANNE HEATH

Counselors are increasingly confronted with culturally different clients who challenge their basic assumptions about counseling. It is important to begin by examining these assumptions. First, consumer demand for awareness of special counseling needs from many cultural perspectives has resulted in a growing multicultural perspective among counselors and from within the field of counseling. Publications have begun to acknowledge the importance of cultural variables in all counseling activities (Ahia 1984; Atkinson, Morten, and Sue 1983; Lefley and Pedersen 1986; Marsella and Pedersen 1981; Marsella and White 1982; Pedersen 1985; Sue 1981a).

Second, counseling has also been influenced by the developing field of cross-cultural psychology (Brislin 1981; Landis and Brislin 1983; Segall 1979; Triandis and Draguns 1980). Other disciplines outside the field of counseling have also influenced the trend toward multiculturalism (Driver 1965; Favazza and Oman 1977; Hsu 1972; Leininger 1978; McGoldrick, Pearce, and Giordano 1982), emphasizing anthropological, sociological, psychiatric, and medical perspectives.

Third, it is increasingly apparent that all counselors have an ethical responsibility to know their client's cultural values (Fields 1979; Ibrahim and Arredondo 1986). It is also apparent that multicultural counseling is not limited to the study of exotic populations but must include the inculcation of multicultural awareness in all competently trained counselors.

Fourth, the field of counseling is growing larger than the Euroamerican context in which it was developed. Non-Western, alternative modes of counseling are gaining prominence (Higginbotham 1979; Marsella 1979; Pedersen 1981; Tart 1975; Torrey 1986; Watts 1961). The multicultural and international perspective has highlighted a cultural bias in counseling based on dominant Euroamerican assumptions that do not

23

apply outside that cultural context (Diaz-Guerrero 1977; Pande 1969; Sampson 1977). (A discussion of non-Western and, more particularly, Asian approaches to counseling and therapy is, however, beyond the scope of this chapter.)

We will attempt to meet the needs of counselors to learn more about this new multicultural perspective in counseling by addressing the following areas: (1) the development of cross-cultural counseling; (2) client variables; (3) counselor variables; (4) environmental variables; (5) training issues; and (6) future trends. We hope to acquaint the reader with an overview of multicultural counseling literature, drawing from both international and domestic sources. All behaviors are based on culturally learned expectations. Consequently, the multicultural perspective is essential to an accurate assessment of behaviors for counseling.

A Historical Perspective

Historically, the interrelationship between culture and personality has been systematically studied more often by anthropologists than by psychologists (Favazza and Oman 1977). To understand the history of multicultural counseling it is important to discuss the two separate but related traditions of anthropology and psychology in their approach to culture. The psychological position is that there is a fixed state of mental health whose observation is obscured by cultural distortions and which relates cultural behaviors to some *universal* definition of normative behavior. This position assumes that there is a single, universal definition of mental health, whatever the person's cultural origin.

A contrasting anthropological position views cultural differences as clues to divergent attitudes, values, and assumptions that differentiate one culture from another in a *comparative* framework based on culture-specific perspectives (Berry 1969, 1980). This perspective assumes that different groups or individuals have somewhat different definitions of mental health as a result of their own unique cultural contexts.

Anthropologists have tended to take a relativist position when classifying and interpreting behavior. Typically, they have identified diverse behaviors as specific to each culture. Multiple interpretations of acceptable behavior are allowed to coexist with one another in the intercultural situation. Each culture becomes a separate configuration (Sears 1970).

Psychologists, in contrast, have tended to link social characteristics and psychological phenomena, giving only minimum attention to the different multicultural values. Typically, they have applied the same interpretation to the same behavior regardless of the cultural context in which that behavior was displayed.

Unfortunately, the history of counseling may be more typified by cultural blindness. In working with minorities, counselors have occasionally been accused of maintaining or protecting the status quo (Halleck 1971). These attitudes toward culturally different groups can be traced to "scientific racism" (Guthrie 1976; Williams 1978) and Euroamerican ethnocentrism in psychology (White 1984). Sue (1981a) has described the "genetic deficiency" model that promoted the idea that whites were superior to blacks and other nonwhite populations through biological reasons. These beliefs have been traced to the early writings of Charles Darwin (*On the Origin of Species by Means of Natural Selection*, 1859), Sir Francis Galton (*Hereditary Genius: An Inquiry into Its Laws and Consequences*, 1909), and G. Stanley Hall (cited in Williams 1978). Although archaic in concept, this model has persisted in psychology up to recent times (e.g., Jensen 1969). Additionally, psychological tests have been shown to be culturally biased (Lonner 1985; Lonner and Sundberg 1985).

The genetic deficiency model was followed by a "cultural deficit" model in which social scientists described culturally different ethnic minority persons as "deprived" or "disadvantaged" merely because they were not behaving according to middle-class values, language systems, and customs. Seen from a class perspective, there has been an implicit assumption by white middle-class society that other cultures do not advance themselves because of this "cultural deficit." Cole and Bruner (1972) discussed the misperception that lower-class communities were disorganized and culturally deprived. They have refuted this deficit hypothesis as a distortion. Both the genetic deficiency model and the culturally deprived model failed to state the implicit cultural biases that shaped these negative perceptions and inhibited the understanding of the role of sociopolitical forces (Jenkins 1982; Jones 1980). White (1984) has described this bias as "Euro-American ethnocentricity." The genetic and cultural deficiency models have been refuted and replaced by the "culturally different" model (Sue 1981a).

Psychology as a field has paid little attention, until recently, to minority clients. Casas (1984, 785) explains, "Though various reasons could be given to explain this lack of attention, some of the major reasons include: (1) a blatant and irresponsible lack of interest in these groups; (2) the continued existence in subtle yet complex forms of racism, biases and prejudices relative to specific racial/ethnic minorities; (3) the prevalence of an ethnocentric perspective which seeks to downplay cultural differences and pushes for assimilation and mainstreaming of the culturally different; and (4) a preference for working with clients whose characteristics are similar to those of the counselor and correlated with successful counseling outcomes."

The underrepresentation of minority views was also evident in the allocation of program time to cross-cultural issues by the American Psychological Association (APA) (Lee et al. 1981; Inouye and Pedersen 1985). Ethnic and cultural content in the APA convention program ranged from 3% to 5% across divisions for the period from 1977 to 1982. Since 1982, however, the APA convention directory index has included "cross-cultural" as a category, and a greater number of APA programs include the mention of culture in their titles.

Russo, Olmedo, Stapp, and Fulcher (1981) surveyed the representation of ethnic minority groups and women among psychologists generally. Ethnic minorities and women are extremely underrepresented at all levels and especially at the more professionally advanced levels of the profession. Likewise, in their tabulation of faculty ethnicity, whites greatly outnumbered nonwhites, and white males especially outnumbered all females.

Many other studies document how minorities are underrepresented as students and faculty in clinical and counseling programs both recently and historically (Casas 1984; Kennedy and Wagner 1979; Parham and Moreland 1981). Atkinson, Morten, and Sue (1983), however, reported data from 305 counselor education programs that ethnic minorities are progressively gaining representation among students and presumably will gain more in the future as these students become faculty members.

The perspective of multicultural counseling has widened from one in which culture was considered largely irrelevant to a broader perspective in which the cultural aspect of human behavior has become significant. Pressure from special interest groups to have their viewpoints represented has resulted in a political awareness of culture. Pressure from groups who consider their interests to be underrepresented has resulted in an economic awareness of culture. Pressure from continuing research on the accurate interpretation of culturally learned behavior has resulted in an academic awareness of culture. The influence of the multicultural perspective is growing throughout the social sciences as a fourth force that will significantly change the way counseling is viewed. It may not be an exaggeration to say that this multicultural perspective is one of the few really new developments in the past decade of counseling.

Client Variables in Multicultural Counseling

Early studies of the counseling dyad found that racial similarities are a factor in forming the counseling relationship. Carkhuff and Pierce (1967) concluded that counselors and clients who are similar in ethnicity and social class or gender have a greater potential for empathic interpersonal relationships. Stranges and Riccio (1970) found that counselor trainees preferred counselors of the same racial and cultural backgrounds. Mitchell (1970) likewise asserted that the white counselor cannot counsel the "Black psyche." Levine and Campbell (1972) reviewed the literature on ethnocentrism and concluded that groups or individuals who perceive themselves as similar are more likely to relate harmoniously than groups who perceive themselves as different. Muliozzi (1972) discovered that white counselors felt more genuine and empathic with white than with black clients, however black clients did not see white counselors as less understanding, less genuine, or less unconditional in their regard. Black clients did not feel that white counselors "liked them as much" compared with white clients.

Since 1970 the number of studies in the area of counselor-client matching has expanded greatly. Atkinson (1985a, 1985b) and Atkinson and Schein (1986) have analyzed this body of research in which are found four major literature reviews on race effects in psychotherapy (Abramowitz and Murray 1983; Atkinson 1983; Harrison 1975; Sattler 1977). We will summarize their analysis by highlighting the general trends, limitations, and recommendations of the research.

The research on the preference of minority clients for counselor ethnicity has typically involved three types of research design: the analogue study with simulated counseling interviews, survey questionnaires, and field research in naturalistic settings, such as archival retrieval of records. The results of the above-mentioned review articles concluded that the available evidence is mixed on counselor preference, ranging from same-race preference to no preference to cross-racial preference. Harrison (1975) and Atkinson (1983) found support for a black preference for black counselors over white counselors. Berman (1979) demonstrated how blacks were more expressive but attended less well than whites. Sattler's (1977) review of the research found a preference for black therapists by black clients but also noted that counseling style or technique was a more important variable than race. Abramowitz and Murray (1983) suggested that Sattler may have understated the effects of therapist ethnicity, and other reviewers (Griffith 1977; Griffith and Jones 1979; Jones 1974) have noted support for racial or ethnic similarity between client and counselor as a factor in successful counseling. Ewing (1974) indicated that black students tended to react more favorably than white students to black or white counselors, suggesting that racial similarity by itself was not a crucial factor.

Atkinson (1983) extended his review to include ethnic groups other than blacks (American Indians, Asian Americans, and Hispanics) but found little support for same-ethnicity preferences in these groups from the few studies reviewed. Acosta and Sheehan (1976) provided data indicating that both Mexican Americans and Anglo-Americans attributed more skill, understanding, and trustworthiness to therapists who were either Anglo-American professionals or Mexican-American nonprofessionals. Research studies on Native Americans have indicated some support for differences in preferences (see the Trimble and Fleming chapter in this volume).

Some studies have even shown a preference for cross-racial pairing in counseling. Gambosa, Tosi, and Riccio's (1976) analogue study found that white delinquent girls preferred a black counselor for personal and social assistance. Bernstein, Wade, and Hofmann (1987) reported in a survey study of urban university students that both black and white students tended to prefer black counselors regardless of problem type. Black and white participants in this study expressed counselor preferences for sex, age, experience, and race in similar proportions.

The other studies suggested that racial or ethnic preferences may be a function of within-group differences rather than of ethnicity per se. For example, Jackson and Kirschner (1973) found that subjects who identified themselves as "Black" or "Afro-American" had a stronger preference for black counselors than those who identified themselves as "Negro." Gordon and Grantham (1979) found no racial preference but did find that subjects preferred counselors of the same social class. Morten (1984), however, reported no significant differences between racial self-labeling and counselor preference in a survey of black college students. Parham and Helms (1981) developed a racial identity scale based on Cross' (1971) model and found that black subjects who scored in the preencounter stage preferred white counselors, but those in the encounter, immersion, and internalization stages preferred black counselors. In addition, black students in the encounter stage rated themselves higher on self-esteem (Parham and Helms 1985a) and self-actualization tendencies (Parham and Helms 1985b). (See Helms 1985 for further discussion of cultural identity.)

Pomales, Claiborn, and LaFromboise (1986) tested the hypothesis that racial identity based upon Parham and Helms' (1981) racial identity stages affected counselees' perceptions of the cultural sensitivity of white counselors. Participants saw the culturally sensitive counselor as more competent than the culturally blind counselor, although racial identity differences were marginally supported. Anderson (1983) examined preferences for facilitative versus directive counseling techniques and found that blacks differed in preferences from whites and Mexican-American subjects and that black females preferred a more facilitative approach.

Sanchez and Atkinson (1983) found in a survey study that Mexican-American subjects preferred racially similar counselors depending upon their level of cultural commitment. Those subjects with the strongest commitment to Mexican-American culture expressed the greatest preference for a Mexican-American counselor and were least willing to self-disclose to whites in counseling.

It is possible that other variables, such as the active intervention for positive change through counseling, could be more important than racial similarity in assessing counselor effectiveness (Atkinson, Maruyama, and Matsui 1978; Peoples and Dell 1975).

Lower-income persons were less likely to be in therapy or tended to remain in therapy for shorter periods of time, even though similar symptoms were described as more severe compared to upper-income clients. Likewise, lower-income persons were treated by less experienced staff and were treated with short-term somatic therapies generally considered to be less valuable in terms of provider costs. Norms for adjustment were defined according to the middle-class values favoring conformity, thrift, respectability, control of emotions, and future orientation (Lorion and Parron 1985).

The findings from research on client counseling preferences are mixed and raise more questions than they provide answers. Abramowitz and Murray (1983) discussed several possible reasons for this variance in the research. The differences in methodologies tend to favor certain findings; for example, the analogue study favors the null hypothesis of no effects for ethnicity. Sampling bias is another concern. For instance, an archival study of black patients who have completed therapy may be different from one of black patients who terminate therapy prematurely. Investigator bias (i.e., selective attention to results that confirm the researcher's own political beliefs) and the social desirability of respondents may also influence the conclusions of this research (Abramowitz and Murray 1983).

In summary, the literature on client variables in multicultural counseling has yielded mixed results. The causes for this ambiguous conclusion may be traced to research methodologies and the limitations of using a narrowly defined concept of "race." As researchers have become more aware of the complexities of cross-cultural relationships, they have identified more specific variables that need to be incorporated into research designs. For example, the client's previous counseling experiences have not been considered in the counselor preference literature (Atkinson 1983). In addition, other variables, such as the client's sense of racial identity, social class, within-group differences, and counseling style preferences need to be considered. Existing measures may be inadequate to tap into the dimensions of client preferences in therapy.

Counselor Variables in Multicultural Counseling

Wrenn (1962, 1985) described counselor "encapsulation" as substituting stereotypes for the real world, disregarding cultural variations among clients, and dogmatizing a technique-oriented definition of the

counseling process. Kagan (1964) and Schwebel (1964) further suggested that counselor education programs may actually be contributing
to encapsulation by teaching a cultural bias, however implicitly, in their
curricula. Morrow (1972) introduced but did not develop the metaphor
that counselors tend to become "addicted" to one system of cultural
values in a dependency that is counterproductive to effective counseling.

Given that therapists reflect the same rates of stereotyping and ethnocentrism as the general public (Bloombaum, Yamamoto, and James
1968), it is no surprise, as Vontress (1981) suggests, that few counselors
really want to change to fit other cultural perspectives. Our cultural bias
is not likely to change as the result of brief or superficial contact through
books, lectures, or courses. Change is more likely to occur after sustained immersion or contact with persons or ideas from a variety of different cultures.

Lorion and Parron (1985) and Torrey (1986) have presented evidence
showing how professional mental health services are class-bound, relating the expectancy and type of psychiatric disorder to a person's position in society's class structure. Clients from different social classes were
given different treatments and diagnoses. Some confusion exists in the
literature between social class differences and racial affiliation as they
influence adjustment. Menacker (1971) and Sweeney (1971) have discussed guidance for lower-income persons, emphasizing that years of
neglect, even benign neglect, are not eradicated by a few hours of counseling. A lower-income population must be viewed within the total context of its unique home and community environment. Gordon and
Smith (1971) likewise have maintained that the guidance specialist
should be concerned with changing the environment as well as with
changing the student being counseled. There is a danger that the counselor will stereotype a lower-income client, disregarding individuality.
This tendency is particularly dangerous when the counselor comes from
an upper-class or middle-class background.

Socioeconomic class has been identified as an important cultural
influence. Cultural attributes have been identified with economic class
(Sue 1977), and lower-class culture has been described as different in
values and communication styles from middle-class culture (Daniel
1985). Therefore, it is important to identify socioeconomic status in
understanding the underlying values of a client's worldview.

Counselor expectations of client behaviors has also been identified as
a source of cultural bias. Goldstein (1981) suggests that the *conformity
prescription,* which expects the client to conform in therapy, is less desirable but more frequently encountered than the *reformity prescription,* in
which the treatment is reformulated to fit the client's cultural expectations. Acosta, Yamamoto, and Evans (1982) reported on an effective

psychotherapy program for low-income and minority mental health patients in which the clients were trained through role-plays on how to interact with their therapists prior to entering therapy. In turn, therapists were also sensitized to cultural and class issues through ongoing seminars. The authors in this study recommended role preparation and the clarification of expectations with clients as a means toward more effective psychotherapy.

There is some increased agreement in the literature that therapy should be shaped to fit client expectations (Gomes-Schwartz, Hadley, and Strupp 1978; Higginbotham 1977, 1979; Higginbotham and Tanaka-Matsumi 1981). Previous research suggests that therapy opportunities have favored the YAVIS (youthful, attractive, verbal, intelligent, successful) group and disfavored the QUOID (quiet, ugly, old, indigent, culturally dissimilar) and the HOUND (homely, old, unattractive, nonverbal, dumb) (Krumboltz, Becker-Haven, and Burnett 1979). Similarly, Gourash (1978) reported that most help seekers, which included medical, social, legal, or self-help, tended to be young, white, educated, middle class, and female.

Higginbotham (1977) developed a model describing the individually diverse role expectations, client preferences, forms of anticipated support, types of advice sought, or medical care requested from the client's "expectancy" perspective as indicated in the Tanaka-Matsumi and Higginbotham chapter of this book. For example, Chien and Yamamoto (1982) suggested that new Chinese immigrants would present psychological problems in the form of physical symptoms and expect a medical solution from a doctor or herbalist of their own culture. Kleinman and Kleinman (1985) document in some detail the somatization of psychological stress by presenting physiological rather than psychological symptoms. This well-documented tendency provides an alternative to "talk" therapy as a method of treatment.

Multicultural counseling does not imply, however, that we abandon the rich resources of counseling theory and research. Wohl (1981) is critical of the "super-flexible" counselor with "elastic modifications" of counseling principles. Likewise, Patterson (1974, 1978) is rightly critical of cross-cultural counselors who urge students to abandon the fundamentals of counseling and therapy in favor of unproven and unorthodox culturally defined alternatives. The task is rather to effectively adapt the skills of traditional counseling to the perspectives of culturally different clients. Genuineness, warmth, and empathy can and must be demonstrated differently in different cultural settings.

There are many qualities that can positively influence the multicultural counseling process. Lambert (1981) describes research that relates the personal qualities of counselors to their effectiveness in counseling and therapy. Those factors that contribute to a positive relationship in counseling also contribute to its effectiveness. Kemp (1962) and Mezzano (1969) found that open-minded and flexible counselors excel in the supportive understanding and self-exploration that are usually associated with counseling effectiveness. Russo, Kelz, and Hudson (1964), Millikan (1965), and Millikan and Patterson (1967) discovered that prejudice or factors related to prejudice are associated with less effective counseling as assessed by counseling supervisors (see Ridley chapter on racism). The personal qualities required of multicultural counselors are complex, and each cultural context requires different combinations of skills.

The literature has included counselor credibility as an important facilitator in the counseling relationship. Sue (1981b) describes counselor credibility as an important precondition for trust and understanding between counselor and client. Credibility includes both expertise and trustworthiness. An expert counselor should be perceived as informed, capable, and intelligent. A counselor is trustworthy to the extent that clients believe what the counselor says.

Westermeyer (1976) suggests that the therapist can best develop credibility when working with culturally different clients by learning from the children in the host society. Sue (1978) suggests that cross-cultural counselors must integrate the client's worldview without losing their own cultural identity. The counselor experiences a great variety of alternative roles. Some of these alternatives include the roles of outreach consultant, ombudsman, change agent, and facilitator of indigenous support systems, any or all of which might be appropriately matched to the culturally different client's need (Ivey 1977).

Atkinson (1983) found only a few research studies that examined the effects of ethnicity on perceived counselor credibility. Most studies used measures of perceived counselor expertness, trustworthiness, and attractiveness. Only two studies reported a significant effect for counselor-client ethnic similarity in samples of Asian Americans (Atkinson, Maruyama, and Matsui 1978) and American Indians (Dauphinais, Dauphinais, and Rowe 1981). Unfortunately, most of these studies were limited to an analogue design with simulated interviews and the use of college students to simulate actual counseling situations. Neimeyer and Gonzales' (1983) archival study on counselor-client similarity and perceived effectiveness reported no differences in perceived effectiveness per se but found that white clients attributed change more to counseling than to other factors and that nonwhite clients expressed less overall satisfaction with counseling.

The research on matching clients and counselor according to similar ethnicity raises several issues: (1) The preference for counseling style may be more important than ethnic matching; (2) Matching clients and counselors suggests stereotyping; (3) Some minority clients will respond to matching with anger; (4) Other alternatives, such as bringing in a cultural broker or mediator, are more promising in bridging ethnic differences; and (5) Counselors who are bilingual themselves have a great advantage.

Understanding *counselor* racial identity development is important for the multicultural counselor and trainer. Helms (1984) outlined a model of racial consciousness for whites as well as blacks and focused on the interactional dynamics of cross-racial dyads. She has recommended that future research in this area examine the cross-racial dyad in order to understand how best to treat culturally diverse clients (Helms 1986). Similarly, Jones and Seagull (1983) discussed relationship issues between the black client and white therapist. They stressed the importance of the white therapist examining his or her feelings aroused by the cross-racial interaction, including such issues as white guilt, countertransference, and the need to be powerful.

The client's cultural background is significant as one aspect in perceived similarity or shared identity. Although counselors cannot change their cultural identity, they can learn the styles appropriate for working with culturally different clients and enhance the degree of perceived similarity between themselves and their clients. The development of culturally appropriate styles for counseling culturally different clients is therefore an important aspect of counseling. It may be possible to train counselors in the styles appropriate to different cultures even though the counselor and client come from different cultures with different personal constructs (Kelly 1955). Training in cross-cultural counseling workshops has changed counselor's perceptions (Neimeyer and Fukuyama 1984) and attitudes (Fukuyama and Neimeyer 1985).

In sum, the counselor variables in multicultural counseling are as complex and as important as the client variables. Further study is needed on the topics discussed in this section. While barriers exist such as cultural bias, stereotyping, and prejudice, there are also positive counselor qualities that can promote successful multicultural relations.

The Cultural Context of Psychological Helping

Many of the basic assumptions of counseling and therapy reflect the social, economic, and political context of the Western Euroamerican cultures in which they developed. These dominant cultural assumptions are not universally applicable (Pedersen 1977, 1979). Sampson (1977) and Diaz-Guerrero (1977) pointed out how different assumptions reflect their own cultural contexts. Rotenberg (1974) and Draguns (1974) described the influence of the Protestant ethic in developing a scientific, rational approach to counseling and therapy in Western psychology by idealizing active adjustment rather than passive acceptance in striving for success as individuals. In the Chinese context Hsu (1972) rejects individualism and describes mental health in terms of an interpersonal nexus. Hsu's theory of psychosocial homeostasis emphasizes the individual in context and the relationship between persons as more important than individual success.

In addition, ethnic psychologies have developed their own definitions of psychology. Jones and Korchin (1982) also cited the development of specific Third World psychologies, for example, African psychology (Khatib and Nobles 1977), Chinese psychology (Tong 1971), and La Raza psychology (Martinez 1977). White (1984) described cultural values of the Afro-American worldview in contrast to the Euroamerican alternative. Dualism (e.g., good and bad, superior and inferior, health and illness) characterizes the Euroamerican perspective. The individual is more important than the family unit, and power is defined by winning or dominating others. White (1984, 2) further characterizes the psychology of blackness as having seven dimensions: "1) openness to self and others; 2) tragedy and resilience; 3) psychological connectedness and interdependence; 4) the oral tradition; 5) creative synthesis; 6) fluid time perception; and 7) the value of direct experience combined with respect for the elderly." This worldview has its roots in an African heritage and contrasts sharply with the Euroamerican emphasis on individual competition, written traditions, linear time, and youth.

There are many examples of adapting Euroamerican counseling methods to other cultures. There are also some examples of adapting counseling methods familiar to non-Western cultures into the Euroamerican context. Ishiyama (1987) presented a practical application of Japanese Morita therapy in counseling Western clients for shyness. Watts' (1961) Oriental prescription, which provides a "way of liberation," resembles the process of liberation described by Jung, self-actualization described by Maslow, functional autonomy described by Allport, and creative selfhood described by Adler. Watts, a Westerner writing about Asia, pointed out that each individual is a participant in a social game that is based on conventional rules and that defines the boundaries between the individual and the environment—a hostile and alien world. Watts went on to say that the duty of the therapist is to involve the participant in a "counter-game" that restores a unifying perspective of ego and environment and that results in the liberation of the person. In many ways the skills required of a counselor parallel the insights resulting from Zen training (Leung 1973). Whereas Western psychology has studied the psyche or mind as a clinical entity, Eastern cultures have regarded mind and matter, soul and body, as interdependent. Many Asians have written on Eastern thought and culture from the point of view of Asian culture and religion (Pedersen 1977, 1981;

Lebra 1982; Murase 1982). Oriental religious training shares some similar goals with counselor education in our culture. Fromm, Suzuki, and
Martino (1960) described some of these similarities, as did Watts (1961)
and Pande (1969). Asian perspectives emphasize the importance of balance as a construct. The most familiar example of this concept is the
symbol of yin and yang in which light and darkness are combined to
form a circle. Applied to counseling this might suggest that the goal of
counseling is not a one-directional emphasis on happiness, pleasure, or
goodness but a two-directional perspective in which both happiness and
sadness, both pleasure and pain, both goodness and badness are important to the discovery of meaning in a balanced perspective.

Sinclair (1967) described the sequence of indigenous healing rituals
in New Guinea. First, at the impact of a crisis, the victim becomes fearful and anxious. Second, a cause of the misfortune is sought through
divination in the supernatural. Third, the responsibility for the crisis is
transferred to a supernatural agent so that the personal anxiety that
threatens the psychological equilibrium of the victim becomes identified
as the energy of that agent. There are many other examples of societies
in which the supernatural is seen to contain hostile forces capable of act-
ing upon the individual (Weidman 1969; Weidman and Sussex 1971;
Yap 1969). Wittkower and Weidman (1969) described the psychologically integrative function of magic in which something that is ill-
defined, anxiety-arousing, and disruptive is given a name. Torrey
(1986) claims that both psychiatrists and witch doctors use the same
basic approach. Both depend on naming the problem, the personal
qualities of the therapist, and the client expectancies to get better.

There is a tendency to look for the pathology in the client while overlooking the pathology of the surrounding environment (King 1978) and
to neglect the larger network of persons within which the client is
located (Sampson 1977). Our goal should be to maintain the natural
support system in the client's environment to mediate mental health.
The alternative approach ignores the client's cultural context and allows
culturally encapsulated counselors to assume that their limited views
can accommodate the broad range of cultural variations with validity.

In much of the world, professional counseling is available only to the
economic and social elite (Drapela 1977). Psychological help to other
segments of the population is supplied through informal networks of
family and friends (Brammer 1978). Counselors can learn a great deal
through these informal networks to facilitate outreach services and to
identify modal characteristics of the informal helper who is accessible,
credible, empathic, caring, practical, and in direct touch with the client.

Many healers and healing institutions build on the self-righting
mechanisms of the client's natural support system but also provide
alternative supports when these endogenous mechanisms break down.

Prince (1976) describes the importance of these frequently overlooked endogenous elements of healing as opposed to the more popularly studied exogenous factors. Under conditions of stress, these self-healing mechanisms might take the form of altered states of consciousness such as dreams, dissociated states, religious experiences, or even psychotic reactions. Hispanic cultures have variations of folk illnesses caused by sociopsychological and spiritual disturbances (Levine and Padilla 1980). Torrey (1986) in his comparison of witch doctors and psychiatrists provides numerous examples of these self-righting approaches including the study of *curanderas* and *espiritismo*.

Counseling can occur in an informal as well as a formal context. The place or environment where counseling occurs and the method by which counseling is provided are defined differently in different situations. Pearson (1985) developed a model for studying natural support systems in counseling to meet the basic needs for affiliation and attachment. Green (1982) developed a model for help-seeking behavior in social services that incorporates both the client's cultural framework for labeling problems and the provider's way of offering help. Counselors must be able to transcend their own biases and examine the strength of a client's network of support resources and incorporate those resources in counseling.

Pedersen (1986) matches formal and informal counseling methods with formal and informal counseling contexts to describe the range of support systems that apply to counseling. In many cultures the informal method or context or both is the preferred source of help and support. A formal method of counseling in a formal setting is frequently a threatening and less valuable source of help and support among culturally different client populations.

Pedersen and Pedersen (1985) are developing a "Cultural Grid" that integrates a full range of ethnographic, demographic, status, and affiliation variables into social systems that apply to each person and context. These social systems on one dimension of the grid are matched with personal cognitive variables of behavior, expectations, and values on the grid's second dimension. By matching social systems with person variables, the grid illustrates a personal-cultural orientation to a particular decision in a dynamic rather than a static framework that allows for the complexity of cultural differences.

In many cultures indigenous helpers, such as *curanderas,* medicine men and women, shamans, psychics, or voodoo practitioners (Green 1982), are often sought for assistance during illnesses. Indigenous practices need not take the place of psychological or physical treatments but may be used in conjunction with these treatments. Without understanding the origins and functions of folk healing methods, the chances of cultural misunderstandings are high and sometimes tragic. For example, the *Journal of the American Medical Association* reported that a Vietnamese father who had practiced *cao gio* (coin rubbing) on his child was falsely accused of child abuse. *Cao gio* involves rubbing the skin (back, neck, chest areas) with a coin to alleviate common cold or flu symptoms. Although the lesions that result from *cao gio* resemble those inflicted in traumas, there are no known harmful effects. An unfortunate outcome of this incident was that the father committed suicide (Yeatman and Dang 1980).

To prevent such cultural misconceptions, it is important for the counselor to respect the client's worldview. A worldview is a holistic concept that ties together the belief systems, values, lifestyles, and modes of problem solving of a particular cultural group. The concept of worldview is a complex one, and models for describing it are needed. Several paradigms have been proposed that we will discuss briefly.

Sue (1977, 1978) defined a worldview as the way in which the individual perceives his or her relationship to the world, including other people, institutions, nature, and things. One dimension of this worldview is based on Rotter's (1966, 1975) distinction between internal control (IC), in which reinforcement is contingent on a person's own actions, and external control (EC), in which consequences are perceived to result from luck, chance, fate, or powerful others. Next Sue has added the dimension of an internal locus of responsibility (IR), where success is attributed to a person's skills, resulting in "person blame," and an external locus of responsibility (ER), where the sociocultural environment is more potent than the individual, resulting in "system blame." In Sue's classification the IC-IR worldview exemplifies white middle-class cultural values, the EC-IR view describes minority persons likely to have little control over how others define them, the EC-ER view is prevalent among minorities who blame their problems on an oppressive social system in which they are powerless, and the IC-ER view assumes the belief in one's ability to achieve personal goals if given a chance (see Sue 1981a for discussion). Helms and Giorgis (1980) tested Sue's worldview model on white, black, and African male college students. Their findings provided some support for different cultural groups exhibiting different worldviews. The worldview of black students was consistently an "external locus of control, external locus of responsibility" (EC-ER), and that of white students was the opposite (IC-IR). Worldviews of African students varied between three orientations depending on how the locus of responsibility was measured.

Kluckhohn and Strodtbeck (1961) defined worldview through a value orientation concept derived from existential categories such as human nature, the relationship of humans to the natural world, time perspective, activity orientation, and interpersonal relations. Helpers need to understand both the client's values and their own to develop appropriate problem-solving strategies (Ibrahim 1985). Ibrahim and Kahn (1987) reported on a 45-item Likert-type scale designed to assess the five value orientations of the Kluckhohn model. Their findings indicated adequate reliability and construct validity of their Scale to Assess World Views Across Cultures (SAWVAC). Carter and Helms (1987) studied black American racial identity attitudes and value orientations. Carter (1984) had reported moderate reliability for the Intercultural Values Inventory used in this study. The authors found differences in value orientation as related to gender and various stages of racial identity.

Multicultural Training Issues

Counseling professionals are not trained to meet the mental health needs of ethnic minorities (e.g., Dillard 1983; Sue 1981a; Sue et al. 1982; Pedersen 1981). Two important training recommendations that came out of psychology conferences held at Austin (1975) and Dulles (1978) were that psychological education and training programs should include an evaluation of cross-cultural competency and that continuing professional development should occur beyond the advanced degree (Sue et al. 1982).

In a study assessing the status of minority curricula and training in accredited clinical psychology programs, Bernal and Padilla (1982) mentioned many reasons for preparing mental health professionals to provide services to ethnic minorities. For example, minority groups are underserved, and there is a severe shortage of ethnic minority mental health professionals. A large proportion of nonminority graduates will be employed in settings serving minorities. The need reaches a critical state in light of the 1980 census figures that show that minorities now make up 23% of the U.S. population (U.S. Bureau of the Census 1985).

Current multicultural training programs are described as experimental and scarce (Lefley 1985), lacking an established constituency (Pedersen 1981), and inadequate in addressing skill development (Sue 1981a). Ibrahim and Thompson's (1982) survey of counselor education programs revealed that only 3% of the respondents reported having cross-cultural counseling as part of their core curriculum. Similarly, the American Psychological Association's (APA) Subcommittee on Culturally Sensitive Models of the Board of Ethnic Minority Affairs (BEMA) conducted a nationwide survey to assess the specific types of culturally relevant course material and experiences that are offered in training graduate students. Results indicated that only 4.2% of the programs offered culturally relevant training material in a format in which it could be comprehensively covered.

There is disagreement on how counseling programs can best meet the needs of minority clients (McDavis and Parker 1977). Some believe that existing strategies are effective for all people, while others believe that existing models are based on middle-class, dominant cultural values and are thus ineffective with other cultures. Bernal and Padilla (1982) pointed out that the training that is available is concentrated in a few programs. Their survey revealed that minority-related courses were taught in only 16 out of 76 accredited clinical psychology programs.

Several authors have expressed concern that cross-cultural issues in counseling are analyzed from a white middle-class perspective (Atkinson, Staso, and Hosford 1978; Smith 1977; Sue 1981a). This is one of several problems that have hindered the training of culturally skilled counselors. Other problems include a lack of direction, a haphazard approach, and a low priority for program development. There is also little emphasis on skills development and inadequate sharing of successful training programs (Ponterotto and Casas 1987).

Members of the APA's Division 17 (Counseling Psychology) Education and Training Committee (see Sue et al. 1982) concurred that a cross-cultural training curriculum should incorporate beliefs and attitudes, knowledge, and skills. It should also focus on immediate social needs and problems and present a balanced positive picture of minority groups. The committee felt "a strong responsibility to bring to the membership's attention the need for developing minimal cross-cultural counseling competencies to be incorporated into training programs" (Sue et al. 1982, 48–49). General guidelines were presented and endorsed by the Executive Committee of Division 17 (Smith 1982). For example, counselors should be aware of their own values and biases and how they may affect minority clients; counselors should be aware of institutional barriers that prevent minorities from using mental health services; and counselors should be able to send and receive accurate and appropriate verbal and nonverbal messages.

Vontress (1981) and Korchin (1980) viewed direct "experiential" exposure of counselors to culturally different populations as a necessary part of training. Copeland (1983) suggested that such exposure would be desirable in a supervised practicum after preparation. Direct contact can only happen when culturally different persons are accepted as resources and eventually as colleagues (Helms 1984). Pedersen, Holwill, and Shapiro (1978) stressed the necessity for training programs to consider culturally different people as relevant resources for both minority and majority trainees.

Ultimately, the numbers of minority students and tenure-track minority faculty should be increased (Bernal and Padilla 1982; Myers

1982). Increasing the minority faculty may serve to counterbalance stereotyping and misinterpretation, increase the credibility of graduate training programs, and present viable role models to minorities interested in psychology careers (Smith 1982). Unfortunately, minority students frequently anticipate a nonsupportive environment and will not apply to counseling programs in which they notice a scarcity of course offerings on nonwhite perspectives and a low representation of minority faculty (Parham and Moreland 1981).

Training programs should include at least four components (Copeland 1983; Helms 1984; Sue 1981a): (1) consciousness raising, (2) cognitive development, (3) affective awareness, and (4) skills development. Helms (1984) has created a cognitive development model that responds to the trainee's level of racial consciousness. She proposes that trainees start with historical and sociocultural information, then proceed to skill building, cognitive and affective self-awareness, and finally to cultural immersion. Similarly, Carney and Kahn (1984) devised a developmental training model that consists of five stages of development, each responding to an appropriate training environment. Other models have been formulated for training culturally effective counselors that could be matched to a trainee's level of cultural awareness (e.g., Arredondo-Dowd and Gonsalves 1980; Copeland 1982; McDavis and Parker 1977; Sue 1973).

Lefley and Pedersen (1986) describe three major training projects supported by the National Institute of Mental Health: Brandeis University's Training Program in Ethnicity and Mental Health, the University of Hawaii's Developing Interculturally Skilled Counseling (DISC) program, and the University of Miami's Cross-Cultural Training Institute for Mental Health Professionals. In an attempt to systematically describe and organize curricula for graduate programs, Ridley (1985) has also developed a three-dimensional model, with an emphasis upon population, intervention, and curriculum target at Fuller Theological Seminary.

Copeland (1983) suggested that training models could be divided into four types: (1) a separate course added to an existing program; (2) a core of courses with skill-building activities and a practicum or internship; (3) an interdisciplinary approach in which students enroll in courses outside their department; and (4) an integration model in which the entire department is committed to addressing cross-cultural issues in every aspect of the program. Copeland concluded that the integration model is the most desirable, yet most difficult, to implement. More recently, Margolis and Rungta (1986) suggested that the best and most feasible model integrates specialized knowledge (of ethnic minorities and other special populations) into a single course, insuring that relevant knowledge, awareness, and skills are generalized across populations. Clearly, training programs in cross-cultural counseling are still in the process of development.

Future Trends in Multicultural Counseling

A Delphi study among 53 identified experts in the field of cross-cultural counseling was conducted by Heath, Neimeyer, and Pedersen (1987) to predict the course of cross-cultural counseling during the next 10 years. Using a 48-item questionnaire, the panel anticipated developments in the area of training and preparation, theory and research, and social organization.

Results of this Delphi poll showed that increases were predicted in every area of cross-cultural training and preparation. The most probable change predicted is a 45% or greater increase in the number of cross-cultural training programs that incorporate skills development. Smith (1982) and Brammer (1985) made similar speculations.

Increases were also anticipated for all research and theory items. The most probable change is a 47% or higher increase in publications related to Hispanics. Padilla and DeSnyder (1985) also foresaw such a trend. In the area of social organization, the most likely change is that there will be presentations on cross-cultural counseling at all counseling psychology regional and national conferences and conventions.

The 53 Delphi panelists were also asked to nominate the top graduate programs in cross-cultural counseling (see Heath 1987 for discussion). Syracuse University, the University of Hawaii, Western Washington University, and Teachers College, Columbia University, had the highest-ranked programs. These findings were similar to those found by Ponterotto and Casas (1987) in evaluating multicultural training within counselor education programs.

Three major trends emerge from this study. First, although there is considerable optimism about improving the quality of current cross-cultural counseling training and preparation programs, as indicated by the projected increase in incorporating skills development and role-playing, there is less optimism regarding the increase in the number of programs at the doctoral and postdoctoral levels. Second, the research of the future will reflect the tremendous need to better understand the specific ethnic groups that are increasing most rapidly (i.e., Hispanics, Asians, refugees). Comparably less emphasis will be on how various cultural differences affect the client-counselor dyad. The third trend reveals positive changes in the area of professional networking and acknowledgment of multicultural issues (e.g., association effectiveness and conference presentations) but continued difficulty in transferring the ideals and awareness into better services.

Conclusion

The cultural bias in counseling has become more visible as alternative mental health services have been developed by a variety of culturally different groups. Each special population maintains a unique perspective with its own cultural identity. Increased attention to minority needs has helped the counseling profession move toward increased multicultural awareness.

This chapter has outlined the historical factors behind this increase in multicultural awareness. Contemporary research on client, counselor, and environmental variables further documents the importance of multicultural awareness for accuracy in counseling communication. There are indications that the level of multicultural awareness is likely to increase still further in the future.

The cultural variable has been difficult to study because of its complexity and political volatility. The lack of a clear constituency has inhibited counselor education and training programs in their allocation of resources toward multicultural awareness. In the last few years, however, an expanding literature on multicultural research and more courses and programs with cross-cultural emphasis have emerged. In searching for significant developments in counseling as a profession during the last several decades, the impact of multicultural awareness may emerge as the single most important development.

The motivation for increased multicultural awareness in counseling has been based on an ethical obligation to treat all clients fairly and humanely. There is another equally strong argument to be made for multicultural development to improve the measurement of psychological data and the provision of appropriate and effective services to a multicultural population. We may choose to ignore cultural variables in counseling. However, the multicultural dynamics of counselors and clients will continue to shape the delivery of counseling services with or without our cooperation. It is therefore essential that all intentional counselors prepare themselves for a multicultural future in which all significant and salient variables of counseling are considered.

References

Abramowitz, S. I., and Murray, J. 1983. Race effects in psychotherapy. In J. Murray and P. R. Abramson (eds.), *Bias in psychotherapy*, 215–255. New York: Praeger.

Acosta, F., and Sheehan, J. 1976. Preferences toward Mexican American and Anglo American psychotherapists. *Journal of Consulting and Clinical Psychology* 44:272–279.

Acosta, F., Yamamoto, J., and Evans, L. A., eds. 1982. *Effective psychotherapy for low-income and minority patients.* New York: Plenum Press.

Ahia, C. E. 1984. Cross-cultural counseling concerns. *Personnel and Guidance Journal* 62:339–341.

Anderson, J. W. 1983. The effects of culture and social class on client preferences for counseling methods. *Journal of Non-White Concerns* 11 (3): 84–98.

Arredondo-Dowd, P. M., and Gonsalves, J. 1980. Preparing culturally effective counselors. *Personnel and Guidance Journal* 58:657–662.

Atkinson, D. R. 1983. Ethnic similarity in counseling: A review of research. *Counseling Psychologist* 11:79–92.

————. 1985a. A meta-review of research on cross-cultural counseling and psychotherapy. *Journal of Multicultural Counseling and Development* 13 (4): 138–153.

————. 1985b. Research on cross-cultural counseling and psychotherapy: A review and update of reviews. In P. B. Pedersen (ed.), *Handbook of cross-cultural counseling and therapy,* 189–197. Westport, CT: Greenwood Press.

Atkinson, D. R., Maruyama, M., and Matsui, S. 1978. The effects of counselor approach on Asian Americans' perceptions of counselor credibility and utility. *Journal of Counseling Psychology* 25:76–83.

Atkinson, D. R., Morten, G., and Sue, D. W. 1983. *Counseling American minorities: A cross-cultural perspective.* 2d ed. Dubuque, IA: William C. Brown.

Atkinson, D. R., and Schein, S. 1986. Similarity in counseling. *Counseling Psychologist* 14 (2): 319–354.

Atkinson, D. R., Staso, D., and Hosford, R. 1978. Selecting counselor trainees with multi-cultural strengths: A solution to the Bakke decision crisis. *Personnel and Guidance Journal* 56:546–549.

Berman, J. 1979. Individual versus societal focus: Problem diagnosis of black and white female counselors. *Journal of Cross-Cultural Psychology* 10 (4): 497–507.

Bernal, M. E., and Padilla, A. M. 1982. Status of minority curricula and training in clinical psychology. *American Psychologist* 37:780–787.

Bernstein, B. L., Wade, P. D., and Hofmann, B. 1987. Students' race and preferences for counselor's race, sex, age, and experience. *Journal of Multicultural Counseling and Development* 15 (2): 60–70.

Berry, J. W. 1969. On cross-cultural compatibility. *International Journal of Psychology* 4:119–128.

————. 1980. Social and cultural change. In H. C. Triandis and J. W. Berry (eds.), *Handbook of cross-cultural psychology.* Vol. 5, *Social psychology,* 211–281. Boston: Allyn and Bacon.

Bloombaum, M., Yamamoto, J., and James, Q. 1968. Cultural stereotyping among psychotherapists. *Journal of Consulting and Clinical Psychology* 32 (1): 99.

Brammer, L. M. 1978. Informal helping systems in selected subcultures. *Personnel and Guidance Journal* 56 (8): 476–479.

————. 1985. Nonformal support in cross-cultural counseling and therapy. In P. B. Pedersen (ed.), *Handbook of cross-cultural counseling and therapy,* 87–92. Westport, CT: Greenwood Press.

Brislin, R. W. 1981. *Cross-cultural encounters: Face to face interaction.* New York: Pergamon Press.

Carkhuff, R. R., and Pierce, R. 1967. Differential effects of therapist race and social class upon patient depth of self-exploration in the initial clinical interview. *Journal of Consulting Psychology* 31 (6): 632–634.

Carney, C. G., and Kahn, K. B. 1984. Building competencies for effective cross-cultural counseling: A developmental view. *Counseling Psychologist* 12:111–119.

Carter, R. T. 1984. *The relationship between black American students' value-orientations and their racial identity attitudes.* Typescript. University of Maryland, College Park.

Carter, R. T., and Helms, J. E. 1987. The relationship of black value-orientations to racial identity attitudes. *Measurement and Evaluation in Counseling and Development* 20:183–193.

Casas, J. M. 1984. Policy, training, and research in counseling psychology: The racial/ethnic minority perspective. In S. D. Brown and R. W. Lent (eds.), *Handbook of counseling psychology,* 785–831. New York: John Wiley and Sons.

Chien, C., and Yamamoto, J. 1982. Asian-American and Pacific Islander patients. In F. X. Acosta, J. Yamamoto, and L. A. Evans (eds.), *Effective psychotherapy for low-income and minority patients,* 117–145. New York: Plenum Press.

Cole, M., and Bruner, J. S. 1972. Cultural differences and inferences about psychological processes. *American Psychologist* 26:867–876.

Copeland, E. J. 1982. Minority populations and traditional counseling programs: Some alternatives. *Counselor Education and Supervision* 2:187–193.

———. 1983. Cross-cultural counseling and psychotherapy: A historical perspective, implications for research and training. *Personnel and Guidance Journal* 62:10–15.

Cross, W. E. 1971. The Negro-to-black conversion experience. *Black World* 20:13–27.

Daniel, J. 1985. The poor: Aliens in an affluent society: Cross-cultural communication. In L. A. Samovar and R. E. Porter (eds.), *Intercultural communication: A reader,* 128–135. Belmont, CA: Wadsworth Publishing.

Dauphinais, P., Dauphinais, L., and Rowe, W. 1981. Effects of race and communication style on Indian perceptions of counselor effectiveness. *Counselor Education and Supervision* 21:72–80.

Diaz-Guerrero, R. 1977. A Mexican psychology. *American Psychologist* 32:934–944.

Dillard, J. M. 1983. *Multicultural counseling: Toward ethnic and cultural relevance in human encounters.* Chicago: Nelson-Hall.

Draguns, J. G. 1974. Values reflected in psychopathology: The case of the Protestant ethic. *Ethos* 2:115–136.

Drapela, V. J., ed. 1977. *Guidance in other countries.* Tampa: University of South Florida.

Driver, E. D. 1965. *The sociology and anthropology of mental illness.* Amherst: University of Massachusetts Press.

Ewing, T. N. 1974. Racial similarity of client and counselor and client satisfaction with counseling. *Journal of Counseling Psychology* 21:446–449.

Favazza, A. R., and Oman, M. 1977. *Anthropological and cross-cultural themes in mental health: An annotated bibliography 1925–1974.* Columbia: University of Missouri Press.

Fields, S. 1979. Mental health and the melting pot. *Innovations* 6 (2): 2–3.

Fromm, E., Suzuki, D. T., and Martino, R. 1960. *Zen Buddhism and psychoanalysis.* New York: Harper and Row.

Fukuyama, M. A., and Neimeyer, G. J. 1985. Using the Cultural Attitudes Repertory Technique (CART) in a cross-cultural counseling workshop. *Journal of Counseling and Development* 63:304–305.

Gambosa, A. M., Tosi, D. J., and Riccio, A. C. 1976. Race and counselor climate in the counselor preference of delinquent girls. *Journal of Counseling Psychology* 23:160–162.

Goldstein, A. P. 1981. Expectancy effects in cross-cultural counseling. In A. J. Marsella and P. B. Pedersen (eds.), *Cross-cultural counseling and psychotherapy: Foundations, evaluation, and cultural considerations,* 85–101. Elmsford, NY: Pergamon Press.

Gomes-Schwartz, B., Hadley, S. W., and Strupp, H. H. 1978. Individual psychotherapy and behavior therapy. *Annual Review of Psychology* 29:435–472.

Gordon, E. W., and Smith, P. M. 1971. The guidance specialist and the disadvantaged student. In D. R. Cook (ed.), *Guidance for education in revolution.* Boston: Allyn and Bacon.

Gordon, M., and Grantham, R. J. 1979. Helper preference in disadvantaged students. *Journal of Counseling Psychology* 26:337–343.

Gourash, N. 1978. Help-seeking: A review of the literature. *American Journal of Community Psychology* 6 (5): 413–424.

Green, J. W. 1982. *Cultural awareness in the human services.* Englewood Cliffs, NJ: Prentice-Hall.

Griffith, M. S. 1977. The influence of race on the psychotherapeutic relationship. *Psychiatry* 40:27–40.

Griffith, M. S., and Jones, E. E. 1979. Race and psychotherapy: Changing perspectives. In J. H. Masserman (ed.), *Current psychiatric therapies.* Vol. 8. New York: Grune and Stratton.

Guthrie, R. 1976. *Even the rat was white: A historical view of psychology.* New York: Harper and Row.

Halleck, S. L. 1971. Therapy is the handmaiden of the status quo. *Psychology Today* 4:30–34, 98–100.

Harrison, D. K. 1975. Race as a counselor-client variable in counseling and psychotherapy: A review of the research. *Counseling Psychologist* 5 (1): 124–133.

Heath, A. E. 1987. *The future of cross-cultural counseling: A Delphi poll.* Master's thesis, University of Florida, Gainesville.

Heath, A. E., Neimeyer, G. J., and Pedersen, P. B. 1988. The future of cross-cultural counseling: A Delphi poll. *Journal of Counseling and Development* 67 (2): 27–30.

Helms, J. E. 1984. Toward a theoretical explanation of the effects of race on counseling: A black and white model. *Counseling Psychologist* 12 (4): 153–165.

———. 1985. Cultural identity in the treatment process. In P. B. Pedersen (ed.), *Handbook of cross-cultural counseling and therapy*, 239–245. Westport, CT: Greenwood Press.

———. 1986. Expanding racial identity theory to cover the counseling process. *Journal of Counseling Psychology* 33 (1): 62–64.

Helms, J. E., and Giorgis, T. W. 1980. A comparison on the locus of control and anxiety level of African, black American, and white American college students. *Journal of College Student Personnel* 21:503–509.

Higginbotham, H. N. 1977. Culture and the role of client expectancy. In R. W. Brislin and M. P. Hamnett (eds.), *Topics in culture learning*, Vol. 5:107–124. Honolulu: East-West Center Press.

———. 1979. Culture and the delivery of psychological services in developing nations. *Transcultural Psychiatric Research Review* 16:7–27.

Higginbotham, H. N., and Tanaka-Matsumi, T. 1981. Behavioral approaches to counseling across cultures. In P. B. Pedersen, J. G. Draguns, W. J. Lonner, and J. E. Trimble (eds.), *Counseling across cultures,* 247–274. Honolulu: University of Hawaii Press.

Hsu, F. L. K., ed. 1972. *Psychological anthropology.* Cambridge, MA: Schenkman.

Ibrahim, F. A. 1985. Effective cross-cultural counseling and psychotherapy: A framework. *Counseling Psychologist* 13:625–638.

Ibrahim, F. A., and Arredondo, P. M. 1986. Ethical standards for cross-cultural counseling: Counselor preparation, practice, assessment, and research. *Journal of Counseling and Development* 64:349–352.

Ibrahim, F. A., and Kahn, H. 1987. Assessment of world views. *Psychological Reports* 60:163–176.

Ibrahim, F. A., and Thompson, D. L. 1982. Preparation of secondary school counselors: A national survey. *Counselor Education and Supervision* 22:113–120.

Inouye, K. H., and Pedersen, P. B. 1985. Cultural and ethnic content of the 1977 to 1982 American Psychological Association Convention programs. *Counseling Psychologist* 13:639–648.

Ishiyama, F. I. 1987. Use of Morita therapy in shyness counseling in the West: Promoting client's self-acceptance and action taking. *Journal of Counseling and Development* 65:547–551.

Ivey, A. E. 1977. Toward a definition of the culturally effective counselor. *Personnel and Guidance Journal* 55:296–302.

Jackson, G. C., and Kirschner, S. A. 1973. Racial self-designation and preference for a counselor. *Journal of Counseling Psychology* 15:226–236.

Jenkins, A. H. 1982. *The psychology of the Afro-American: A humanistic approach.* Elmsford, NY: Pergamon Press.

Jensen, A. R. 1969. How much can we boost IQ and scholastic achievement? *Harvard Educational Review* 39:1–123.

Jones, A., and Seagull, A. A. 1983. Dimensions of the relationship between the black client and the white therapist: A theoretical overview. In D. R.

Atkinson, G. Morten, and D. W. Sue (eds.), *Counseling American minorities: A cross-cultural perspective,* 2d ed., 156–166. Dubuque, IA: William C. Brown.

Jones, E. E. 1974. Social class and psychotherapy: A critical review of the research. *Psychiatry* 37:307–320.

Jones, E. E., and Korchin, S. J., eds. 1982. *Minority mental health.* New York: Praeger.

Jones, R. T. 1980. *Black psychology.* 2d ed. New York: Harper and Row.

Kagan, N. 1964. Three dimensions of counselor encapsulation. *Journal of Counseling Psychology* 11 (4): 361–365.

Kelly, G. 1955. *The psychology of personal constructs.* New York: Norton.

Kemp, C. 1962. Influence of dogmatism on the training of counselors. *Journal of Counseling Psychology* 9:155–157.

Kennedy, C. D., and Wagner, N. N. 1979. Psychology and affirmative action: 1977. *Professional Psychology* 10:234–243.

Khatib, S. M., and Nobles, W. W. 1977. Historical foundations of African psychology and their philosophical consequences. *Journal of Black Psychology* 4:91–101.

King, L. M. 1978. Social and cultural influences on psychopathology. *Annual Review of Psychology* 29:405–533.

Kleinman, A., and Kleinman, J. 1985. Somatization: The interconnections in Chinese society among culture, depressive experiences, and the meanings of pain. In A. Kleinman and B. Good (eds.), *Culture and depression: Studies in the anthropology and cross-cultural psychiatry of affect and disorder,* 429–490. Berkeley: University of California Press.

Kluckhohn, F. R., and Strodtbeck, F. L. 1961. *Variations in value orientation.* New York: Harper and Row.

Korchin, S. J. 1980. Clinical psychology and minority problems. *American Psychologist* 35:262–269.

Krumboltz, J. D., Becker-Haven, J. F., and Burnett, K. F. 1979. Counseling psychology. *Annual Review of Psychology* 30:555–602.

Lambert, M. J. 1981. The implications of psychotherapy outcome research on cross-cultural psychotherapy. In A. J. Marsella and P. B. Pedersen (eds.), *Cross-cultural counseling and psychotherapy: Foundations, evaluations, and cultural considerations,* 126–158. Elmsford, NY: Pergamon Press.

Landis, D., and Brislin, R. W., eds. 1983. *Handbook of intercultural training.* Vols. 1–3. New York: Pergamon Press.

Lebra, T. S. 1982. Self-reconstruction in Japanese religious psychotherapy. In A. J. Marsella and G. M. White (eds.), *Cultural conceptions of mental health and therapy,* 269–283. Boston: D. Reidel Publishing.

Lee, J. D., Trimble, J. E., Cvetkovich, G., and Lonner, W. J. 1981. Exploring ethnic cultural content of APA conventions. *APA Monitor* 12 (2): 3.

Lefley, H. P. 1985. Mental health training across cultures. In P. B. Pedersen (ed.), *Handbook of cross-cultural counseling and therapy,* 259–266. Westport, CT: Greenwood Press.

Lefley, H. P., and Pedersen, P. B., eds. 1986. *Cross-cultural training for mental health professionals.* Springfield, IL: Charles C. Thomas.

Leininger, M. 1978. *Transcultural nursing: Concepts, theories and practices.* New York: John Wiley and Sons.

Leung, P. 1973. Comparative effects of training in external and internal concentration on two counseling behaviors. *Journal of Counseling Psychology* 20 (3): 227–234.

Levine, E. S., and Padilla, A. M. 1980. *Crossing cultures in therapy: Pluralistic counseling for the Hispanic.* Monterey, CA: Brooks-Cole.

Levine, R., and Campbell, D. T. 1972. *Ethnocentrism: Theories of conflict, ethnic attitudes and group behavior.* New York: John Wiley and Sons.

Lonner, W. J. 1985. Issues in testing and assessment in cross-cultural counseling. *Counseling Psychologist* 13:599–614.

Lonner, W. J., and Sundberg, N. D. 1985. Assessment in cross-cultural counseling and therapy. In P. B. Pedersen (ed.), *Handbook of cross-cultural counseling and therapy,* 200–205. Westport, CT: Greenwood Press.

Lorion, R. P., and Parron, D. L. 1985. *Counseling the countertransference: A strategy for treating the untreatable.* In P. B. Pedersen (ed.), *Handbook of cross-cultural counseling and therapy,* 79–87. Westport, CT: Greenwood Press.

McDavis, R. J., and Parker, M. 1977. A course on counseling ethnic minorities: A model. *Counselor Education and Supervision* 17:146–149.

McGoldrick, M., Pearce, J. K., and Giordano, J., eds. 1982. *Ethnicity and family therapy.* New York: Guilford Press.

Margolis, R. L., and Rungta, S. A. 1986. Training counselors for work with special populations: A second look. *Journal of Counseling and Development* 64:642–644.

Marsella, A. J. 1979. Cross-cultural studies of mental disorders. In A. J. Marsella, R. Tharp, and T. Ciborowski (eds.), *Perspectives on cross-cultural psychology,* 233–262. New York: Academic Press.

Marsella, A. J., and Pedersen, P. B., eds. 1981. *Cross-cultural counseling and psychotherapy: Foundations, evaluation, and cultural considerations.* Elmsford, NY: Pergamon Press.

Marsella, A. J., and White, G. M., eds. 1982. *Cultural conceptions of mental health and therapy.* Dordrecht, Holland: D. Reidel.

Martinez, J. L., Jr. 1977. *Chicano psychology.* New York: Academic Press.

Menacker, J. 1971. *Urban poor students and guidance.* Boston: Houghton Mifflin.

Mezzano, J. 1969. A note on dogmatism and counselor effectiveness. *Counselor Education and Supervision* 9 (1): 64–65.

Millikan, R. L. 1965. Prejudice and counseling effectiveness. *Personnel and Guidance Journal* 43:710–712.

Millikan, R. L., and Patterson, J. J. 1967. Relationship of dogmatism and prejudice to counseling effectiveness. *Counselor Education and Supervision,* 6:125–129.

Mitchell, H. 1970. The black experience in higher education. *Counseling Psychologist* 2:30–36.

Morrow, D. L. 1972. Cultural addiction. *Journal of Rehabilitation* 38 (3): 30–32.

Morten, G. 1984. Racial self-labeling and preference for counselor race. *Journal of Non-White Concerns* 12 (3): 105–109.

Muliozzi, A. D. 1972. *Inter-racial counseling: Does it work?* Paper presented at an American Personnel and Guidance Association meeting. Chicago.

Murase, T. 1982. *Sunao:* A central value in Japanese psychotherapy. In A. J. Marsella and G. M. White (eds.), *Cultural conceptions of mental health and therapy,* 317–329. Boston: D. Reidel Publishing.

Myers, R. A. 1982. Education and training: The next decade. *Counseling Psychologist* 10:39–45.

Neimeyer, G. J., and Fukuyama, M. 1984. Exploring the content and structure of cross-cultural attitudes. *Counselor Education and Supervision* 23 (3): 214–224.

Neimeyer, G. J., and Gonzales, M. 1983. Duration, satisfaction, and perceived effectiveness of cross-cultural counseling. *Journal of Counseling Psychology* 30:91–95.

Padilla, A. M., and DeSnyder, N. S. 1985. Counseling Hispanics: Strategies for effective interaction. In P. B. Pedersen (ed.), *Handbook of cross-cultural counseling and therapy,* 157–164. Westport, CT: Greenwood Press.

Pande, S. K. 1968. The mystique of "Western" psychotherapy: An Eastern interpretation. *Journal of Nervous and Mental Disease* 146:425–432.

Parham, T. A., and Helms, J. E. 1981. The influence of black students' racial identity attitudes on preference for counselor's race. *Journal of Counseling Psychology* 28:250–257.

———. 1985a. Attitudes of racial identity and self-esteem of black students: An exploratory investigation. *Journal of College Student Personnel* 26 (2): 143–147.

———. 1985b. Relation of racial identity attitudes to self-actualization and affective states of black students. *Journal of Counseling Psychology* 32 (3): 431–440.

Parham, W., and Moreland, J. R. 1981. Non-white students in counseling psychology: A closer look. *Professional Psychology* 12:499–507.

Patterson, C. H. 1974. *Relationship counseling and psychotherapy.* New York: Harper and Row.

———. 1978. Cross-cultural or intercultural psychotherapy. *International Journal for the Advancement of Counseling* 1:231–248.

Pearson, R. E. 1985. The recognition and use of natural support systems in cross-cultural counseling. In P. B. Pedersen (ed.), *Handbook of cross-cultural counseling and therapy,* 299–306. Westport, CT: Greenwood Press.

Pedersen, A., and Pedersen, P. B. 1985. The cultural grid: A personal cultural orientation. In L. Samovar and R. Porter (eds.), *Intercultural communication: A reader,* 50–62. Belmont, CA: Wadsworth Publishing.

Pedersen, P. B. 1977. Asian theories of personality. In R. Corsini and A. J. Marsella (eds.), *Contemporary theories of personality.* Itasea, IL: Peacock.

———. 1979. Non-Western psychologies: The search for alternatives. In A. J. Marsella, R. Tharp, and T. Ciborowski, (eds.), *Perspectives in cross-cultural psychology,* 77–98. New York: Academic Press.

———. 1981. The cultural inclusiveness of counseling. In P. B. Pedersen, J. G. Draguns, W. J. Lonner, and J. E. Trimble (eds.), *Counseling across cultures,* rev. ed., 22–58. Honolulu: University of Hawaii Press.

———, ed. 1985. *Handbook of cross-cultural counseling and therapy.* Westport, CT: Greenwood Press.

———. 1986. The cultural role of conceptual and contextual support systems in counseling. *Journal of the American Mental Health Counselor Association* 8 (1): 35–42.

Pedersen, P. B., Holwill, C. F., and Shapiro, J. A. 1978. A cross-cultural training procedure for classes in counselor education. *Counselor Education and Supervision* 17:146–149.

Peoples, V. Y., and Dell, D. M. 1975. Black and white student preferences for counselor roles. *Journal of Counseling Psychology* 22:529–534.

Pomales, J., Claiborn, C. D., and LaFromboise, T. D. 1986. Effects of black student's racial identity on perception of white counselors varying in cultural sensitivity. *Journal of Counseling Psychology* 33:57–61.

Ponterotto, J. G., and Casas, J. M. 1987. In search of multicultural competence within counselor education programs. *Journal of Counseling and Development* 65:430–434.

Prince, R. H. 1976. Psychotherapy as the manipulation of endogenous healing mechanisms: A transcultural survey. *Transcultural Psychiatric Research Review* 13:115–134.

Ridley, C. R. 1985. Imperatives for ethnic and cultural relevance in psychology training programs. *Professional Psychology* 16:611–622.

Rotenberg, M. 1974. The Protestant ethic versus people-changing sciences. In J. Dawson and W. J. Lonner (eds.), *Readings in cross-cultural psychology.* Hong Kong: University of Hong Kong Press.

Rotter, J. 1966. Generalized expectancies for internal versus external control of reinforcement. *Psychological Monographs* 80 (1, Whole no. 609).

———. 1975. Some problems and misconceptions related to the construct of internal versus external control of reinforcement. *Journal of Consulting and Clinical Psychology* 43:56–67.

Russo, N. F., Olmedo, E. L., Stapp, J., and Fulcher, R. 1981. Women and minorities in psychology. *American Psychologist* 36:1315–1363.

Russo, R. J., Kelz, J. W., and Hudson, G. 1964. Are good counselors open-minded? *Counselor Education and Supervision* 3 (2): 74–77.

Sampson, E. 1977. Psychology and the American ideal. *Journal of Personality and Social Psychology* 11:767–782.

Sanchez, A. R., and Atkinson, D. R. 1983. Mexican-American cultural commitment, preference for counselor ethnicity and willingness to use counseling. *Journal of Counseling Psychology* 30:215–220.

Sattler, J. M. 1977. The effects of therapist-client racial similarity. In A. S. Gurman and A. M. Razin (eds.), *Effective psychotherapy: A handbook of research,* 252–290. New York: Pergamon Press.

Schwebel, M. 1964. Ideology and counselor encapsulation. *Journal of Counseling Psychology* 11 (4): 366–369.

Sears, R. R. 1970. Transcultural variables and conceptual equivalence. In T. Al-Issa and W. Dennis (eds.), *Cross-cultural studies of behavior.* New York: Holt, Rinehart and Winston.

Segall, M. H. 1979. *Cross-cultural psychology: Human behavior in global perspective.* Monterey, CA: Brooks-Cole.

Sinclair, A. 1967. *Field and clinical survey report of the mental health of the indigenes of the Territory of Papua and New Guinea.* Port Moresby: Government Publication.

Smith, E. M. J. 1977. Counseling black individuals: Some stereotypes. *Personnel and Guidance Journal* 55:390–396.

———. 1982. Counseling psychology in the marketplace: The status of ethnic minorities. *Counseling Psychologist* 10 (2): 61–68.

Stranges, R., and Riccio, A. 1970. A counselee preference for counselors: Some implications for counselor education. *Counselor Education and Supervision* 10:39–46.

Sue, D. W. 1978. World views and counseling. *Personnel and Guidance Journal* 56 (8): 458–463.

———. 1981a. *Counseling the culturally different: Theory and practice.* New York: John Wiley and Sons.

———. 1981b. Evaluating process variables in cross-cultural therapy. In A. J. Marsella and P. B. Pedersen (eds.), *Cross-cultural counseling and psychotherapy: Foundations, evaluation and cultural considerations,* 102–125. Elmsford, NY: Pergamon Press.

Sue, D. W., Bernier, J. E., Durran, A., Feinberg, L., Pedersen, P. B., Smith, E. J., and Vasquez-Nuttall, E. 1982. Position paper: Cross-cultural counseling competencies. *Counseling Psychologist* 10 (2): 45–52.

Sue, D. W., and Sue, D. 1977. Barriers to effective cross-cultural counseling. *Journal of Counseling Psychology* 24:420–429.

Sue, S. 1973. Training of "Third World" students to function as counselors. *Journal of Counseling Psychology* 20:73–78.

Sweeney, T. J. 1971. *Rural poor students and guidance.* Boston: Houghton Mifflin.

Tart, C. 1975. Some assumptions of orthodox Western psychology. In C. Tart (ed.), *Transpersonal psychologies,* 59–113. New York: Harper and Row.

Tong, B. 1971. The ghetto of the mind: Notes on the historical psychology of Chinese Americans. *Amerasia Journal* 1:28.

Torrey, E. F. 1986. *Witchdoctors and psychiatrists: The common roots of psychotherapy and its future.* New York: Harper and Row.

Triandis, H. C., et al., eds. 1980. *Handbook of cross-cultural psychology.* Vol. 6. *Psychopathology.* Boston: Allyn and Bacon.

U.S. Bureau of the Census. 1985. *Statistical abstract of the United States: 1986.* Washington, DC: Government Printing Office.

Vontress, C. E. 1981. Racial and ethnic barriers in counseling. In P. B. Pedersen, J. G. Draguns, W. J. Lonner, and J. E. Trimble (eds.), *Counseling across cultures,* 87–107. Honolulu: University of Hawaii Press.

Watts, A. W. 1961. *Psychotherapy east and west.* New York: Mentor Press.

Weidman, H. H. 1969. The self-concept as a crucial link between social sciences and psychiatric theory. *Transcultural Psychiatry Research Review* 6:113–116.

Weidman, H. H., and Sussex, J. N. 1971. Cultural values and ego functioning in relation to the typical culture-bound reactive syndromes. *International Journal of Social Psychiatry* 17 (2): 83–100.

Westermeyer, J. 1976. Clinical guidelines for the cross-cultural treatment of chemical dependency. *American Journal of Drug and Alcohol Abuse* 3 (2): 315–322.

White, J. L. 1984. *The psychology of blacks: An Afro-American perspective.* Englewood Cliffs, NJ: Prentice-Hall.

Williams, L. N. 1978. *Black psychology: Compelling issues and views.* 2d ed. Washington, DC: University Press of America.

Wittkower, E. D., and Weidman, H. H. 1969. Magic, witchcraft and sorcery in relation to mental health and mental disorder. *Social Psychiatry* 8:169–184.

Wohl, J. 1981. Intercultural psychotherapy: Issues, questions, and reflections. In P. B. Pedersen, J. G. Draguns, W. J. Lonner, and J. G. Trimble (eds.), *Counseling across cultures,* 133–159. Honolulu: University of Hawaii Press.

Wrenn, C. G. 1962. The culturally encapsulated counselor. *Harvard Educational Review* 32 (4): 444–449.

————. 1985. Afterward: The culturally encapsulated counselor revisited. In P. B. Pedersen (ed.), *Handbook of cross-cultural counseling and therapy,* 323–329. Westport, CT: Greenwood Press.

Yap, P. M. 1969. The culture-bound reactive syndromes. In W. Caudill and T. Y. Lin (eds.), *Mental health research in Asia and the Pacific.* Honolulu: East-West Center Press.

Yeatman, G. W., and Dang, V. V. 1980. *Cao gio* (coin rubbing): Vietnamese attitudes toward health care. *Journal of the American Medical Association* 244:2748–2749.

PART TWO

General Considerations

The study of counseling across cultures is controversial and challenges a number of well-established assumptions in the field of counseling generally. This section seeks to integrate the priorities of multicultural counseling with traditional perspectives with a minimum of heat and a maximum of light.

Charles R. Ridley's chapter is challenging in its reference to racism, prejudice, and stereotyping. He approaches the topic systematically in a sequence of sections to help the majority culture readers realize that the chapter is about them, without at the same time offending or discouraging them. The prevalence of institutional racism throughout U.S. culture includes the traditional institutions of counseling as well. Ridley demonstrates clearly the extent of our cultural encapsulation and suggests approaches to reduce that error.

Julian Wohl applies counseling across culture to a more international perspective, integrating the literature from psychiatry, anthropology, and other disciplines to increase our awareness of multicultural counseling. Counseling must now be viewed in an international world-context perspective outside the Euroamerican context in which it was conceived. Wohl provides guidelines for developing an adequate worldview for multicultural counseling.

Teresa D. LaFromboise and Sandra L. Foster provide an excellent review of the widely scattered literature on ethics as it is influenced by cultural differences. Professional associations have increasingly emphasized the importance of fairness and equity across culturally different populations. This chapter provides essential reading for those attempting to design and develop equitable approaches.

3

Racism in Counseling as an Adversive Behavioral Process

CHARLES R. RIDLEY

Consider the following adverse outcomes in counseling and other mental health services. Compared to white clients, ethnic minority clients are more likely to receive inaccurate diagnoses; be assigned to junior professionals, paraprofessionals, or nonprofessionals rather than senior professionals; receive low-cost, less preferred treatment consisting of minimal contact, medication, or custodial care rather than individual psychotherapy; be disproportionately represented in mental health facilities; show a much higher rate of premature termination; and have more unfavorable impressions regarding treatment (Hollingshead and Redlich 1958; Jackson 1976; Jones and Korchin 1982; Ridley 1978; S. Sue 1977). These findings vary somewhat across the various ethnic minority groups and in different treatment settings. However, the picture generally reveals that majority group clients consistently receive preferential treatment over minority group clients in counseling settings. Why?

My purpose in this chapter is to answer that question by delineating the nature of racism in counseling. To accomplish this objective, I have organized this chapter into four major sections. The first section explores two common explanations of racism. Both of these are shown to be inadequate to account for consistent inequitable outcomes. The second section operationally defines several concepts with a view toward clarifying the nature of racism. Racism is shown to be the most likely source of adverse impact in counseling. The third section illustrates seven variables that negatively influence the counseling experience for ethnic minorities. In the fourth section I provide some recommendations to assist the cross-cultural counselor.

Explanations of Adverse Minority Experiences in Counseling

There are at least three possible reasons for the negative experiences of minorities in counseling. Two of these are ruled out as valid explanations, making it easier to accept as valid a third explanation—racism.

Chance or Random Occurrence

This explanation assumes that there are no compelling forces that cause the negative outcomes described. Rather, those outcomes are thought to occur as natural phenomena or events without outside interference. The implication is that there is nothing inherently faulty about the persons (in this case ethnic minority clients) or the settings (in this case the counseling settings and mental health delivery systems). According to this perspective, for example, ethnic minority clients could more often be assigned to custodial care simply because of chance.

To challenge this explanation, consider the following probability experiment. A barrel contains 100 balls, 20 of which are red and 80 of which are white. Each ball is drawn individually and not replaced. This act is called an elementary event. Successive drawings are made, without replacement, until all of the balls are drawn. In addition, each fifth selection is tossed into the trash.

Assuming that the balls are thoroughly mixed (unbiased), a probability of 1/100 is assigned to the elementary events. That is, each ball has an equal chance of being selected. Although a hundred possible outcomes exist, there is no way (or should be no way) to predict with certainty which outcomes will result. During the experiment it is observed that every fifth selection happens to be a red ball. Thus, all 20 red balls are tossed away, but all 80 white balls remain as prized property. The experimenter concludes that white balls are luckier than red balls.

Theoretically, it is absolutely possible for white balls to be selected favorably over red balls. According to the rules of probability, however, such experimental outcomes are highly unlikely or improbable. The chance occurrence or recurrence of an event or set of events in a given sample space (situation) is measured by the ratio of the number of cases or alternatives favorable to the event to the total number of cases or alternatives. In other words, it is statistically improbable that white balls could be repeatedly selected over red balls, all things being equal.

Similarly, the repeated negative outcomes for ethnic minorities in mental health delivery systems are improbable. Repeated premature termination, for example, simply defies the laws of probability as a natural phenomenon. This consistent adverse recurrence is highly unlikely to be accidental. Therefore, if we are willing to rule out chance as an explanation, two other causes remain: faultiness in the ethnic clients themselves or faultiness in the counseling setting.

Deficit Hypothesis

The deficit hypothesis claims that there are predetermined deficiencies in ethnic minorities that relegate them to an inferior status (Thomas and Sillen 1972). There are two major variations of the deficit hypothesis. The first variation is the genetic deficit hypothesis. The genetic deficit hypothesis has a long history, and it can be divided into two categories. One category, the intellectual deficit model, claims that genes play a predominant role in the determination of intelligence. Ethnic minorities are claimed to be born with inferior brains and have a limited capacity for mental development compared to whites (Stanton 1960). Another category, the personality deficit model, claims that ethnic minorities tend to be abnormal in character and behavior whether by nature or nurture.

The second variation is the cultural deficit hypothesis. It also has two categories. The cultural deprivation category states that ethnic minorities have an inferior culture or no culture at all. The blame in this model shifts to the lifestyles of various ethnic groups. In contrast, the cultural stress category states that ethnic minorities have broken down emotionally and have become debilitated under cultural stress. Consequently, they cannot compete as effectively as their white counterparts.

The deficit hypothesis has gained some acceptance on one level or another. The psychological and sociological literature has often viewed ethnic minorities from a deficit perspective. Support for the theory comes from such writers as Jensen (1969), Riessman (1962), and Dreger and Miller (1960). Considerable research, however, has challenged the hypothesis as scientifically untenable (Cole and Bruner 1972; Scarr and Weinberg 1976). Unfortunately, this chapter cannot devote attention to the arguments against the deficit hypothesis. However, students of counseling would benefit from reading the critiques of Jones and Korchin (1982) and Thomas and Sillen (1972).

The Concept of Racism

If chance occurrence and the deficit hypothesis are disqualified as valid explanations for the negative outcomes of ethnic minorities in counseling, then we must conclude that the problem lies within the social context, and in this case, the treatment settings. I would like to argue that the cause of adverse impact in counseling is racism and that racism is a social problem. To develop my argument, I want to examine five assumptions regarding racism and then define relevant terms related to the concept.

Assumptions about Racism

1. Racism is reflected in behavior. Racism is evident in what a person does as opposed to how a person feels or thinks. Although feelings

and attitudes are often important in motivating people to behave preferentially, racism is not in the feeling but in the behavior. Various individuals may have different motives for the same actions. Racist consequences occur as the result of behavior.

2. Racist acts can be performed by prejudiced as well as nonprejudiced people. Prejudice (which will be defined later) is often confused with racism, but it is not itself racism. Another misconception is that prejudice always precedes racism and discrimination as a learned condition (Lum 1986). Such a view is unfortunately propagated by some social scientists (e.g., Leigh 1984). The position assumes a causal relationship in which the presence of racism is contingent upon prejudice as an antecedent.

These arguments certainly sound convincing. Yet, consider the fact that well-intentioned people can still behave to the detriment of others, especially when they are misinformed. During earlier eras medical practitioners mistakenly treated patients in unclean facilities, which often led to further declines in health because of serious infections. Some of the most insidious acts of racism are performed with the best of intentions. Conversely, malevolent intentions may not always get translated into destructive behavior. Prejudiced people, for instance, do not always have the ability or capacity to carry out their negative intentions. In this case someone is prejudiced but not racist.

3. Racism is not the sole responsibility of a single ethnic group. Anyone is capable of behaving in a racist manner, including ethnic minorities themselves. Unfortunately, people are often unknowing participants in racism. Their unawareness, however, does not prevent them from causing adverse consequences for the victims of racism. Black, Asian, Hispanic, and other ethnic professionals may be unwittingly responsible for individual acts of racism. Many acts of racism occur because people lack valid information or are misinformed about other cultural groups.

4. The criteria for judging whether or not a behavior is racist lies in the consequences, not the causes, of the behavior. The notion of intentionality in racism begs the issue. The insistence on merely finding motivations turns needed attention away from developing constructive solutions to eliminate or, at least, minimize racist acts. During the past couple of decades, spurred by the civil rights movement, tremendous emphasis has been placed on consciousness raising, but limited appreciable change has occurred in terms of the way people actually behave.

5. Power is a force that is absolutely essential to perpetuate racism. Power is the ability to control ourselves and others as a means of altering problem situations or reducing environmental stress. Powerlessness is the inability to control ourselves or others (Leigh 1984).

People in power can control access to opportunities and privileges of people without power. Ethnic minorities are extremely limited in power as evidenced by their disproportionately small number in positions of power in major social systems. Representational inequity of professionals in mental health delivery systems is well documented (Ridley 1985a). Therefore, the majority of power influences upon ethnic minority clientele comes from white professionals.

Relevant Terms

Prejudice. Prejudice literally means a preconceived judgment or opinion without justification or sufficient knowledge (Axelson 1985). Prejudices can be positive or negative; people can have preconceived judgments for or against something without any just grounds. However, I define prejudice as an attitude expressing unfavorable feelings and behavioral intentions toward a group or its individual members (Davis 1978).

There have been numerous theoretical attempts to explain the nature of prejudice. Jones (1972) suggested that prejudice is based upon a social comparison process in which an individual's own group is used as the positive reference point. Brislin (1981), taking a somewhat different perspective, suggested that prejudiced people blame the out-group, fail to admit uncomfortable feelings about themselves, and organize and structure the world around their own rationale. Regardless of the perspective, there is general agreement that prejudice involves negative attitudes and intentions. Also, prejudice tends to be tenacious, resisting extinction (Selznick and Steinberg 1969).

Stereotyping. Stereotyping is a simplified, generalized labeling of certain people or social groups. A common stereotype is that people who wear thick wire-rim glasses are intellectual and socially awkward. The term is distinguished from prejudice, which is a special category of stereotyping and implies bigotry. Prejudiced people stereotype, but people who stereotype are not necessarily prejudiced. In fact, it has been argued that stereotypes are inevitable and necessary coping mechanisms that allow people to avoid cognitive overload (Brown 1965). Stereotyping (or generalizing) provides a way for people to package a variety of stimuli impinging upon them into a manageable number of categories. Although many stereotypes are inaccurate, some stereotypes contain a "kernel of truth."

Stereotyping becomes faulty when characteristics assigned to a social group are assumed to be genetically or ethnocentrically negative or inferior; the stereotypes lead to a "self-fulfilling prophesy"; or the stereotyper is dogmatic in his or her beliefs and unwilling to open the beliefs to new information. The salient feature is that stereotyping produces a fixed or overly general mental picture, and once adopted it is highly resistant to change (Axelson 1985). Counselors especially need to ana-lyze their stereotypes of other people and relinquish their inaccurate ones.

Ethnocentrism. Ethnocentrism is the belief that one's own group is the center of everything and the standard by which all other groups are measured. Ethnocentric people behave in the interest of their in-group. Ethnocentrism does not necessarily involve prejudice. It is possible to think positively about one's social group without having a negative atti-tude toward the out-group (although this often does not occur). Ethno-centrism is also not in itself racist. It does not have to result in racist consequences, although at times it may. Ethnocentric people may be-have in ways that block privilege to other groups, though their motiva-tional intent is simply the welfare and protection of their own in-group.

Racism

Racism is defined as any behavior or pattern of behavior that systemati-cally tends to deny access to opportunities or privilege to one social group while perpetuating privilege to members of another group. The key words in this definition are *behavior* and *systematic.* Behavior means human action and motor activity that are observable, measurable, and verifiable. Systematic means that the consequences of racist behavior are predictable and occur repeatedly over time. Racism then confers benefits upon the dominant group. Benefits are gains in terms of psy-chological feelings, social privilege, economic position, or political power (Axelson 1985).

Racism can be classified into individual and institutional racism. Individual racism involves the adverse behavior of one person or small group of people. Institutional racism involves the adverse behavior of social systems or institutional structures. Both categories of racism can be broken down into small units of analysis. Overt racism, which may be either individual or institutional, is behavior in which the intentionality is defined by the behavior. Overt acts of racism are always intentional. Covert racism, on the other hand, which also may be indi-vidual or institutional, hides or masks the motive behind the behavior. Covert acts of racism may be either intentional or unintentional. Inten-tional covert racism occurs when the consequences of the behavior are consistent with the practitioner's motives. Unintentional covert racism occurs when the behavioral effects are unintended or even contradictory to the person's motives. Table 1 provides a behavioral model of racism including examples of racism in mental health delivery systems.

Based upon this description of racism, practically everyone has the capacity for engaging in racist behavior. Mistakenly, racism is often

Table 1. A Behavioral Model of Racism in Mental Health Delivery Systems

	Individual Racism	Institutional Racism
Overt	e.g., therapist who believes that ethnic minorities are inferior and on this basis refuses to accept them as clients.[1]	e.g., mental health agency openly denies treatment to ethnic minority clientele.[1]
Covert		
Intentional	e.g., senior psychologist assigns a minority client to an intern because of social discomfort but claims to have a schedule overload.	e.g., mental health agency deliberately sets fees above the affordable range of most ethnic minority clients, thus excluding them from treatment.
Unintentional	e.g., therapist, functioning under the illusion of color blindness, erroneously diagnoses pathology.	e.g., mental health agency routinely uses standardized psychological tests without consideration of subcultural group differences and biases in test construction and interpretation.

[1] These practices are now illegal according to federal civil rights legislation.

equated with prejudice, and solutions to the problem are generally limited to attitude change and consciousness raising. Certainly, these concerns are important. However, such a focus distracts from the more basic problems of identifying and modifying the specific types of behavior that systematically produce adverse consequences for ethnic minorities.

According to Sedlacek and Brooks (1976), most racism is unknowing or unintentional. Most people are unaware of the damaging effects of their behavior upon ethnic minority groups. Because of this unawareness, unintentional covert forms of racism are the most insidious. These are the practices that are consistently adverse but operate inconspicuously.

Racism Process Variables

The following seven counseling process variables adversely affect therapy for minority clients. They fall into the category of individual unintentional covert racism; counselors are unlikely to recognize them or regard them as adverse behaviors.

Color Blindness

Color blindness is an illusion based on the erroneous assumption that the minority client is simply another client (Bernard 1953; Block 1981; Griffith 1977; Thomas and Sillen 1972). Comments from the therapist such as "We're all the same," "I don't see you as being a black person, just another human," or "It is as though you are white" signal that the therapist is color blind.

There are several causes of color blindness. The counselor may need to feel impartial. The counselor may be uncomfortable in discussing ethnic issues or may feel insecure about his or her own views on race or may have unresolved issues about race. Also, the counselor may fear hurting the client by discussing race or fail to understand the idioms of the client's cultural background.

Color-blind counselors abstract minority clients from the specific conditions of their history and experience. Their denial of color disregards the central importance of color in the psychological experience of the client. It also simultaneously disregards the undeniable influence of the counselor's whiteness upon the client (Sager, Brayboy, and Waxenburg 1972).

The adverse consequence of color blindness is the automatic labeling of deviations from white middle-class standards and norms as evidence of pathology. Therapists who fail to understand the culture of their minority clients tend to regard the clients' values and cultural idioms as inherently inferior to their own values. For example, some cultures have a time orientation different from that of Western culture. Clinicians may mistakenly judge a client's tardiness as resistance when the client is authentically behaving according to the customary norms of his or her culture. Color blindness is one of the dominant contributing factors to the disproportionate representation of ethnic minorities in pathological diagnostic categories. This also represents a Type I diagnostic error, designating pathology where none exists (Edwards 1982; Ridley 1984).

Color Consciousness

Color consciousness is an illusion based on the erroneous assumption that all of the client's problems come from being an ethnic minority (Adams 1950; Bernard 1953; Block 1981; Griffith 1977; Thomas and Sillen 1972). This is the opposite illusion of color blindness. A therapist who surmises, "If you were not a Native American, these problems would not exist," is probably color conscious.

The illusion stems from the correct view that ethnic minorities have been subjected to a lifelong history of oppression and control. The incorrect conclusion, however, is that they have developed an "irreversible mark of oppression" that is essentially a permanently crippled personality (Kardiner and Ovesey 1951). Other contemporary terms that often represent psychological deficits resulting from oppression include "culturally deprived," "underprivileged," and possibly "minority" (Griffith 1977).

A major cause of color consciousness is the therapist's guilt about the mistreatment of ethnic minorities in society. In some ways they bear the burden of guilt for the total majority group whether or not they themselves have been overtly racist. Neurotic guilt often underlies their attempt to atone for racism for which they are not directly responsible.

The primary adverse consequence of color consciousness is the overlooking of what may be real psychopathology. The failure to identify pathology when, in fact, a pathological condition exists represents a Type II diagnostic error (Edwards 1982; Ridley 1984). This problem is probably less pervasive than the Type I error. Nevertheless, its toll on the mental health of ethnic minority communities is enormous. A secondary consequence is that minority clients are given special privileges and relaxed standards of treatment (Cooper 1973). Paradoxically, the people who may most need treatment are often released and comprise many of the "walking wounded." The crisis of color consciousness is the unintentional failure to treat significant mental health needs.

Cultural Transference

Freud (1949) provided some original ideas on the quality of the counselor-client relationship and its effect upon the client's treatment. During the course of therapy he noticed that clients often transferred to the therapist either positive or negative feelings and attitudes originally felt about the client's parents or other significant people in the client's life. These clients, he noticed, reacted in a similar fashion to the therapist or as though the therapist was a parent or significant other.

As an intern in a Veterans Administration Hospital, I observed this phenomenon in action. One afternoon a fellow intern was conducting a therapy session with a female client. Suddenly, the client yelled, "You remind me of my father." She then jumped out of her chair and attempted to physically assault the therapist. According to the Freudian viewpoint, the patient's anger and frustration toward her father were vented onto my colleague. Certainly, the example is dramatic, but transference reactions frequently occur in less obvious forms.

Freud felt that the development of transference could be used to successfully promote therapy. As clients reenact their emotions and experiences, the counselor has a unique opportunity to work with emotional material otherwise inaccessible to therapy. The role of the counselor is to clarify and interpret the transference dynamics. Clients benefit by gaining insight into unconscious conflicts and the effect of these conflicts on current behavior and attitudes.

Cultural transference refers to the emotional reactions of a client of one ethnic group transferred to the therapist of a different ethnic group. The client has had previous significant experiences with members of the therapist's ethnic group outside of therapy. In some cases the client's feelings toward the therapist may have little to do with how the therapist actually treats the client. Instead, negative feelings (and in some cases positive feelings) are evoked in the client simply because the therapist represents the majority group.

Although not the original source of the client's frustration, the counselor may show incompetence by not adequately handling the transference. The unskilled or uninsightful therapist either fails to recognize the transference or minimizes its significance if it is recognized. A further difficulty is the therapist's inability to employ constructive interventions to resolve the conflicts underlying the transference. Cross-cultural counselors need to be especially alert to these client reactions since they can be of tremendous therapeutic importance. The skilled counselor might correctly ascertain that insecurity with whites is causing extremely intimidating or challenging behavior in a client. Cultural transference can reveal a client's racial motivations. Counselors who disregard cultural transference will fail to help their clients resolve important conflicts.

Cultural Countertransference

Countertransference, like transference, has tremendous impact on the quality of therapy and on its outcome. Countertransference refers to the emotional reactions and projections of the therapist toward the client. Counselors react to their clients in the way they have previously reacted to someone else. The phenomenon is caused by the therapists' anxiety. They do not fully understand their feelings, and as a result their perception of the client is distorted.

Cultural countertransference refers to the emotional reactions of the therapist of one ethnic group projected onto the client of another ethnic group. The mere presence of the client may evoke intense emotions in the therapist similar to those experienced in past interactions with other members of the client's ethnic group. Also, unfamiliar cultural mannerisms, idioms, expressions, and values may elicit intense feelings in the therapist.

Regardless of the stimulus, the therapist is unaware that these feelings and projections are irrational. These projections are also reinforced because they are shared by members of the therapist's own group.

Because of this shared experience, therapists are hindered in their ability to do objective reality testing. Therefore, they will more likely accept these feelings as rational responses rather than as personal or group idiosyncrasies. Essentially, the therapist does not have an objective basis from which these reactions can be judged as irrational. Furthermore, the client is extremely vulnerable because of a history of being negatively stereotyped. This vulnerability almost precludes many clients from having the ability to challenge or reject the negative stereotypes.

The adverse consequence of cultural countertransference is that psychological deficiencies that belong to the therapist are ascribed to the client. Distrust, sexual promiscuity, hostility, and Machiavellianism are examples of culturally countertransferred characteristics. The emphasis of therapy becomes oriented toward treating the therapist's projections rather than actual problems in the client. Many clients may even accept an invalid assessment. Other clients who reject the assessment are penalized for being "uncooperative and indifferent." The net effect is that the client's real presenting problems remain untreated.

Cultural Ambivalence

White counselors often have ambivalent motives in treating ethnic minority clients. On the one hand, they exhibit a high need for power and dominance (Jones and Seagull 1977). These counselors have a need to maintain absolute control over their ethnic clients. Their need for power is motivated by insecurity, intimidation, and perhaps the perception that the client may seek reprisal for injustice. Concerning this issue, Pinderhughes (1973, 104) states:

> One problem area for many patients lies in the unconscious needs of many psychotherapists to be in helping, knowledgeable, or controlling roles. Unwittingly they wish to be initiators and have patients accommodate to them or their style or approach. More Black patients than White perceive in this kind of relationship the basic ingredients of a master-slave pattern.

The high power need of the white counselor fittingly has been named "The Great White Father Syndrome" (Vontress 1981). The syndrome leads counselors to behave in a condescending, paternalistic, and ultimately enraging manner. The danger is that the counselor reinforces learned helplessness and passivity in the client. Paradoxically, the ideal goals of therapy are not achieved because the client has not acquired effective problem-solving skills. The client is likely to continue avoiding problems rather than asserting personal responsibility.

On the other hand, white counselors may simultaneously exhibit a high dependency need. In this case counselors may expend considerable energy in seeking security or gaining acceptance in the relationship with the minority client. In reality the white counselor wishes to be absolved of any guilt, real or imagined, for being racist. Some white professionals, in fact, are motivated to counsel minorities almost completely out of their guilt about racism (Jones and Seagull 1977).

By attempting to gain the client's approval, the therapist engages in subtle manipulation to appear "OK" as a white person. The counselor attempts to prove that he or she is really different from "other white people." Unknowingly, the therapist is more susceptible to counter-manipulation by the client, who is keenly perceptive of the dependency of the therapist (Ridley 1984).

In both the cases of dominance and dependency, the adverse consequence is that the real focus of counseling becomes counselor-centered rather than client-centered. The psychological conflicts and unresolved issues of the client in a subtle way take a back seat to the needs of the counselor. Although the client may remain in treatment, much of the effort is nontherapeutic. Therapeutic resources are misdirected toward the counselor, the so-called helper. As a result the minority client does not receive the appropriate assistance to resolve personal problems.

Evoking Pseudotransference

Pseudotransference occurs when the ethnic minority client responds defensively to racist attitudes and behaviors in the white therapist. The client's behavior is then misinterpreted and subsequently labeled by the therapist as a form of pathology (Thomas 1962; Thomas and Sillen 1972). What the therapist may ignore is the possibility that the client's critical reactions have a reality base. On this subject Thomas (1962, 899) states:

> Disturbed, unhealthy responses of the patient in the therapeutic situation cannot, however, be assumed to be necessarily transference phenomena. They may be "pseudo-transference" responses to unhealthy attitudes or behavior of the therapists, and therefore not an accurate reflection of the patient's neurosis. The well-known counter-transference phenomena caused by an unhealthy pattern of individual origin in the therapist can produce such pseudo-transference reactions.

Thomas (1962) also contended that clients may be especially sensitive to stereotypic attitudes, since they are repetitions of the many similar experiences of everyday life. Ridley (1985b) added that the client's susceptibility to pseudotransference is accentuated because of both the increased power of the therapist and the vulnerability of the client.

A hypothetical example can illustrate the problem. During the course of therapy the therapist remarks, "Why, we have a very fine black psychologist from Harvard on our staff." The remark implies white superiority despite the "good" intentions of the therapist. In response the client becomes visibly annoyed but avoids self-disclosure. The client perceives the therapist as patronizing. The therapist takes careful note of the client's annoyance and avoidance, concluding erroneously that the client has an anxiety disorder or some other sort of individual pathology. Pseudotransference is another source of Type I diagnostic errors.

Misinterpreting Client Nondisclosure

Despite the acknowledged therapeutic importance placed upon client self-disclosure, considerable research has indicated the difficulty ethnic minority clients have in being disclosive (Ridley 1984, 1986b; Sue and Sue 1983). The socialization of ethnic minorities in America has conditioned them to be cautious and mistrusting of majority group therapists. The expectation and thrust of the white therapist for disclosure by the ethnic minority client create a paradoxical situation for the client. On the one hand, the client can remain invulnerable but forfeit the potential benefits of the therapy. On the other hand, the client can choose to self-disclose but risk being misunderstood by the therapist. The paradox creates a no-win situation that is antithetical to the goals of therapy (Ridley and Tan 1986).

Ridley (1984) has described two dimensions of interpersonal functioning due to self-disclosure. Although his discussion was directed specifically toward the black client, the dynamics are applicable to other ethnic minority groups as well. "Cultural paranoia" is defined as a healthy psychological reaction to racism. "Functional paranoia" is defined as an unhealthy condition that is itself an illness. A four-mode typology that categorizes clients according to two dimensions is presented in figure 1.

Mode one, the intercultural nonparanoiac discloser, includes clients who are low on both functional and cultural paranoia. This client can be expected to disclose in any therapy setting, regardless of the therapist's ethnicity. Mode two, the functional paranoiac, includes clients for whom the problem of nondisclosure lies primarily in their personal pathology. These clients are nondisclosing to both white therapists and therapists from their own ethnic minority group. Mode three, the healthy cultural paranoiac, includes clients whose nondisclosure is evidence of a protection against the negative consequences of racism and oppression. These clients are nondisclosing to white therapists but are likely to disclose to therapists from their own ethnic minority group. Mode four, the confluent paranoiac, includes clients whose problem is both a reaction to racism and part of a personal pathology. This is the most difficult client to treat because of the complex interaction of cultural and functional paranoia in the client. These clients, like the func-

Cultural Paranoia	Functional Paranoia: Low	Functional Paranoia: High
Low	MODE 1 Intercultural Nonparanoiac Discloser • Disclosive to either ethnic minority or white therapist	MODE 2 Functional Paranoiac • Nondisclosive to both ethnic minority and white therapists
High	MODE 3 Healthy Cultural Paranoiac • Disclosive to ethnic minority therapist • Nondisclosive to white therapist	MODE 4 Confluent Paranoiac • Nondisclosive to both ethnic minority and white therapists

Figure 1. Typology of Ethnic Minority Client Self-Disclosure

tional paranoiac, are nondisclosing in any therapy setting, regardless of the therapist's ethnicity.

According to Ridley, the intercultural nonparanoiac is a rarity, and the great majority of ethnic minority clients fall into mode three, the healthy cultural paranoiac. Ironically, many mode three clients often are categorized as mode two, functional paranoiacs. Misclassification results from the clinician's incompetence and inability to differentiate cultural from pathological dynamics. This is another major contribution to the overrepresentation of minorities in pathological categories and is yet another source of the Type I diagnostic error.

Recommendations

Counseling for the Cross-Cultural Counselor

Cross-cultural counselors may find it useful and even essential to undergo personal therapy themselves. Rogers (1961), for example, has long asserted the need for congruence in the therapist as a condition for facilitating client self-exploration. Congruent counselors are aware of their own feelings, attitudes, and perceptions at a conscious level. Because ethnicity is such an emotionally charged issue in our society, therapists may need to look within themselves for attitudes and behaviors that may interfere with their ability to do effective therapy. Two white psychiatrists, Rosen and Frank (1962), have claimed that few people are free from racial prejudice. Indeed, the importance of self-awareness in intercultural psychotherapy has been previously emphasized (Wintrob and Harvey 1981). Moreover, it has been suggested as the only means of preventing a therapist's personal reactions from intruding in unhelpful ways (Jones 1985).

Individual counseling with a therapist of another ethnic group who is skilled in cross-cultural therapy may be especially beneficial. Ideally, the therapist of choice should come from the ethnic group that represents the counselor's largest client population. The major goal of this counseling endeavor would be to identify, understand, and overcome the counselor's prejudices, stereotypes and biases. Cross-cultural pairing in a counseling dyad can illuminate derogatory stereotypes by analyzing resistance or overcompensation in the counselor. Successful counseling would result in therapists who are more culturally sensitive and congruent about their own ethnicity and attitudes about other groups. Congruent and self-aware counselors are less likely to project their unresolved cultural conflicts onto their clients. Essentially, developing awareness of hidden prejudices is the first step in promoting an open-minded counseling relationship (Axelson 1985).

Training the Cross-Cultural Counselor

There is a well-documented need to train counselors in cross-cultural skills (Arredondo 1985; Ibrahim 1985; Ridley 1985a; Sue et al. 1982). Counselors need skills that will enable them to function more effectively in an increasingly multicultural world. In addition, indigenous professionals need to recognize the limitations of their ethnocentric perspectives on treatment within their own cultures (Ridley 1986a).

A key consideration is that training should be planned and intentional. There are two reasons for this suggestion. First, it is easy for professional training programs to ignore or minimize the role of cross-cultural training. Hicks and Ridley (1979) argued for "academic legitimacy," and later Brislin (1983) cautioned against cross-cultural training becoming of fringe interest. Fringe interest develops out of the low priority given to ethnic concerns relative to other curriculum concerns.

Second, cross-cultural training could place additional demands upon the client. The expectation is that the culturally different client will assist in facilitating the counselor trainee's cultural awareness. This deviates somewhat from traditional training paradigms that rely less on active client contributions to the counselor's development. It also calls for a reciprocal learning paradigm that benefits both the counselor and the client—the counselor in developing professional competence and the client in exploring personal issues (Ridley 1986a).

An inherent danger in cross-cultural training is that the counselor, not the culturally different client, will benefit from the experience. Certainly, such an outcome is to be avoided. It raises an ethical issue. Ethically, the concern is for the welfare of the consumer (AACD 1981; APA 1981). Mental health professionals are required to respect the integrity and protect the welfare of the clients they serve. Effective training programs will implement adequate procedures and quality control to prevent abuse of cross-cultural consumers. Simultaneously, it is essential to get people thoroughly trained. Carefully implemented training should overcome the pitfalls of client abuse and counselor incompetence.

Facilitating Healthy Ethnic Identity

It should now be obvious that ethnicity and culture can play an important role in counseling. Emotionally charged, the topic is often threatening even to experienced counselors. Ethnicity has been equated with sex and death as a subject that touches off deep unconscious feelings in most people (McGoldrick, Pearce, and Giordano 1982). Even the attitudes of ethnic minority clients toward their own ethnicity can have significant emotional overtones. Their ethnic attitudes may have a direct bearing upon their mental health. Like majority group counselors, minority clients may distort reality by overemphasizing or minimizing their ethnicity.

Added to an already complicated process, ethnic and cultural dynamics ensure that the counselor has no small task. Nevertheless, the need for effective counseling remains. But how are counselors to sift through all of the psychological nuances to determine the significance of ethnicity to the client? How are counselors to distinguish distortions due to cultural transference from realistic reactions to the counselor? How are counselors to ascertain if there is a major conflict over ethnic identity? To answer these questions, counselors can take the following steps.

First, counselors must recognize that initially many ethnic minority clients probably have some fear and anxiety in relating to a white counselor. In an earlier writing I demonstrated how a hostile transference may occur because the client views the counselor as a symbol of the white power structure (Ridley 1984). Clients may be unaware of their real feelings. To deal with this problem, counselors must accept their clients' anxiety as legitimate. They must allow their clients to express their anxieties and, if necessary, "act out" their fears in therapy. Counselors should be especially careful not to penalize their clients for self-expression. Accepting a client's anxiety also means that counselors recognize and accept their own anxiety and discomfort brought about by the client's anxiety. Counselors must admit to themselves that the emotional intensity also makes them feel apprehensive and uncomfortable. At the same time, they must be careful not to allow their anxiety to interfere with providing a psychologically safe and secure treatment setting.

Second, counselors should explore their clients' attitudes toward their own ethnicity during the early stages of counseling. Ethnic difference probably has its greatest impact early in treatment, particularly at the first session (Jones and Seagull 1977; Jones 1979). Counselors should be willing to explore these issues in depth. Failing to initiate in depth exploration can pose an important block to therapy progress and minimize the possibility of positive interracial experiences for the client in the future (Ridley 1984).

The counselor in this situation has a most challenging job. Because of the initial sense of wariness, the client is likely to test the therapist's degree of acceptance (Jones 1979). It is instructive for the counselor again to provide an open environment and teach the client "disclosure flexibility" (Chelune 1977). Ethnic minority clients need to learn that they can be vulnerable with a concerned white therapist and not to generalize all white people as unhelpful (Ridley 1984). They need to discriminate social cues, recognizing when it is in their best interest to be disclosive.

Third, counselors may need to confront the client once trust has been established. Confrontation is not an attack or verbal assault on the client. Confrontation is rather a basic counseling skill used to identify discrepancies or inconsistencies in a client's behavior (Evans et al. 1984). For example, a counselor might say to a culturally different client, "I've noticed that every time you bring up a new problem—whether it's your academic studies, part-time job in the bookstore, or intramural basketball—you end up saying that your failures are due to the racist system. I don't want to make light of the real injustices that exist on campus. But isn't it possible that your constant focus on racism actually distracts from some deep feelings you have about being an ethnic minority?"

In this "confrontation" the counselor is attempting to establish whether or not the client is overemphasizing racism. The possible discrepancy is that the client is blaming the system for personal inadequacies when, in reality, the client may have unresolved conflicts about his or her ethnicity. These conflicts lead the client to create situational or interactional problems regardless of the initial dynamics of the situation. As long as the inadequacies are unrecognized and untreated, the client's prognosis is poor.

Confrontation requires counselor sensitivity. Counselors must be as accurate as possible in interpreting the client's behavior. Once the confrontation is made, counselors must avoid imposing mistaken interpretations onto the client or prematurely backing off at the first sign of client resistance. In summary, effective confrontation helps the client to achieve a deeper level of self-understanding. The ultimate goal is to help clients move toward a healthy self-esteem without overemphasizing or minimizing their ethnicity.

Treatment Flexibility

There is a need for individualized treatment plans such that each client is treated as a unique person and not merely as a member of an ethnic category. Sue (1983) has restated the necessity of considering within-group differences as well as between-group differences when dealing with ethnic minorities. This position recognizes that all persons from an ethnic group are not similar in all psychological characteristics. In fact, within-group differences have been found to be larger than between-group differences (Lewontin 1972). The range of personalities, behavioral styles, and temperaments supports the rich diversity within a group.

By recognizing the tremendous variability among members from similar backgrounds, it becomes imperative that counselors employ flexible and balanced treatment methods. Counseling goals and techniques must be based upon the unique needs and problems of the client. Several techniques in some cases could be used in treating a single presenting problem. Different techniques, in other cases, could be beneficially used to treat various problems. The skillful counselor will have the ability to identify correct treatment goals, employ a broad repertoire of techniques, remain flexible, and apply techniques appropriately to specific presenting problems.

One common view held by many counselors is that identical treatments should be provided to clients from all ethnic populations. The assumption underlying this view is that equal treatment means equitable treatment. D. W. Sue (1977) poignantly dispelled this position, arguing that equal treatment in counseling might mean discriminatory treatment. According to Sue, differential treatment may not necessarily imply discriminatory treatment. Since having equal access and opportunity is the real issue, he favors the use of differential techniques that are nondiscriminatory. I wholeheartedly endorse Sue's suggestion.

Multimodal behavior therapy (Lazarus 1976) has been recommended as a framework that allows treatment flexibility (Ridley 1984). According to Lazarus, multimodal therapy uses a variety of techniques without identifying itself with a specific therapeutic orientation. Instead, its techniques appeal to six modalities: behavior, affect, sensa-

Table 2. Hypothetical Modality Profile

Modality	Problem	Proposed Treatment
Behavior	Avoidance of interracial encounters	Reeducation; desensitization
	Nondisclosure	Therapist self-disclosure; modeling; teaching disclosure flexibility
	Inability to maintain employment	Career assessment and counseling
	Habitual procrastination	Time management training; operant techniques
Affect	Fear in the presence of whites	Desensitization; confrontation of fear stimuli by assigning a sensitized white therapist
	Compliance and pent-up anger	Assertiveness training
Sensation	Muscular tension	Relaxation training
Imagery	Recurring images of violence during civil rights demonstrations	Thought stopping
Cognition	Irrational self-talk: "All whites are oppressors." "All of my problems are because of my blackness." "Blacks are inferior to whites."	Rational disputation and corrective self-talk; bibliotherapy
Interpersonal relationships	Pseudotransference reactions	Modification of therapist's behavior
	Secondary gains from "gaming" and manipulating white therapist	Paradoxical procedures; interracial group therapy with black and white co-therapists
Drugs	Hypertension	Medical evaluation; chemotherapy

tion, imagery, cognition, and interpersonal relationships. These six modalities are said to constitute human personality. A seventh modality, drugs (or medication), is also used. Lazarus coined the acronym BASIC ID, derived from the first letter of each modality. See table 2 for a hypothetical modality profile.

In using the multimodal framework, cross-cultural counselors can systematically employ a broad repertoire of interventions. It reduces the possibility of being confined to interventions that are not always appropriate or helpful. Flexibility of therapeutic techniques is probably the most important assumption for effective treatment with ethnic minority clients.

Conclusion

Like other major social systems, mental health care is an active participant in a larger system of racism. The counseling and therapy enterprise in particular accounts for a tremendous amount of the adverse
impact upon ethnic minority clientele. The past and present conditions
in the counseling profession reveal a strange irony. Racism in counseling is an enigma. Counseling is supposed to help and heal, not hurt, the
consumer. Despite their best intentions, counselors often end up exacer-
bating the disturbing conflicts and confusion in ethnic minority clients.
Effective intervention is often nonexistent. What can be said of this
dilemma? "Physician, heal thyself!" By availing themselves of the recommendations found in this chapter, counselors should find that they
can more easily attain cross-cultural competence. Ultimately, the counseling professional will be able to provide more equitable services and
live up to one of its most valued ethical principles: the welfare of the
consumer.

References

Adams, W. 1950. The Negro patient in psychiatric treatment. *American Journal
of Orthopsychiatry* 20 (2): 305–310.

American Association for Counseling and Development (AACD). 1981. *Ethical
standards.* Rev. ed. Alexandria, VA: American Association for Counseling and Development.

American Psychological Association (APA). 1981. Ethical principles of psychologists. *American Psychologist* 36:633–681.

Arredondo, P. M. 1985. Cross-cultural counselor education and training. In
P. B. Pedersen (ed.), *Handbook of cross-cultural counseling and therapy,* 281–
289. Westport, CT: Greenwood Press.

Axelson, J. A. 1985. *Counseling and development in a multicultural society.* Monterey,
CA: Brooks-Cole.

Bernard, V. 1953. Psychoanalysis and members of minority groups. *Journal of
the American Psychoanalytic Association* 1:256–267.

Block, C. 1981. Black Americans and the cross-cultural counseling and psychotherapy experience. In A. J. Marsella and P. B. Pedersen (eds.), *Cross-
cultural counseling and psychotherapy: Foundations, evaluation, and cultural considerations.* Elmsford, NY: Pergamon Press.

Brislin, R. W. 1983. Cross-cultural studies in social psychology of relevance to
ethnic group research: Examples and recommendations. Paper presented at the annual meeting of the American Psychological Association,
Anaheim, CA.

Brown, R. 1965. *Social psychology.* New York: Free Press.

Chelune, G. 1977. Disclosure flexibility and social-situational perceptions.
Journal of Consulting and Clinical Psychology 45:1139–1143.

Cole, M., and Bruner, J. S. 1972. Cultural differences and inferences about psychological processes. *American Psychologist* 26:867–876.

Cooper, S. 1973. A look at the effect of racism on clinical work. *Social Casework* 54:76–84.

Davis, F. J. 1978. *Minority-dominant relations: A sociological analysis.* Arlington Heights, IL: AHM Publishing.

Dreger, R. M., and Miller, K. S. 1960. Comparative psychological studies of Negroes and whites in the United States. *Psychological Bulletin* 57:361–402.

Edwards, A. 1982. The consequences of error in selecting treatment for blacks. *Social Casework: The Journal of Contemporary Social Work* 63:429–433.

Evans, D., Hearn, M., Uhlemann, M., and Ivey, A. 1984. *Essential interviewing: A programmed approach to effective communication* 2d ed. Monterey, CA: Brooks-Cole.

Freud, S. 1949. *An outline of psycho-analysis.* New York: W. W. Norton.

Griffith, M. S. 1977. The influence of race on the psychotherapeutic relationship. *Psychiatry* 40 (1): 27–40.

Hicks, L., and Ridley, S. 1979. Black studies in psychology. *American Psychologist* 34:597–602.

Hollingshead, A., and Redlich, F. 1958. *Social class and mental illness.* New York: John Wiley and Sons.

Ibrahim, F. A. 1985. Effective cross-cultural counseling and psychotherapy: A framework. *Counseling Psychologist* 13 (4): 625–638.

Jackson, A. 1976. Mental health center delivery systems and the black client. *Journal of Afro-American Issues* 4 (1): 28–34.

Jensen, A. R. 1969. How much can we boost I.Q. and scholastic achievement? *Harvard Educational Review* 39:1–123.

Jones, A., and Seagull, A. A. 1977. Dimensions of the relationship between the black client and the white therapist: A theoretical overview. *American Psychologist* 32:850–855.

Jones, E. E. 1979. Race and psychotherapy: Changing perspectives. In J. H. Masserman (ed.), *Current psychiatric therapies,* vol. 18, 225–235. New York: Grune and Stratton.

———. 1985. Psychotherapy and counseling with black clients. In P. B. Pedersen (ed.), *Handbook of cross-cultural counseling and therapy,* 173–179. Westport, CT: Greenwood Press.

Jones, E. E., and Korchin, S. J. 1982. Minority mental health: Perspectives. In E. E. Jones and S. J. Korchin (eds.), *Minority mental health,* 3–36. New York: Praeger.

Jones, J. 1972. *Prejudice and racism.* Reading, MA: Addison-Wesley Publishing.

Kardiner, A., and Ovesey, L. 1951. *The mark of oppression: Explorations in the personality of the American Negro.* Cleveland: World Publishing.

Lazarus, A. 1976. *Multimodal behavior therapy.* New York: Springer.

Leigh, J. W. 1984. Empowerment strategies for work with multi-ethnic populations. Paper presented at the annual meeting of the Council on Social Work Education, Detroit.

Lewontin, R. C. 1972. The apportionment of human diversity. In. T. Dobzhansky, M. K. Hecht, and W. C. Steere (eds.), *Evolutionary biology,* vol. 6, 381–398. New York: Appleton-Century-Crofts.

Lum, D. 1986. *Social work practice and people of color: A process-stage approach.* Monterey, CA: Brooks-Cole.

McGoldrick, M., Pearce, J. K., and Giordano, J., eds. 1982. *Ethnicity and family therapy.* New York: Guilford Press.

Pinderhughes, C. A. 1973. Racism and psychotherapy. In C. Willie, B. Kramer, and B. Brown (eds.), *Racism and mental health,* 61–121. Pittsburgh: University of Pittsburgh Press.

Ridley, C. R. 1978. Cross-cultural counseling: A multivariate analysis. *Viewpoints in Teaching and Learning* 54:43–50.

———. 1984. Clinical treatment of the nondisclosing black client: A therapeutic paradox. *American Psychologist* 39 (11): 1234–1244.

———. 1985a. Imperatives for ethnic and cultural relevance in psychology training programs. *Professional Psychology Research and Practice* 16 (5): 611–622.

———. 1985b. Pseudo-transference in interracial psychotherapy: An operant paradigm. *Journal of Contemporary Psychotherapy* 15 (1): 29–36.

———. 1986a. Cross-cultural counseling in theological context. *Journal of Psychology and Theology* 14 (4): 288–297.

———. 1986b. Optimum service delivery to the black client. *American Psychologist* 41 (2): 226–227.

Ridley, C. R., and Tan, S. Y. 1986. Unintentional paradoxes and potential pitfalls in paradoxical psychotherapy. *Counseling Psychologist* 14 (2): 303–308.

Riessman, F. 1962. *The culturally deprived child.* New York: Harper and Row.

Rogers, C. R. 1961. *On becoming a person.* Boston: Houghton Mifflin.

Rosen, H., and Frank, J. D. 1962. Negroes in psychotherapy. *American Journal of Psychiatry* 119:456–460.

Sager, C. J., Brayboy, T. L., and Waxenberg, B. R. 1972. Black patient—white therapist. *American Journal of Orthopsychiatry* 42:415–423.

Scarr, S., and Weinberg, R. A. 1976. I.Q. test performance of black children adopted by white families. *American Psychologist* 3:726–739.

Sedlacek, W. E., and Brooks, J. C. 1976. *Racism in American education: A model for change.* Chicago: Nelson-Hall.

Selznick, G. J., and Steinberg, S. 1969. *The tenacity of prejudice.* New York: Harper and Row.

Stanton, W. 1960. *The leopard's spots: Scientific attitudes toward race in America, 1815–1859.* Chicago: University of Chicago Press.

Sue, D. W. 1977. Counseling the culturally different: A conceptual analysis. *Personnel and Guidance Journal* 55:422–425.

Sue, D. W., Bernier, J. E., Durran, A., Feinberg, L., Pedersen, P. B., Smith, E. J., and Vasquez-Nuttall, E. 1982. Position paper: Cross-cultural counseling competencies. *Counseling Psychologist* 10 (2): 45–52.

Sue, D. W., and Sue, S. 1983. Counseling Chinese Americans. In D. R. Atkinson, G. Morten, and D. W. Sue (eds.), *Counseling American minorities: A cross-cultural perspective,* 2d ed., 97–106. Dubuque, IA: William C. Brown.

Sue, S. 1977. Community mental health services to minority groups: Some optimism, some pessimism. *American Psychologist* 32:616–624.

———. 1983. Ethnic minority issues in psychology: A reexamination. *American Psychologist* 38:583–592.

Thomas, A. 1962. Pseudo-transference reactions due to cultural stereotyping. *American Journal of Orthopsychiatry* 32 (5): 894–900.

Thomas, A., and Sillen, S. 1972. *Racism and psychiatry.* Secaucus, NJ: Citadel Press.

Vontress, C. E. 1971. Racial differences: Impediments to rapport. *Journal of Counseling Psychology* 18:7–13.

——. 1981. Racial and ethnic barriers in counseling. In P. B. Pedersen, J. G. Draguns, W. J. Lonner, and J. E. Trimble (eds.), *Counseling across cultures,* 2d ed., 87–107. Honolulu: University of Hawaii Press.

Wintrob, R. M., and Harvey, Y. K. 1981. The self-awareness factor in intercultural psychotherapy: Some personal reflections. In P. B. Pedersen, J. G. Draguns, W. J. Lonner, and J. E. Trimble (eds.), *Counseling across cultures,* 2d ed., 108–132. Honolulu: University of Hawaii Press.

4

Cross-Cultural Psychotherapy

JULIAN WOHL

Shortly after establishing a date for a forthcoming wedding, an otherwise healthy male university student notices an increasingly strong sense of tension. He has difficulty concentrating on his studies. He frequently feels frustrated and irritable. A painful sensation in his abdomen, difficulty in breathing, and irregularity in elimination develop. Bewildered and frightened by these changes, the student consults some friends, one of whom advises that he seek professional help.

Among the sources available are a Gestalt counselor in the university counseling center, a pastoral counselor in the local church, and a psychoanalytic psychotherapist in the community. Also available is an array of assorted other local healers, such as shamans, diviners, astrologers, readers, advisers, and fortune tellers, who provide services to distressed people.

Our unhappy student could be found in any university around the world. But whatever the location, and regardless of the particular method or system of helping that is employed by any of these socially defined "experts in interpersonal relations" (Sullivan 1954), much of what they do will be identical. All the practitioners will emit an air of confidence, convey concern and helpful intent, listen with careful attention and compassion. They will assess the situation, try to understand the problem, formulate some reflections, and prescribe some course of action intended to relieve distress. Furthermore, wherever the helping encounters occur, in each instance it will be identified as a special place that is reserved for such activities. Despite their particular differences of theory and method, these varied practitioners, whether they employ modern, scientifically rooted approaches, folk methods, or supernatural ones, all will have the capacity to make careful, acute appraisals and exert psychological influence upon a supplicant eager and ready for relief.

The systematic, formal use of psychological influence to help people may well occur in all human societies (Draguns 1975) and throughout human history (McNeill 1965; Bromberg 1959). Whether all such activities should be referred to as psychotherapy is a question that cannot be answered without argument. There is arbitrariness in any definition, as Prince (1980) notes, and danger in either a too liberal definition or a too restrictive one. Regardless of the personal preferences of any user of the term, in practice in cross-cultural contexts it tends to be used broadly and loosely to encompass all manner of psychological influencing methods, including some that involve even physical contact or drug and herb use.

Depending upon how it is defined, psychotherapy is either an ancient art that has existed in all societies or is a creation of nineteenth-century Europe that has been exported to much of the world. In the broadest sense it is a generic concept that refers to a wide range of activities having in common the use of words to incite change in someone else.

In this chapter psychotherapy refers to an activity that occurs in a specially created professional situation in which a recognized, qualified expert and a claimant for help have agreed formally to meet, usually on a regular and continuing basis, and talk about the claimant in an effort to reduce psychological distress and improve functioning in the help-seeker. Although this definition seems inclusive, it is also restrictive, emphasizing several distinguishing characteristics of psychotherapy. The idea of a "specially created professional situation" excludes serendipitous encounters, for example, such as are experienced in long-distance travel or in briefer stops in taverns, with people who are troubled and need to express themselves to the stranger who will never be seen again. Such meetings may be helpful, but for the occasion to be psychotherapy the situation must be defined as one in which psychotherapy occurs, the meetings must be regularly scheduled, the therapist must be culturally defined as one qualified in that art, and both parties must acknowledge that psychotherapy is what they are doing. It is thus formalized.

Finally, the primary medium of psychotherapy is speech, although, of course, nonverbal communication is included in the interaction of therapist and client. Many non-Western healing rituals include symbolic forms in addition to speech and some observers include these in the psychotherapy category. Clearly, in their own cultural contexts such activities are the functional equivalents of psychotherapy, regardless of the label attached. In many societies these activities are not framed in psychological terms but are formulated in the language of magic, religion, the occult, philosophy, or education. The dominant languages in North America are those of medicine, science, and technology, but considerable controversy exists as to the suitability of each of those frameworks. It is wisest not to be too insistent on a definition but to acknowledge that if a special sociocultural mechanism does what psychotherapy does, using methods that are psychological, then it is functionally psychotherapy. This is clearly the practice among scholars in cross-cultural psychotherapy (Frank 1974, 1982; Prince 1980; Torrey 1986), and it has resulted in a substantial advance in knowledge about psychological helping practices around the world as well as a more objective perspective for examining our own.

Meanings of Cross-Cultural Psychotherapy

A psychotherapeutic situation is cross-cultural (or intercultural) when any of its basic components is culturally variant from any other. In this section I present a taxonomy of the more commonly found arrangements to systematize and order what Draguns (1981) referred to as the "semi-autonomous areas" that fit the rubric of cross-cultural psychotherapy. In effect, this comprises a series of operational meanings of the term.

As a prelude we might note two controversial points. First, all psychotherapy is cultural; and second, all psychotherapy is cross-cultural. Psychotherapy is inherently cultural because wherever it occurs it is a human invention. As such, and as a helping procedure, that is, an interpersonal, communicative relationship, psychotherapy deals with meanings, interpretations of reality, values, standards of right and wrong, health and illness, and norms of conduct. All psychotherapy that remains in its culture of origin is in the "indigenous" or folk category (Draguns 1981) or the "cultural psychotherapy" category of Wittkower and Warnes (1974). Each psychotherapy is a reflection of the culture that produces it, and because of the harmony of their relationship, the cultural part of a psychotherapy operating on home ground is not usually noticed. Draguns (1975) notes that culture is always a silent participant and that psychotherapy can be understood as a culture learning or relearning situation. Only when there sounds a blaring discordant cultural note does "culture" become a conscious factor. But noticed or not, it is useful to keep in mind that all psychotherapy is cultural and that each psychotherapy is a cultural product that requires relativistic assessment and understanding. When certain cultural components of psychotherapy become blatant, the psychotherapy becomes cross-cultural. Generally, cultural differences are not analyzed very closely in the literature but are taken at face value. Gross categories such as ethnicity, religion, socioeconomic status, language, nationality, and political ideology are taken as indicators of fundamental underlying differences in such psychological categories as cognition, attitudes, beliefs, worldviews, values, and motivations.

Not all cultural sources of trouble in psychotherapy are obvious. Culture includes a great deal of what is automatic, habitual, assumptive, and unwitting in conduct and thought. It provides a backdrop of conventional ideas about reality and human action. To the extent that both parties share these conventions they remain unquestioned, even though from another frame of reference they may be prejudices, stereotypes, or even shared delusions. The traditional middle-class Viennese would probably expect to shake hands at the beginning and at the end of each psychotherapy session. Confronted with this, the American psychotherapist or client might experience the mild trauma of a cultural difference. Differences and their effects can be even more subtle. Each of us creates an idiosyncratic interpretation of culture, a private unique understanding of the apparently common culture. For this reason each of us is culturally different from anyone else in our own culture. We implicitly assume that the other person is, as Leach (1978) says, "like us," but we are only partly correct in that assumption. The patient is, in ways unknown at the outset, a member of the "other" group, made up of people who differ from "us." Each person carries some private, individualized conception of cultural reality, what Walter Lippmann in 1922 referred to as "the pictures in our heads" (Lippmann 1965). There are always cultural differences, and therefore all psychotherapeutic communication must traverse a cultural gap.

Fortunately, not all such cultural gaps are insurmountable or even troublesome. Significant cultural variation in a psychotherapeutic situation can come from any or all of its four components: the therapist, the patient, the location or setting, and the method. Generally, the cultural difference will involve one or two of these; for example, an Arab Moslem studying in America might be treated in a clinic by a white Protestant American using experiential psychotherapy. On the face of it cultural congruence prevails among therapist, locale, and method, with the patient a cultural anomaly. The extreme of cultural heterogeneity could be the (fortunately hypothetical) instance of a Greek businessman in Singapore being treated psychoanalytically by a Korean psychiatrist.

The following scenarios describe eight of the most typical cross-cultural psychotherapeutic situations and thus provide operational meanings of cross-cultural psychotherapy.

Representatives of one culture study the therapeutic modes and practices of another. This is essentially a pure research activity, usually carried out by anthropologists and anthropologically informed psychiatric or psychological clinicians (Kennedy 1973; Kleinman 1980). It does not entail practicing psychotherapy across a cultural gap but involves observing the indigenous practices of local healers on their home territory. From such studies can come a sense of the relativity of our own theories and practices. Similarities and differences in form and content, including methods, techniques, and values, can be detected. Looking from the outside at a substantially different culture can provide an appreciation of relationships between psychological disorders and psychotherapeutic practices that are not apparent to those immersed in the culture. Such observations have inspired the search for transcultural universality and cultural individuality in psychotherapy (Frank 1974; Pluk and Wojciechowski 1985; Torrey 1986). Many studies of so-called culture-specific disorders, traditional healers, and folk treatment practices fall into this category (Kiev 1964; Lebra 1976; Marsella and White 1982).

Cultural heterogeneity: a member of one subculture engages in psychotherapy with the patient of another subculture, both of whom are also participants in a larger, superordinate culture. With the increasing recognition of the cultural pluralism that exists in many areas of the world, this domain attracts great interest. Much of the literature on this subject is based upon work in the United States and is related to the relatively recent "discovery" of American minorities and their mistreatment by the mental health system. While there is no question that special problems are associated with psychotherapeutic work with certain "nontraditional" patients, some members of minority groups, or other special populations, the use of the term "culture" to characterize all such groups has been criticized (DeVos 1982). Nevertheless, this is an area of great and accelerating interest as demonstrated by several chapters in this volume and a number of other recent books targeted on treatment issues with American subcultural or special populations (Chunn, Dunston, and Ross-Sheriff 1983; Dana 1981; Jones and Korchin 1982; Levine and Padilla 1980).

Cultural pluralism is not of course restricted to the United States. In addition, Canada, India, Sri Lanka, Singapore, Malaysia, Burma, and Indonesia come readily to mind as other societies that are culturally pluralistic and therefore could experience problems in serving the psychotherapeutic needs of the subcultural minority segments of their populations. In the typical arrangement in the United States a white middle-class psychotherapist treats a nonwhite or ethnic minority person of lower socioeconomic status. One major problem in this area is stereotyping: an individual is prejudged as having characteristics based upon generalizations applied to a group such as "lacks psychological mindedness," "not suitable for talking therapy." Another serious problem is the confounding of ethnic membership with socioeconomic class, which leads to ascribing characteristics to the ethnic group that are derived from social class membership. It is encouraging that much of the more recent literature is sensitive to these issues as well as to the danger of confusing righteous outrage over ethnic and racial injustice with the understanding of cultural differences (Atkinson 1985; Beutler, Crago, and Arizmendi 1986; Jones 1985; Jones and Korchin 1982; Lorion 1978; Lorion and Felner 1986). This literature and substantially more (e.g., Jones and Matsumoto 1982; Bluestone and Vela 1982; and Lerner 1972 [a major study in this field]) vigorously attack and seriously damage the myths that minorities and the poor cannot be treated with exploratory psychotherapy and that members of minority groups can be treated only or better by members of those same groups.

The non-Western sojourner in a Western land receiving psychotherapy. Foreign students constitute a large segment of this group. Most of the thousands of students who come to North America each year adapt to their new circumstances without recourse to mental health services. Some use those services on their campuses, and some use other resources. A number of studies have been made of issues related to clinical and subclinical problems of foreign students. Excellent surveys are available (Alexander et al. 1981; Hull 1978).

The non-Western sojourner in a Western land training in psychotherapy. This situation has two possible conclusions that are of interest. In one the individual remains in the culture where the training occurred. In the other the trainee returns to the culture of origin to practice the newly acquired skill.

In the early days of this century traffic moved across the Atlantic from West to East as Americans went to learn from Freud and his colleagues. Since those early days, and with greatly increased frequency since World War II, it has flowed the other way. People from all parts of the world come to Great Britain and to North America to study in the mental health disciplines, including psychotherapy. It is remarkable that only a limited and nonsystematic body of literature seems to have developed on training people to work with systems of psychotherapy that are culturally foreign to them. Yet anyone who has watched the struggles of a non-Western student clinician to understand the inner workings of Western psychotherapy knows that the culturally based difficulties are pronounced. The student must operate with a psychotherapeutic conceptual framework that is pervaded with assumptions about life and people that are remarkably different from those that the student therapist's cultural experience has provided and that have become part of that person's basic character makeup. The therapist must assimilate a new, culturally foreign system of thought with its associated assumptions about expectable or normative motivation, feeling, and conduct. Furthermore, this is being accomplished while, and through, working at applying this system to a patient who is culturally different from the trainee. If that is not enough, the student must also cope with being supervised during clinical training (at least in better programs) and the way in which this special teaching-learning situation is structured in the West.

Supervisors will of course have culturally based problems in managing the supervision. Consider the case of a male Korean second-year psychiatric resident applying psychoanalytic psychotherapy to an American patient. Having in hand the process notes he prepared immediately after the session, he sits in his American supervisor's office to review the previous hour.

Confined compactly in this situation are many of the most pervasive and sensitive issues found in cross-cultural psychotherapy. A practitioner from a foreign culture is working with a client in the client's cultural milieu. To what extent need the client's culture be known and understood by the practitioner? How at home in the client's culture need the practitioner be? The abstract notions of "unconscious," "overdetermination," "resistance," "therapeutic relationship," and "dynamics," to name but a few, will have to be given concrete meaning, and the communication of the patient will have to be made comprehensible in the framework of those meanings. The therapist also will need to handle the amenities of the interaction while managing and controlling the structure of the therapeutic relationship to foster the "therapeutic alliance."

The supervisory listening method is analogous to the therapeutic one. Given the cultural differences, can the supervisor be expected to gather accurately data from within the supervisory interaction and convey it effectively to the student? Since supervision follows the model of therapy to some degree, would not the cultural difficulties that the therapeutic relationship creates also be generated by the supervisory relationship? Would the supervisor be able to analyze the therapeutic situation in the typical way given its foreignness to the student? To what extent would effective use of it demand from the supervisor a knowledge of the supervisee's culture and particularly of how teacher-learner relationships work there?

The questions are many, but little systematic examination of these issues seems to have been undertaken. In a relatively recent paper Desai (1982) discusses some of the training questions with respect to problems of the Hindu Indian learning Western psychodynamic psychotherapy. He identifies certain Hindu assumptions about human relationships, which in their clash with Western ideas create difficulties for these novice psychotherapists. One that he notes is the collaboration versus individuation contrast. The Hindu healer moves the client toward societal integration and harmony not individual growth. The Indian, he says, finds it hard to empathize with aspirations in patients for individuality and autonomy. He finds that Hindu Indian trainees tend to be uncomfortable with the expression of hostility or anger within a family and would be inclined naturally toward suppression rather than expression of these feelings. Among other problems, he named the difficulty Indians have with appreciating the notion of an unconscious mental life. They understand suppression well but have significant difficulty in understanding restraint in the framework of unconscious defensive activity.

Newly trained psychotherapists return home having successfully endured the cultural stresses of the foreign culture with its peculiar learning arrangements, having learned how to use that framework with patients culturally different from themselves. Then those therapists are faced with the challenge of applying the new knowledge to patients more or less culturally similar to themselves but to whom the therapeutic approach is remote and strange. This challenge constitutes a new source of stress of which several components can be identified.

First is the cultural readjustment required by the move back home. Therapists who have learned the new system well enough to use it on American patients probably have also internalized other aspects of the host culture besides the narrowly construed therapeutic ones. Bringing what amounts to a new partial identity transformation back to the source of the original identity can create conflict, the tensions of which can require some substantial effort to resolve. A new synthesis may be required before they can again feel comfortable enough to function freely and effectively.

Beyond the problems of personal adjustment are the difficulties of applying a foreign therapeutic modality to patients unfamiliar with it. Rarely, it appears from the literature, is a method transportable without considerably modifying or adapting it to make it palatable in a new context. To change a method with discrimination demands from the practitioner a thorough understanding of what is essential to it and what is relatively superfluous. Such an eclecticism requires a thorough and deeply ingrained comprehension of the system in question. The cultural transformation required of the practitioner in learning the system must be profound enough to achieve that level of understanding.

Cultural outsiders practice their form of therapy with members of a different culture in that group's locale. Here a visitor, sojourner, or immigrant attempts to apply methods that are foreign to the host culture. The primary role of the visitor may be research, training, or service. From the viewpoint of the host society, direct service by a temporary resident has little practical significance. Unless the training of local people occurs, little valuable residue of the visit remains, beyond whatever help has been provided the few who received and benefited from the psychotherapy. A classic example of this is the work of Devereux, who treated psychoanalytically a Plains Indian (Devereux 1951, 1953, 1980). His main interest was research, but as he engaged in psychotherapy he came to realize that tension between his scientific curiosity and his therapeutic activity required careful monitoring to protect the therapeutic endeavor.

In situations where outsiders use outside methods, we cannot answer the question of whether the method itself can be employed by locals on a local clientele. In fact, it is unlikely that a method or system of psychotherapy can be separated from the "person of the patient and the person of the therapist" (Strupp 1982, 45). Nevertheless, there still remain the problems associated with efforts to carry over a psychotherapeutic approach from the culture that conceived, bore, and nurtured it to an alien cultural context.

Transferring a method to a new cultural locale. Ultimately, a therapeutic practice must be performed by local persons who have been trained in the foreign methods. The criterion of success will not be that outsiders can claim success with local clients but rather that local practitioners can be trained to use the foreign methods competently and effectively. While no definitive answer to this question can be provided, a good-sized body of literature, albeit some of it is political and strident conveying more heat than light, points toward an increase in our understanding of this issue. These studies encompass the practices of both Western and Western-trained local therapists who apply Western methods to a population substantially foreign to that to which the methods are traditionally applied. In addition, much of this research looks at problems in using "traditional" psychotherapies with "nontraditional" patient populations. This body of work dealing with problems of transferring methods of psychotherapy will be considered later in this chapter.

Members of a Western culture who have lived for some time in a non-Western developing society and associate to a great extent with select members of that culture. This is a special but not necessarily rare cultural situation (Useem and Useem 1967; Useem, Useem, and Donaghue 1963). Through their frequent interaction, dictated usually by the nature of their jobs, the members of the two cultures develop social rules and interpersonal patterns that, although rooted in their respective original cultures, synthesize a new, binational, third culture. As examples, the authors cited in India the Indo-British carryover from the colonial era and an Indo-American hybrid culture based upon the American commercial and aid complex. More recently, Oyewumi (1986), a Western-trained practitioner returned to Nigeria, suggests that Western methods can be used in relatively unmodified form only with Westernized Nigerians who are university trained and, by implication, more a part of a Western culture. These "third culture" situations find the Western practitioner or Western-trained local practitioner working with local Westerners or "Westernized" non-Westerners.

Cultural differences among healers. This is a special cross-cultural issue that has become a subject of interest and controversy (Torrey 1986). As traditional societies develop into modern ones, the question of the role of folk or traditional healers and their methods in relation to modernization is posed. Supernatural, magical, and religious healing modes play important roles (Ehrenwald 1976; Kiev 1964). Considerable dispute about the position of these practices has arisen as Western, scientific methods are introduced. An extreme position would be that these practices should be eliminated as quickly as possible because they are useless or fraudulent at best and harmful to patients at worst. Most observers, however, do not express such a strong negative attitude. Prince (1980) summarizes the arguments in favor of and against local, indigenous healers: they are effective; they are necessary to the extent that Western facilities are not available; they have prestige and are acceptable to local populations; and Western methods may be neither acceptable nor workable within a particular cultural context. The opposition arguments are that their use perpetuates antimodern, nonscientific views; they may be harmful to patients in some instances; and they may exploit and intimidate people. Prince's summary shows the controversial nature of this question.

Some writers unenthusiastically acknowledge the use of traditional healers and their methods and suggest that it might be helpful to work with them because they are accepted and functional in their cultures (Bolman 1968).

A forceful argument against integrating traditional American Indian healing systems with modern ones is presented by Bates (1981). He says that natural evolution will bring about a synthesis of what are now two complementary, and not necessarily oppositional, systems. It has been noted by others that people will take advantage of what their opportunities are, and if both systems are available they will use both as they see fit.

A number of observers advocate a positive effort to understand their value and to work with traditional healers, because they are culturally syntonic and respected and accepted by local populations (Jilek and Jilek-Aall 1981; Ness and Wintrob 1981; Oyewumi 1986; Salan and Maretzki 1983; Wessels 1985). Lefley (1984) provides a careful, comprehensive survey and analysis of the arguments, issues, and directions in this domain. She notes a number of programs under way in which traditional helpers are being used, although in some quarters this is still strongly opposed. Torrey (1986) devotes a chapter to the question of traditional healers and argues for the wisdom of using their skills. The issue seems no longer to be whether indigenous healers and their methods are to be accepted as part of a treatment system but rather how their talents can be exploited in the interest of providing the best care possible while still protecting patients against ineffective, harmful, or fraudulent healers.

Doubts about Cultural Transplants

Psychotherapy, although perhaps a limited and frail manifestation of Western technology when compared with such achievements as electronic communication, high-powered fertilizer, and life-preserving pharmaceuticals, no less represents a technological intervention developed in Western society as a response to Western problems. As with the implantation of any body part, the risk of rejection is real. Psychotherapy's universal functionality cannot be safely assumed, and knowledgeable observers, both Western and non-Western, are skeptical about this peculiar institution of Western culture surviving a transplant unless it undergoes drastic change.

Torrey (1986) in his broad survey judged certain attempts at transplantation as failures or exceptionally difficult. Neki (1975) found Western psychotherapy at best suitable only for the few highly Westernized Indians. Lambo's (1974) description of the cultural context of African psychotherapy leads one to conclude that Western individual psychotherapy would barely be recognizable to the Western practitioner observing it in Africa, if it could be applied at all; and Olatawura (1975) used case material also to argue its unsuitability, without considerable modification, for Nigerian patients. Penningroth and Penningroth (1977) listed a number of modifications that make psychotherapy feasible in Guam, but the degree and kind of change suggested was substantial. An optimistic picture was presented of Korea by Chang and Kim (1973) and Kim and Rhi (1976), but there was more evidence of hope than accomplishment in their surveys. For Greece, the literature presents a generally negative picture of individual psychotherapy (Kokantzis and Ierodiakonou 1975; Ierodiakonou 1983; Hartcollis 1983), although it has been observed that in selected urban areas, such as Athens, and among more cosmopolitan populations, the situation is brighter (Draguns 1987). Pande (1968) was decidedly negative in his claim that psychotherapy was a Western reaction to peculiarly Western problems rooted in the Western style of life. Kakar (1985) has pointed out contrasts between assumptions in psychoanalysis and in Indian thought that interfere with the carryover of the former. Sharp contrasts between Western and non-Western ways of thought have been summarized concisely by Pedersen (1982). Generally, cautions, strictures, and modification requirements were so abundant with respect to Chinese patients (Hsu and Tseng 1972; Singer 1976; Tseng 1978; Tung 1984) that one must wonder how much of Western psychotherapy remains and how much is a residue of psychiatric wisdom or common sense, sometimes characterized as "eclectic." Schumacher and Guthrie (1984) make a good case for nontransferability to the Philippines as does Connor (1982) to Bali. The literature on Indochinese immigrants in the United States also seems to argue that psychotherapy must be dramatically different if it is to be useful with patients from that group (Kinzie 1985; Tung 1985).

It appears that a sound basis in clinical and scholarly research exists for questioning the cultural portability of psychotherapy. While all foreign forms can have far-reaching and complex ramifications within the societies into which they are introduced, the impact upon lives is indirect. A new fertilizer is intended to transform an economy, and its immediate or even long-term effects upon the lives of individual farmers are incidental. But psychotherapy is intended to change directly the lives of those who avail themselves of it. Although it might ultimately affect many aspects of the culture into which it is introduced, such macrocultural effects are secondary to its immediate microcultural purpose.

Psychotherapy does not only impinge directly upon its clients but it strikes at the center of individuals, not at the periphery. It confronts and arouses fundamental personal attitudes, values, feelings, beliefs, and standards about the conduct of life and the interrelationships of people. Draguns' (1975) observation about the centrality of sociocultural purposes and interpersonal methods in psychotherapy is particularly apt. He conceives of psychotherapy as a means of facilitating the return of alienated persons into more complete societal participation and functioning, a position that highlights psychotherapy's cultural focus. But it also highlights the obstacle that pronounced cultural differences in the psychotherapy situation present.

Psychotherapy as a Cultural Universal

Earlier it was stated that psychotherapy can be thought of as present in all, or at least most, human societies without doing violence to any reasonable definition of it. Activities that are the functional equivalents of psychotherapy are found historically and contemporaneously in all societies although they may be performed by people not narrowly defined as mental health experts.

In his exhaustive study of the "cure of souls" in religious and philosophic traditions, McNeill (1965) notes that healing includes caring and concern on the part of the healer, features considered intrinsic to most psychotherapies today. These caring activities have not always been the specialized, discrete functions that they are in the Westernized world today. McNeill observed that the separation of mental healing from its source in religious and philosophic thought and its conversion to a specialized, scientific discipline are relatively recent developments. "Soul healers" have functioned as negotiators or mediators between claimants for help and forces that can release them from suffering. Meadows, referring to ancient Greece, itemizes such methods as "divination, exorcism, absolution, expiation, orgiastic dance, ritual mysteries, teaching, revealing, directing," (1968, 497), all of which are used in psychological healing practice around the world today. Universal in its manifestation in all cultures, while unique in its shape and color in each culture, psychotherapy appears to qualify as a cultural universal (Lonner 1980).

That activities or functions that we refer to as psychotherapy appear to be universally performed provides some hope to those who assert that Western psychotherapy can be useful in non-Western societies. This is qualified, however, by a consensus expressed in the literature (Draguns 1975; Torrey 1986) that the specific form psychotherapy takes in any culture must harmonize with the broader cultural ethos. It should not violate those implicit values and unarticulated presuppositions that constitute the culture's "worldview."

In summing up his collection of papers, which nicely demonstrates the great variety of psychological ways of healing and helping people, Kiev (1964) suggested that we should be working at identifying the essential and universal features of psychotherapy. His recommendation came relatively early, but it was not the first to promote an interest in discovering the common or shared aspects of different psychotherapies.

One of the first comments, at least in the modern era, came from Freud in 1904 (Freud 1953). He noted that psychotherapy is an ancient form of healing and that the suggestibility of the patient can be manipulated in treatment. He reminds his audience of an old dictum that cure is effected through the personal influence of the physician not by the medicine he administers. Much later, Rosenzweig (1936) added emotional catharsis to the personal influence factor and noted that an explanation or interpretation of the patient's problems is provided. Later, Strunkard (1961) focused upon the power inherent in the emotional relationship in psychotherapy, an emphasis that has been maintained throughout work on this topic.

Frank's *Persuasion and Healing* (1974), which appeared originally in 1961, became the foundation for much of the increased interest in common factors. He laid out a model of psychotherapy that incorporated all of the previously discussed characteristics but centered them in a well-organized, clear framework. His approach was to look at psychotherapy as one among many ways to get people to change their minds or mend their ways. Since there is perhaps nothing in human affairs as ubiquitous as the wish to change others, Frank had hit upon a useful approach. His work is frequently cited in the cross-cultural literature, and indeed many recent papers seem to use or paraphrase his definition of psychotherapy.

Frank emphasizes the power conveyed by the personal influence of the helping person in the special situation socioculturally defined as psychotherapeutic. He attributes the major curative value to the contextual arrangements, to the socially defined power, and to the emotional arousal in the relationship. From this point of view what therapists do (techniques and methods) is less important than what they are endowed with; that is, they need to have culturally defined therapeutic qualities and conduct themselves as their clientele expects that they will (relationship factors). In a number of other publications since the 1961 edition of *Persuasion and Healing,* Frank has restated his original views (Frank 1971, 1975, 1982).

For Frank it seems that the most universal feature of effective psychotherapy is the charismatic potency of the therapist to inspire the confidence, trust, hope, and faith of the patient. Universal and essential elements are the emotional bolstering provided by the relationship and the suggestibility of the patient. Relief emerges out of the strength of the therapist, and the readiness of the patient is intensified by the context of treatment. Psychodynamically, the model Frank describes, and which is generally repeated in much of the literature, is that of a transference distortion in which the clients, no matter what their age, experience themselves as children in relation to a powerful, benevolent parent. Sociologically, it reflects the traditional paternalistic doctor-patient or priest-penitent relationship. This conception aptly characterizes healing-helping relationships in many cultural contexts, probably in most. Markedly divergent from it, however, are two other Western traditions, one that comes from the work of Carl Rogers (Patterson 1978) and the other, the psychoanalytic tradition that argues against supporting the infantilization of the patient and proposes using the analytic method to work through and eliminate transference distortions over time as therapy proceeds (Greenson 1967; Langs 1982).

The importance of the factors emphasized by Frank, such as faith, suggestion, and expectation of help, is recognized in much of the literature following his seminal work. Calestro (1972) in an extensive, scholarly survey of non-Western methods argued for the importance of suggestibility and the therapist's capacity to arouse this internal state. Prince (1976) took the same general position but placed emphasis forthrightly upon "endogenous" factors. He first summarized what by then had become the conventional universal factors described variously since Frank's original work by Torrey (1972), Calestro (1972), Draguns (1975), Mendel (1972), Tseng and McDermott (1975), and Singer (1976). These factors included the "special relationship," "shared world view," "expectant hope of the patient," "naming the illness," "attribution of cause and prescription of treatment by the healer," and the "central role of suggestion" (Prince 1976, 115). He characterized these factors as "exogenous" and contrasted them with internal mechanisms and processes, among which he included dreams, mystical and ecstatic states, trance and dissociation phenomena, and other altered states of consciousness. Prince asserted that these latter experiences may themselves provide cures if the therapist can activate them. The material that he provided from non-European societies is used to argue that the manipulation of such mechanisms offers an opportunity for successful intervention where more conventional Western approaches are not feasible.

Working within a pancultural framework, Torrey (1986) has tried to obliterate any distinctions among psychotherapies, arguing that there are a few basic features that all psychotherapies share. But at the same time, he notes that cultural commonality is so critical that a cultural gap of any distance between the participants in a therapeutic interaction provides almost overwhelming barriers to the therapeutic work. His universals include a worldview shared by therapist and patient, personal qualities of the therapist that foster a close interpersonal relationship, the patient's emotionally powered anticipation of being helped, and a growing sense of competence in the patient. To these four general factors he adds that of specific techniques. These operate to strengthen the effects of the general factors. His position, which is well known as evidenced by the frequency with which this work is cited, is one of the most extreme with respect to its assertion of the universal existence of psychotherapy and its insistence on common factors throughout the world.

The search for features shared by all psychotherapies has been a prominent part of studies in cross-cultural psychotherapy since the 1960s (Prince 1980; Pluk and Wojciechowski 1985; Wohl 1976). A parallel line of inquiry has been pursued in the literature on psychotherapy apart from the cross-cultural segment. Strupp has undertaken a close and systematic scrutiny of psychotherapy aimed at isolating its essential, basic, and shared features. In a series of important studies (1973a, 1973b, 1982), he has defined clearly two themes emerging in psychotherapy's recent history. One emphasizes the "nonspecific" healing aura hovering over the psychotherapeutic relationship. Since all psychotherapy involves a therapist and a client interacting in some special way, one is tempted to identify the common factors in this relationship as the essential ingredients. This can help to account for why all therapies can rightfully claim to be helpful (Karasu 1977). The emphasis upon the curative power of the relationship itself has been greatest in the work of Carl Rogers and followers of the "humanistic" approaches. In what is now viewed as a classic paper, Rogers (1957) described conditions he considered "necessary and sufficient" for therapeutic change. For the past 30 years his followers elaborated upon this work. In a recent formulation, accurate empathy, positive regard, nonpossessive warmth, and congruence or genuineness were said to be the requisite therapist characteristics (Lambert, Shapiro, and Bergin 1985). But the relationship is itself complex, and probably not all of the elements of the relationship are equally essential. In general, psychotherapists who favor applying methods cross-culturally, follow the trend that supports universal features and that focuses heavily on the significance of the relationship and various facets of it.

The second major theme is the emphasis upon technical skill and specific therapeutic methods combined with a relative de-emphasis of the "human relationship" in psychotherapy. This theme is prominent in the other two major contemporary approaches to psychotherapy: the behavioral, which is rooted in the tradition of research in learning and cognition of experimental psychology, and the psychodynamic, which emerged from the development of psychoanalysis by Freud. Both emphasize the techniques or procedures used by the therapist rather than the therapeutic climate created by the personal qualities of the therapist. Behavioral techniques encompass various ways of inducing learning such as modeling, selective reinforcement, and conditioning. The primary psychoanalytic technique, interpretation, is designed to enlarge and deepen the client's self-understanding (Karasu 1977).

Strupp has sought to identify the specific features of therapeutic influence, originally with the hope that it would be possible to devise specific techniques for individual persons and their unique symptoms. He relinquished this mechanical conception when he wrote that "we are beginning to recognize and take seriously the extraordinary complexity of the therapeutic influence" (1973b, 275). With some reluctance he acknowledged that generally "the search for highly specific techniques is probably futile" (1973b, 313). His final position was that the therapeutic influence is composed of two fundamental factors: one consists of the nonspecific, basic, or general effect, which inheres in the interpersonal relationship; the other consists of specific techniques employed by the therapist. The techniques, however, are operative only through the medium of the relationship.

In a more recent summing up of the problem, Strupp (1982) emphasizes the inherent inseparability of the therapist's technical skill from the therapist's personality but also notes the importance of technical skill. Finally, while Strupp's research clearly supports the position of Frank in recognizing the power of the relationship and the importance of the therapist's personality, he is troubled clinically, and it seems morally as well, at the exploitation of this power to manipulate the patient, which is inevitable unless transference is recognized and worked through to its resolution. He argues that the interpretation and resolution of transference (the power of relationship) is not only better for the patient clinically but is in keeping with the cultural value of personal freedom embedded in American society.

Culture and the Therapeutic Relationship

The theoretical and scholarly literature on psychotherapy and its cross-cultural potentialities converges on the therapeutic relationship, where the minimal necessary basis for any psychotherapeutically meaningful work is found. Few people experienced in personal counseling or psychotherapy would take issue with the position that at least one universal, fundamental feature of psychotherapy is the emotionally special interpersonal relationship created and managed to foster personal change in the client. Despite this universality, it is possible, and even probable, that the constituent elements of the "good relationship" are different from one culture to another. Presumably, specific techniques, such as interpreting, advising, or reassuring, would not be equally appropriate in all cultures. Some would be consistent with the norms of a specific culture, but others would be alien. But the greater question remains: To what extent is the general Western conception of the good therapeutic relationship universally valid? Even if in all cultures most people respond well to "acceptance," "respect," "interest," "concern," "wish to help," and the other components, one still must ask whether the outsider can deliver, express, and communicate these in terms understandable and acceptable to the client.

Aside from these "internal" aspects of therapy, there are other aspects that are usually taken for granted when both parties share the same culture. Frank emphasized the requirement that patient and therapist share an acceptance of the social trappings and the framework of meaning within which disorder and treatment are understood and confronted. Strupp followed him in recognizing the necessity for a rational system that both parties can use to make sense out of therapeutic events. Is it possible for two people of different cultures to achieve a reasonable degree of agreement and understanding about this superstructure?

Not always sufficiently explicit in this literature is that the two participants in the therapeutic relationship interact with each other primarily through conversation and that the effectiveness of their communication is a major variable in determining productiveness. Whether the patients change their expectations about therapy or the therapists change theirs to fit those of their patients, the recommendation that they reduce the size of their conceptual difference (Higginbotham 1977) speaks to the same issue expressed in much broader terms by Torrey (1986), who stressed the difficulty of cross-cultural therapy where the participants do not share a common worldview.

White and Marsella (1982) affirm a need for congruence between participants in psychotherapy with respect to conceptions of disorder, treatment, ways of communicating, and a background of language and cultural knowledge. Johnson (1981) also focuses upon psychotherapy as a communicative interaction that requires a common framework of understanding.

An anecdotal study (Vassiliou and Vassiliou 1973) has described difficulties arising in the training of therapists in a foreign culture because of different connotations of the same words. Misunderstanding between Greek trainees and their American instructors occurred with respect to their different conceptions of the teacher-learner relationship. Supervisory "indifference" was considered appropriate neutrality by the Americans but "hostility" by the Greeks. The American supervisors' restraint about inquiring into the private lives of the trainees was perceived by them as a lack of interest. If this happens in training, one can only imagine the difficulties existing in practice. Bickley (1978), although not writing specifically about psychotherapy, demonstrates how misunderstandings can occur in delicate negotiations in which the "same" word has different connotations for speakers from two different cultures.

Seminal work on the language and communication aspects of social class (Bernstein 1964) reinforces one's appreciation of the problems in psychotherapeutic discourse presented by participants who believe they speak the same language but have unconsciously disparate semantic worlds. A series of papers by Marcos and associates (Marcos 1976a, 1976b; Marcos and Alpert 1976; Marcos and Urcuyo 1979) has described problems in psychotherapy associated with bilingualism, even when participants are able to use the same language. A clinical paper by Carlson (1979) reports that in psychoanalytic therapy of three native speakers of German it was very productive to conduct their treatment in German, even though their second language was English. Draguns (1987) describes a practice of asking clients whose native language differed from the language of the psychotherapy to label or describe in their original language an especially noteworthy feeling or experience prior to translating it into the language of the therapy. This was intended to encourage a more direct emotional experiencing and reduce the tendency to intellectualize experience. It was found to be valuable to the client to return the experience to its original linguistic form, even though the therapist did not understand the original language of the patient.

The essence of the psychotherapeutic process is human communication. More importantly, much of the activity in therapy consists of communication about communication. A great deal of psychoanalytic psychotherapy includes efforts directed toward clarifying meanings and making conscious and explicit what is indirect, subtle, and unwitting in the client's communication. Participants in any conversation, therapeutic or otherwise, are able to communicate to the extent that they have common referents. They must achieve agreement on what they are discussing and on the manner in which they are to discuss their subject matter (Sullivan 1954).

Ultimately, communication in a special kind of human relationship is fundamental to achieve the effects that will be seen as psychotherapeutic. If communication is to develop within a tolerable limit of error, the framework of understanding within which it occurs requires the sharing of a set of assumptions about the world and its working, about the nature of humankind and its relation to natural events and supernatural influences, and about the physical and social circumstances under which therapy goes on. The culturally indigenous but modern Japanese therapies, Morita and Naikan, exemplify such a harmony between therapeutic mode and cultural values (Reynolds 1980).

The therapeutic relationship can tolerate some disparity between the participants and, indeed, some always exists. Part of the therapeutic work is the mutual learning about such gaps and the negotiation of them; but if the gaps between the participants are too great, there is no basis for understanding, and the "noise" becomes too loud to permit a working alliance (Greenson 1967). For example, a gap may occur because of personal characteristics of the therapist. It is possible that the much-researched trinity of warmth, empathy, and genuineness might appear in a Burmese context to be evidence of weakness and incompetence; perhaps client-centered or psychoanalytic positions, with egalitarianism, mutuality, and openness as part of their value orientations, will not mesh effectively with the hierarchically ordered Thai society. Alexander et al. (1981) indicate how a fundamental therapeutic stance of the therapist, such as nondirectiveness, can be misinterpreted as lack of interest. Kakar (1985) and Roland (1982–83) discuss conceptions of the therapeutic person's role in India that differ from Western ones and that would have to be taken into account in applying a Western therapy to an Indian patient.

Thus, although a special kind of human relationship is a hallmark of psychotherapy, the particular expression of such a relationship and the distinct qualities required of the therapist to muster the integrative forces within the client may not be universally applicable. Furthermore, the sounds and gestures that are intended to convey certain meanings may actually convey other meanings that do not provoke the desired attitudes in the patient. All of this should give pause to those who argue the case for the cultural transferability of psychotherapy. The problems can be seen in better relief when some of the reports of those who have engaged in intercultural psychotherapy are examined.

Experiences with Cross-Cultural Psychotherapy

This section presents a selective survey of accounts of cross-cultural psychotherapy focused upon technical and procedural problems. They all involve modern, Western-developed psychotherapeutic methods practiced by a Western or Western-trained individual with a person to whom the method is culturally alien.

In a study "devoted specifically to the technical problems of a culturally oriented individual psychotherapy," Devereux (1951, 422) wrote of his experiences in psychoanalytic psychotherapy with Plains Indians (1951, 1953). He concluded that three major features—transference, dream utilization, and therapeutic goals—require a significant appreciation of the patient's cultural background. To understand and interpret appropriately transference communications, the therapist must comprehend the cultural context of the patient's family life. Similarly, to understand dreams in therapy, the therapist must know the cultural framework of dream interpretation. But the greatest problem for Devereux was the therapeutic goals. His solution was that the therapist must want "to restore the patient to himself" (1951, 420).

Elaboration on this description of goals adds some understanding of his dilemma. He states that the "patient must be helped to handle the realities of the reservation, which is his predictable future environment" (1951, 421), as well as to learn selectively to use traditional Indian values and means in the white world.

This issue of appropriate therapeutic goals is especially relevant with a member of a restricted or oppressed group. Devereux's solution was an acceptance of the current social situation, a political act that would seem to reinforce that situation. His decision was especially poignant because his patients were acculturated to the degree that they considered their "Indian heritage peripheral" (1951, 411). Today's "radical therapists" would resolve the dilemma of goal selection by supporting or promoting social change. It was not as obvious to Devereux in 1951 as it is today that psychotherapy has inevitable political implications. In certain societies this could be a particularly sensitive factor requiring careful consideration before an attempt is made to embark on any major programmatic importation of foreign therapy. Aleksandrowicz and Czabala (1982) suggest that political ideological constraints in postwar Poland inhibited interest in psychoanalytic therapy. The same forces virtually prohibit it in the rest of Eastern Europe.

Western psychotherapies that are premised upon personal growth through self-exploration could well lead to increased adaptational difficulties in patients as they become more aware of, and hence more dissatisfied with, oppression in their lives (Halleck 1971). Moreover, counselors working in universities in countries with authoritarian regimes where students may be regarded as a threat to the established order might themselves be seen as subversive in their practice of Western psychotherapy (Wohl 1978). The suspicious police mentality would worry about any private, confidential contacts between people, especially if one of the parties was dissatisfied, which it is reasonable to assume a counselee would be. On a more sophisticated level, an increased self-awareness and critical ability developed in counseling might be seen as intrinsically dangerous to an oppressive regime. Such concern by authorities would be even greater in countries where students have historically been a focal point of political dissent and upheaval.

Devereux's patients were all well educated, relatively well acculturated, and by their own account, partly removed from their Indian heritage. The gap here between the therapist and the patient is less than the unmodified term "Plains Indian" might suggest. Is therapy possible here only to the extent that patients are acculturated and can share the therapist's worldview to a considerable degree?

Bishop and Winokur (1956) reported therapy that took place in the United States between a Japanese male physician and an American female psychiatrist. The authors asserted that, in general, knowledge of the cultural background increases the therapist's understanding of the patient's problems and also helps in goal selection. Such knowledge can help avoid "guiding him into patterns" that although acceptable in the therapist's culture create trouble "when the patient returns to his own group" (1956, 369). The authors admit to enticing the prospective patient into therapy through a three-week warm-up period in which the therapist befriended the patient and expressed interest in Japan and in the patient's current work in an American hospital.

Without going further into this apparently successful treatment, it is evident that the "warm-up period" was a substantial departure from any conventional therapeutic procedure. Furthermore, the East-West cultural gap was narrower than it might have seemed at first glance as "there was practically no difficulty with language," and the patient "had lived so long in a cosmopolitan society and had associated extensively with Americans" (Bishop and Winokur 1956, 372).

Abel (1956) advocated the learning of cultural facts to improve the therapist's understanding of the patient and to present formulations in a useful manner. The argument is supported by clinical illustrations—vignettes of her own and others' experiences with cultural differences. Although the points she makes about the advantage of cultural understanding by the therapist are valuable, it must be noted that all of her material refers to therapy in the United States with indigenous or immigrant subcultural groups, largely European in origin. Her own work with a Chinese patient was done in English, and his degree of acculturation was considerable, as Abel reported in a later article (1962).

The kind of intercultural therapy she discusses is a predecessor to the wave of interest that began in the 1960s in problems faced by middle-class, mainstream, Americanized helpers working with educationally and economically impoverished and discriminated-against members of ethnic minorities. Problems in that domain are today probably the center of activity in cross-cultural counseling and psychotherapy, but as Kinzie (1978) maintains, there are continuities between applying Western psychotherapy in Malaysia and applying it to "nontraditional" target populations within the United States. Ishisaka, Nguyen, and Oki-moto (1985), based on their work with Indochinese patients, advised that with immigrants it is important to assess the degree to which their original, traditional culture contributes to their functioning.

One of the few books on culture and psychotherapy that does not con-sist of a collection of separately authored chapters is a work by Abel, Métraux, and Roll (1987). It treats many of the issues of importance in this domain and contains much wisdom for the student or practitioner.

A paper by Bustamente (1957) is similar to that of Abel in its focus upon patients within one society who are treated by a therapist of differ-ent cultural or subcultural background, and it makes the same reason-able points as does Abel's paper. "A psychiatrist must be able to assess the cultural background of his patient, and have a thorough knowledge of his own culture as well, to be effective with polycultural patients" (1957, 811). (By "polycultural" he meant patients who shared or par-ticipated in Cuban, European, and Afro-Cuban traditions.)

Information gathering, or research rather than therapy, is the inter-view function discussed by Carstairs (1961), whose conclusions derive from work done with villagers in India. He indicates that clinicians engaged in research may be obligated to employ their therapeutic skills. The act of drawing forth information may open up problems for the informant that the clinician cannot ignore. The reverse of this situation is described by Devereux (1953), who wrote that his professional inter-est in culture was an obstacle to therapy when he became too interested in cultural features at the expense of clinical involvement with patients. Such an anthropological preoccupation is dangerous in any intercul-tural endeavor in which service rather than science is the basic purpose. There is always a tendency to use the subject as an informant to provide a window onto the culture; in psychotherapy more than in other fields involvement of this kind can become an impediment.

Carstairs is insistent that interviewing be done in the native language of the informant or in the one that he or she normally uses. The use of an interpreter is not adequate because this interferes with the establish-ment of a relationship. Carstairs also points out that as an outsider one is not expected by the members of the culture to have a full knowledge of cultural facts. This position of acknowledged ignorance can be used to promote openness and clarity of communication because it provides a good justification for asking people to explain themselves. He warns against premature interpretations, formulations, or diagnoses: "It is only after a gradual process of feeling one's way into the accepted values and expectations of the groups that one learns to recognize behavior which they regard as abnormal" (1961, 545).

The problem of goal setting has been raised by Hsu and Tseng (1972). They make the same point that Devereux made—that goals need to fit the cultural realities or what is culturally possible for the patient. They emphasize that the therapist needs to know the patient's cultural context very well so that the patient can engage in this goal-oriented activity. Indeed, if the therapist is to set goals and judge that goals are suitable, then this knowledge must be possessed by the therapist. But a therapist can also display ignorance, like Carstairs' (1961) cultural explorer who made the patient explain the culture to him, and develop goals together with the client.

Hsu and Tseng discuss a fundamental issue of psychotherapy, that of a communication problem beyond the basic knowledge of a common language. Verbal localisms, facial expressions, and special cultural nuances of symbols distort communication even when words and sentences are understood literally. Metaphoric communication illustrates this problem well. Communication in therapy constantly employs metaphor, and metaphor represents an almost impassible cultural barrier. A sad, yet humorous, example of this occurred in connection with a patient admitted to a Midwestern mental hospital. One of the allegations made about him upon admission was that he believed there was a radio in his stomach. Inquiry about this revealed that the admitting physician, a recent immigrant to the United States, had interpreted literally the patient's complaint about his neighbor's constant loud playing of the radio. The patient had said, "I got a belly full."

Hsu and Tseng also point out that beyond the problems of language and communication there can be other complications in the relationship, particularly that of the danger of mutual projection of cultural stereotypes. This was noted with respect to subcultural differences by Thomas (1962). These authors conclude by offering a collection of therapeutic aphorisms. These include awareness of the importance of culture in a general sense, knowledge of the patient's culture, mutual acknowledgment and discussion by patient and therapist of differences as they appear, search for the meaning of a patient's history, and provision of a good relationship. These praiseworthy features of therapy could be used as standards applicable to any psychotherapy. But it seems unrealistic to expect these criteria to be more realizable in intercultural therapeutic ventures than in the simpler intracultural efforts.

Kinzie (1978) supports both hopes and doubts about intercultural psychotherapy. He reiterates many of the items mentioned earlier that are seen as helpful in surmounting the cultural barriers in psychotherapy. These include self-awareness and awareness of the patient's culture, an open attitude, continuing mutual checking on the adequacy of communication, and readiness of the therapist to adjust action and style to the patient's conception of a healer. Jilek-Aall (1976), working with Canadian Indians, provides an enlightening tabular presentation of differences between typical Western psychotherapists and non-Western patients, arguing that successful interaction demands a degree of acculturation by the patient. Her case material shows also substantial modification of Western methods.

In clear detail Ozturk (1978) in Turkey gives an extended description of a case in which the physical circumstances rather than the cultural background of the patient seemed most critical in determining the means of psychotherapy. Essentially, he established a long-term dependent tie that provided direction and support for the patient in a therapy conducted by mail, with only intermittent periods of personal contact. That the treatment was successful is not as relevant as that it was far removed from any conventional Western mode of psychotherapy and that the variations were not particularly "culturally" based but were demanded by geography. The circumstances of treatment could just as easily have occurred in the West. Of special interest is the therapist's reporting of similarities between the patient's background and his own and the importance of this in managing the treatment.

On the topic of goals in therapy, Kinzie approaches most closely the position suggested earlier that goals "will be primarily determined by the patient himself and by his culture" (1972, 226). He notes that after therapy the patients may well have achieved a broader perspective of themselves in their cultural contexts and have better recognition of their choices. The point here is that therapists must recognize the danger of foreign cultural values being imposed as goals or criteria for successful therapy, and they must combine this knowledge with the therapeutic position that such criteria are determined with the patient. Therapists need to worry less about what criteria to set and more about guarding against setting foreign ones or making any other inappropriate interventions. The arbitrary imposition of the therapist's beliefs and values violates the rules for proper conduct of most traditional Western psychotherapy. It should be assumed that the same principle of good technique would apply interculturally as well and that goals therefore are not to be determined unilaterally by the psychotherapist.

The paper by Kinzie provides three case examples of psychotherapy in Malaysia that uniquely exemplify the point that intercultural therapy is possible only if the cultural gap between patient and therapist, especially in language and worldview, is not overly wide. The first case was a rural, uneducated woman who saw her "problem in magical and medical terms" (1972, 227), not in concepts of family and interpersonal stress. She was treated with medication that brought relief. The second patient, who had a moderate degree of Western (English-language) background, asked for hypnosis and advice on his interpersonal inadequacy. He was treated with a hodgepodge of behavioral and medical methods that produced little change until he was able to discuss his feelings openly. From that point on he improved, more because of the relationship than the technique. The third patient was apparently at home in the European world, had already some experience in marital therapy, and was able to participate in a cathartic-supportive, self-exploratory relationship. The author pointed out that "because of his previous experience, this patient quickly became involved in therapy" (1972, 228).

In two of the cases, the patient shared conceptions with the therapist about the usefulness of Western psychological methods of helping, whereas in the other, these methods were not attempted. These examples do not really demonstrate intercultural psychotherapeutics. One could just as well argue that the first case suggests the utility of working with traditional healers to make them more effective or the futility of trying to impose Western therapeutic approaches where they are incomprehensible or unknown. These three cases reveal a continuum of readiness to accept psychotherapy correlated with the patient's previous experiences, which in two of the cases reduced the cultural gap between the Western therapy and the patient's expectations.

Much of the literature argues that the gap can be traversed if the therapist is personally flexible, culturally perceptive and committed enough, and if the gap is not too wide. "Psychotherapy, like any method of treatment, can be effective only if it is flexible enough to adapt to the particular needs and conditions of the patients" (Ierodiakonou 1983, 544). Unfortunately, it is not the therapy that must be "flexible" but the therapist using the therapy. This quotation is a truism that is not limited to the cross-cultural situation but applies to any psychotherapist-psychotherapy combination. Interestingly enough, rarely in this literature is reference made to the professional qualities of psychotherapists. Such factors as experience, training, knowledge, and skill, which might reasonably be thought of as related to effectiveness in practice, are generally not mentioned directly. Yet many of the skills deemed important in cross-cultural work ought reasonably to be expected of a competent performer in any psychotherapy. The general research literature on the outcome of psychotherapy emphasizes the importance of therapist attitudes and relationship skills, and suggests that competence and professional experience make some contribution to good results (Lambert 1981; Lambert, Shapiro, and Bergin 1986).

Expectations of the patient that are discrepant from those of the therapist and the therapist's role conception are often noted to present serious barriers in cross-cultural work. Many observers have identified expectations about therapy and therapist conduct in different cultural groups. Some such characteristics of Indochinese immigrants in the United States are described by Kinzie (1985). They expect the therapist to understand their troubles, they want an explanation that they can understand, they want an active treatment resulting in a quick cure or symptom reduction, they hope medicine will help, they want to feel justified in being sick, and they wish for a reduction in the sociopsychological stress factor. In her survey of psychotherapeutic practices and patient characteristics in the Caribbean, Lefley (1981) says that prospective patients seek help for specific problems, not connected to life circumstances in general. They expect and want direct guidance, advice, or instruction; and they expect to follow advice and promptly recover. Lefley notes astutely that these characteristics could be true of psychotherapeutically naive people anywhere, of lower socioeconomic groups in general, of many minority groups, and of people with limited education. Her comment, which could also apply to Kinzie's description, is reinforced the more reports one sees on this topic. Idowu warns against being "democratic, nondirective" (1985, 509) with Nigerian patients because they will think the therapist is incompetent or not interested. He also warns the Western therapist that eye contact, of which so many seem to have made a fetish, is not a Nigerian priority; in fact, it could mean disrespect. Those issues are raised also with respect to Asian-American and Hispanic patients by Maduro (1982); Roll, Miller, and Martinez (1982); and Yamamoto and Acosta (1982). They identify some group characteristics but recognize also that within an ethnic group socioeconomic class makes for differences. Most critically, as Jones (1985) says in regard to interracial psychotherapy between a black patient and a white therapist, the patient must be treated as an individual, not as a member of a category.

Maduro argues that "Latinos" (his term) can be treated psychoanalytically, that the therapist can modify stance enough to respond to the Hispanic expectation that healers should be warm, personal, friendly, and caring and still be psychoanalytic. He says, as an example of the approach, that the therapist "painstakingly attempts to make understanding statements rather than ask questions" (1982, 626); here again is a general principle of good technique, not something especially reserved for cross-cultural work.

An unusually thorough scrutiny of the expectations held by the patient about therapy has been made by Higginbotham (1977). After a careful, scholarly evaluation he concludes that expectations on the part of the patient about the nature of the treatment can have powerful effects upon the development of the therapeutic relationship. He recommends that because cultural conditioning is a critical determinant of expectations about therapy, psychotherapy across a cultural gap should be preceded by an assessment of those expectations and an attempt to reduce the disparity between what the patient expects and the actual therapeutic procedures.

Cross-cultural psychotherapy, in which there exists a tradition of conflict, fear, bitterness, hatred, violence, and distrust between the two

groups represented by the therapy participants, has a far stronger barrier to demolish. Here the participants are not just foreign to each other
but may carry the history of strife in the form of stronger prejudices,
more deeply carved stereotypes, and covert agendas. Such a situation
must influence black-white psychotherapy in the United States, Arab-
Jew psychotherapy in Israel, or German-Jew psychotherapy anywhere.
It is not surprising then that the first message provided by the literature
about such instances is for therapists to develop an understanding of
their own attitudes, biases, assumptions, and stereotypes about the
patient. A second message is that the therapist must be able to engage
the patient in a discussion of the attitudes each has of the other (Gorkin
1986; Wohl 1983; Block 1981). Gorkin's paper identifies an array of
countertransference difficulties and suggests ways of managing and
using the countertransference to advantage.

Basch-Kahre (1984), a female, Swedish psychoanalyst, while arguing
for the feasibility of using psychoanalytic psychotherapy with her male,
black, African patient, described problematic reactions that she experienced in working with him. She especially noticed a feeling of strangeness or distance, resulting, she says, from the different expectations
each held about treatment, and from the patient's inability to use his
own language to communicate with her. In translating into English he
became overly logical and produced few emotional associations. Self-
explorations by therapists have been sensitively portrayed by Wintrob
and Harvey (1981) and by Tobin (1986). What is most encouraging is
that even under very trying conditions psychotherapy can be effectively
conducted.

Summary and Conclusions

If one employs broad concepts and definitions to describe its fundamental character, then psychotherapy can be reasonably viewed as a cultural universal. Many general elements have been identified. First is
the existence of social support, a cultural context that is generally
known and understood and by which the healers and their activities are
defined. There are societal rules that govern or regulate the healing rituals with respect to their social and physical environments. Second are
the sets of variables internal to the process of therapy. Included here are
concepts dealing with the personal qualities of the therapists and with
the therapeutic relationship. Third are the so-called technique variables, those characteristics traditionally seen as most directly involved in
the change-inducing process but now seen as dependent upon the existence of a working therapeutic relationship

Without a fitting external societal context and without therapist and relationship suitability, the magical power of technique is lost. Not only must these sets of variables coexist, they must be harmoniously related to each other. The physical setting, social rules, the therapist's style, the relationship the therapist tries to establish, and the techniques used must be such as to fit in with the general expectations of the patient concerning what healers do. Finally, all of these fundamentals in their concrete manifestations require that communication occur between the participants. They must be able to achieve some agreement and understanding about what they are doing together.

The literature suggests that intercultural psychotherapy is possible if the patient's expectations, based upon some aspects of cultural, subcultural, or intercultural experiences, make them at least minimally receptive to Western psychotherapy. The most successful clinical examples are generally of people who are inclined toward accepting Western psychotherapy, whose worldviews are, even if very different, open enough to permit some new scenery to be examined. Yet paradoxically, these cases have been used to argue for the feasibility of applying Western psychotherapy to non-Western cultures, and even then always with the stipulation that some highly idealistic standards of therapist quality and competence be met. One could, with at least equal justification, suggest that if the therapist must be a paragon of therapeutic skill to deal with patients who are only marginally definable as intercultural, then the enterprise has very limited value.

In many of these cases both the therapist and the therapy were foreign to the patient. The real test of intercultural psychotherapy, the carryover to a different cultural environment of alien modes of psychotherapy, comes in the effort to work with non-Westernized patients only minimally familiar with Western ways. By this selection criterion, therapeutic communication will have to be in the patient's language with a therapist who is very much at home in that language. If that end is to be achieved in any practical way, members of the local culture must be able to identify with Western culture sufficiently to understand its psychotherapies, and they must be sufficiently flexible in their own culture to sense how these therapies can be made to work.

More and more the major barriers to effective cross-cultural psychotherapy are seen as residing in the therapists, who must first be knowledgeable and competent with whatever modes of psychotherapy are employed. They must come to grips with their own characteristics, their own biases, and stereotypic notions. They must be comfortable enough in their professional functioning to allow themselves flexible interpretations of their therapeutic methods to fit patient requirements without becoming irrationally eclectic.

References

Abel, T. 1956. Cultural patterns as they affect psychotherapeutic procedures. *American Journal of Psychotherapy* 10:728–739.

————. 1962. The dreams of a Chinese patient. In W. Muensterberger and S. Axelrod (eds.), *The psychoanalytic study of society.* Vol. 2. New York: International Universities Press.

Abel, T., Métraux, R., and Roll, S. 1987. *Psychotherapy and culture.* Rev. and expanded ed. of *Culture and psychotherapy.* 1974. Albuquerque: University of New Mexico Press.

Aleksandrowicz, J. W., and Czabala, J. L. 1982. Psychotherapy in Poland. *American Journal of Psychiatry* 139:1051–1053.

Alexander, A. A., Klein, M. H., Workneh, F., and Miller, M. H. 1981. Psychotherapy and the foreign student. In P. B. Pedersen, J. G. Draguns, W. J. Lonner, and J. E. Trimble (eds.), *Counseling across cultures.* Honolulu: University of Hawaii Press.

Atkinson, D. R. 1985. A meta-review of research on cross-cultural counseling and psychotherapy. *Journal of Multicultural Counseling and Development* 13 (4): 138–153.

Basch-Kahre, E. 1984. On difficulties arising in transference and countertransference when analyst and analysand have different socio-cultural backgrounds. *International Review of Psychoanalysis* 11:61–67.

Bates, V. E. 1981. Traditional healing and Western health care: A case against formal integration. Paper presented at the American Psychological Association Convention, Los Angeles.

Bernstein, B. 1964. Social class, speech systems and psychotherapy. In F. Reisman, J. Cohen, and A. Pearl (eds.), *Mental health of the poor.* Glencoe: Free Press.

Beutler, L. E., Crago, M., and Arizmendi, T. G. 1986. Therapist variables in psychotherapy process and outcome. In S. L. Garfield and A. E. Bergin (eds.), *Handbook of psychotherapy and behavior change.* New York: John Wiley and Sons.

Bickley, V. 1978. Cross-cultural, cross-national education: The greatest resource. *Culture Learning Institute Report* 5:1–9.

Bishop, M., and Winokur, G. 1956. Cross-cultural psychotherapy. *Journal of Nervous and Mental Disease* 123:369–375.

Block, C. B. 1981. Black Americans and the cross-cultural counseling and psychotherapy experience. In A. J. Marsella and P. B. Pedersen (eds.), *Cross-cultural counseling and psychotherapy: Foundations, evaluation, and cultural considerations.* Elmsford, NY: Pergamon Press.

Bluestone, H., and Vela, R. M. 1982. Transcultural aspects in the psychotherapy of the poor in New York City. *Journal of the American Academy of Psychoanalysis* 10:268–285.

Bolman, W. M. 1968. Cross-cultural psychotherapy. *International Journal of Psychiatry* 124:1237–1244.

Bromberg, W. 1959. *The mind of man: A history of psychotherapy and psychoanalysis.* New York: Harper and Row.

Bustamente, J. A. 1957. Importance of cultural factors in psychotherapy. *American Journal of Psychotherapy* 11:803–812.

Calestro, K. M. 1972. Psychotherapy, faith healing and suggestion. *International Journal of Psychiatry* 10:83–113.

Carlson, R. J. 1979. The mother tongue in psychotherapy. *Canadian Journal of Psychiatry* 24:542–546.

Carstairs, G. 1961. Cross-cultural psychiatric interviewing. In B. Kaplan (ed.), *Studying personality cross-culturally.* Evanston, IL: Harper and Row.

Chang, S. C., and Kim, K. 1973. Psychiatry in South Korea. *American Journal of Psychiatry* 130:667–669.

Chunn, J. C., Dunston, P. J., and Ross-Sheriff, F. 1983. *Mental health and people of color: Curriculum development and change.* Washington, DC: Howard University Press.

Connor, L. 1982. The unbounded self: Balinese therapy in theory and practice. In A. J. Marsella and G. M. White (eds.), *Cultural conceptions of mental health and therapy.* Dordrecht, Holland: D. Reidel Publishing.

Dana, R. H. 1981. *Human services for cultural minorities.* Baltimore: University Park Press.

Desai, P. N. 1982. Learning psychotherapy: A cultural perspective. *Journal of Operational Psychiatry* 13 (2): 82–87.

Devereux, G. 1951. Three technical problems in psychotherapy of Plains Indian patients. *American Journal of Psychotherapy* 5:411–423.

———. 1953. Cultural factors in psychoanalytic psychotherapy. *Journal of the American Psychoanalytic Association* 1 (4): 629–655.

———. 1980. *Basic problems of ethnopsychiatry.* Chicago: University of Chicago Press.

DeVos, G. 1982. Adaptive strategies in U.S. minorities. In E. E. Jones and S. J. Korchin (eds.), *Minority mental health.* New York: Praeger.

Draguns, J. G. 1975. Resocialization into culture: The complexities of taking a worldwide view of psychotherapy. In R. W. Brislin, S. Bochner, and W. J. Lonner (eds.), *Cross-cultural perspectives on learning.* Beverly Hills: Sage Publications.

———. 1981. Cross-cultural counseling and psychotherapy: History, issues, current status. In A. J. Marsella and P. B. Pedersen (eds.), *Cross-cultural counseling and psychotherapy: Foundations, evaluation, and cultural considerations.* Elmsford, NY: Pergamon Press.

———. 1987. Personal communication.

Ehrenwald, J., ed. 1976. *The history of psychotherapy: From healing magic to encounter.* New York: Jason Aronson.

Frank, J. D. 1974. *Persuasion and healing.* New York: Schocken Books. Original ed. 1961. Baltimore: Johns Hopkins University Press. 1963. New York: Schocken Books.

———. 1971. Therapeutic factors in psychotherapy. *American Journal of Psychotherapy* 25:350–361.

———. 1975. An overview of psychotherapy. In A. Usdin (ed.), *Overview of the psychotherapies.* New York: Brunner-Mazel.

———. 1982. Therapeutic components shared by all psychotherapies. In J. H. Harvey and M. M. Parks (eds.), *The master lecture series.* Vol. 1,

Psychotherapy research and behavior change. Washington, DC: American Psychological Association.

Freud, S. [1904] 1953. On psychotherapy. Vol. 1, *Collected papers.* London: Hogarth Press.

Gorkin, M. 1986. Counter-transference in cross-cultural psychotherapy: The example of Jewish therapist and Arab patient. *Psychiatry* 49:69–79.

Greenson, R. 1967. *The technique and practice of psychoanalysis,* Vol. 1. New York: International Universities Press.

Halleck, S. L. 1971. *The politics of therapy.* New York: Harper and Row.

Hartcollis, P. 1983. Psychoanalysis abroad: A report from Greece. *The Psychoanalytic Quarterly* 52 (2): 250–253.

Higginbotham, H. N. 1977. Culture and the role of client expectancy in psychotherapy. In R. W. Brislin and M. P. Hamnett (eds.), *Topics in culture learning* 5:107–124. Honolulu: East-West Center Press.

Hsu, J., and Tseng, W. 1972. Intercultural psychotherapy. *Archives of General Psychiatry* 27:700–706.

Hull, W. F. 1978. *Foreign students in the United States: Coping behavior within the educational environment.* New York: Praeger.

Idowu, A. I. 1985. Counseling Nigerian students in United States colleges and universities. *Journal of Counseling and Development* 63:505–509.

Ierodiakonou, C. S. 1983. Psychotherapeutic possibilities in a rural community mental health center in Greece. *American Journal of Psychotherapy* 37:544–551.

Ishisaka, H. A., Nguyen, Q. T., and Okimoto, J. T. 1985. The role of culture in the mental health treatment of Indochinese refugees. In T. C. Owan (ed.), *Southeast Asian mental health: Treatment, prevention, services, training, and research.* Washington, DC: National Institute of Mental Health.

Jilek, W., and Jilek-Aall, L. 1978. The psychiatrist and his shaman colleague: Cross-cultural collaboration with traditional American therapists. *Journal of Operational Psychiatry* 9:32–39. Reprint. 1981. In R. H. Dana (ed.), *Human services for cultural minorities.* Baltimore: University Park Press.

Jilek-Aall, L. 1976. The Western psychiatrist and his non-Western clientele. *Canadian Psychiatric Association Journal* 21:353–360.

Johnson, F. A. 1981. Ethnicity and interaction rules in counseling and psychotherapy: Some basic considerations. In A. J. Marsella and P. B. Pedersen (eds.), *Cross-cultural counseling and psychotherapy: Foundations, evaluation, and cultural considerations.* Elmsford, NY: Pergamon Press.

Jones, E. E. 1985. Psychotherapy and counseling with black clients. In P. B. Pedersen (ed.), *Handbook of cross-cultural counseling and psychotherapy.* Westport, CT: Greenwood Press.

Jones, E. E., and Korchin, S. J. 1982. Minority mental health: Perspectives. In E. E. Jones and S. J. Korchin (eds.), *Minority mental health.* New York: Praeger.

———, eds. 1982. *Minority mental health.* New York: Praeger.

Jones, E. E., and Matsumoto, D. R. 1982. Psychotherapy with the underserved: Recent developments. In L. R. Snowden (ed.), *Reaching the underserved: Mental health needs of neglected populations.* Beverly Hills: Sage Publications.

Kakar, S. 1985. Psychoanalysis and non-Western cultures. *International Review of Psycho-Analysis* 12:441–448.

Karasu, T. B. 1977. Psychotherapies-overview. *American Journal of Psychiatry* 134:851–863.

Kennedy, J. 1973. Cultural psychiatry. In J. H. Honigman (ed.), *Handbook of social and cultural anthropology.* Chicago: Rand McNally.

Kiev, A. 1964. *Magic, faith and healing.* New York: Free Press.

Kim, K. I., and Rhi, B. Y. 1976. A review of Korean cultural psychiatry. *Transcultural Psychiatric Research Review* 13:101–114.

Kinzie, J. D. 1972. Cross-cultural psychotherapy: The Malaysian experience. *American Journal of Psychotherapy* 26:220–231.

———. 1978. Lessons from cross-cultural psychotherapy. *American Journal of Psychotherapy* 32:510–520.

———. 1985. Overview of clinical issues in the treatment of Southeast Asian refugees. In T. C. Owan (ed.), *Southeast Asian mental health: Treatment, prevention, services, training, and research.* Washington, DC: National Institute of Mental Health.

Kleinman, A. 1980. *Patients and healers in the context of culture.* Berkeley: University of California Press.

Kokantzis, N. A., and Ierodiakonou, C. S. 1975. Some considerations on the position of psychotherapy in today's Greek culture. *Psychotherapy and Psychosomatics* 25:225–258.

Lambert, M. J. 1981. Evaluating outcome variables in cross-cultural counseling and psychotherapy. In A. J. Marsella and P. B. Pedersen (eds.), *Cross-cultural counseling and psychotherapy: Foundations, evaluation, and cultural considerations.* Elmsford, NY: Pergamon Press.

Lambert, M. J., Shapiro, D. A., and Bergin, A. E. 1986. The effectiveness of psychotherapy. In S. L. Garfield and A. E. Bergin (eds.), *Handbook of psychotherapy and behavior change.* 3d ed. New York: John Wiley and Sons.

Lambo, T. A. 1974. Psychotherapy in Africa. *Psychotherapy and Psychosomatics* 24:311–326.

Langs, R. 1982. *Psychotherapy: A basic text.* New York: Jason Aaronson.

Leach, E. 1978. Culture and reality. *Psychological Medicine* 8:555–564.

Lebra, W. P., ed. 1976. *Mental health research in Asia and the Pacific.* Vol. 4, *Culture-bound syndromes, ethnopsychiatry and alternative therapies.* Honolulu: University Press of Hawaii.

Lefley, H. P. 1981. Psychotherapy and cultural adaptation in the Caribbean. *International Journal of Group Tensions* 11:346.

———. 1984. Delivering mental health services across cultures. In P. B. Pedersen, N. Sartorius, and A. J. Marsella (eds.), *Mental health services: The cross-cultural context.* Beverly Hills: Sage Publications.

Lerner, B. 1972. *Therapy in the ghetto: Political impotence and personal disintegration.* Baltimore: Johns Hopkins University Press.

Levine, E. S., and Padilla, A. M. 1980. *Crossing cultures in therapy: Pluralistic Counseling for the Hispanic.* Monterey, CA: Brooks-Cole.

Lippmann, W. 1965. *Public opinion.* New York: Free Press.

Lonner, W. J. 1980. The search for psychological universals. In H. C. Triandis and W. W. Lambert (eds.), *Handbook of cross-cultural psychology: Perspectives.* Vol. 1. Boston: Allyn and Bacon.

Lorion, R. P. 1978. Research on psychotherapy and behavior change with the disadvantaged: Past, present and future directions. In S. L. Garfield and A. E. Bergin (eds.), *Handbook of psychotherapy and behavior change: An empirical analysis,* 2d ed. New York: John Wiley and Sons.

Lorion, R. P., and Felner, R. D. 1986. Research on psychotherapy with the disadvantaged. In S. L. Garfield and A. E. Bergin (eds.), *Psychotherapy and behavior change,* 3d ed. New York: John Wiley and Sons.

McNeill, J. T. 1965. *A history of the cure of souls.* New York: Harper and Row.

Maduro, R. J. 1982. Working with Latinos and the use of dream analysis. *Journal of the American Academy of Psychoanalysis* 10:609–628.

Marcos, L. R. 1976a. Bilinguals in psychotherapy: Language as an emotional barrier. *American Journal of Psychotherapy* 30:552–560.

————. 1976b. Linguistic dimensions in the bilingual patient. *American Journal of Psychoanalysis* 36:347–354.

Marcos, L. R., and Alpert, M. 1976. Strategies and risks in psychotherapy with bilingual patients: The phenomenon of language independence. *American Journal of Psychiatry* 133:1275–1278.

Marcos, L. R., and Urcuyo, C. 1979. Dynamic psychotherapy with the bilingual patient. *American Journal of Psychotherapy* 33:331–338.

Marsella, A. J., and White, G. M., eds. 1982. *Cultural conceptions of mental health and therapy.* Dordrecht, Holland: D. Reidel Publishing.

Meadows, P. 1968. The cure of souls and the winds of change. *Psychoanalytic Review* 55:491–504.

Mendel, W. 1972. Comparative psychotherapy. *International Journal of Psychoanalytic Psychotherapy* 1 (4): 117–126.

Neki, J. S. 1975. Psychotherapy in India: Past, present and future. *American Journal of Psychotherapy* 29:92–100.

Ness, R. C., and Wintrob, R. M. 1981. Folk healing: A description and synthesis. *American Journal of Psychiatry* 138:1477–1481.

Olatawura, M. O. 1975. Psychotherapy for the Nigerian patient. *Psychotherapy and Psychosomatics* 25:259–266.

Oyewumi, L. K. 1986. Psychotherapy in Nigerian psychiatric practice: An overview. *Psychiatric Journal—University of Ottawa* 11:18–22

Ozturk, O. M. 1978. Psychotherapy under limited options: Psychotherapeutic work with Turkish youth. *American Journal of Psychotherapy* 32:307–319.

Pande, S. K. 1968. The mystique of "Western" psychotherapy: An Eastern interpretation. *Journal of Nervous and Mental Disease* 146:425–432.

Patterson, C. H. 1978. Cross-cultural or intercultural psychotherapy. *International Journal for the Advancement of Counseling* 1:231–248.

Pedersen, P. B. 1982. The intercultural context of counseling and psychotherapy. In A. J. Marsella and G. M. White (eds.), *Cultural conceptions of mental health and therapy.* Dordrecht, Holland: D. Reidel Publishing.

Penningroth, P. S., and Penningroth, B. A. 1977. Cross-cultural mental health practice on Guam. *Social Psychiatry* 12:43–48.

Pluk, P. W. M., and Wojciechowski, F. L. 1985. Culture and healing: A study of comparative and intercultural psychotherapy. In M. A. van Kalmthout, C. Schaap, and F. L. Wojciechowski (eds.), *Common factors in psychotherapy.* Toronto: Hogrefe.

Prince, R. H. 1976. Psychotherapy as the manipulation of endogenous healing mechanisms: A transcultural survey. *Transcultural Psychiatric Research Review* 13:115–134.

———. 1980. Variations in psychotherapeutic procedures. In H. C. Triandis and J. G. Draguns (eds.), *Handbook of cross-cultural psychology*. Vol. 6, *Psychopathology*. Boston: Allyn and Bacon.

Reynolds, D. K. 1980. *The quiet therapies*. Honolulu: University Press of Hawaii.

Rogers, C. R. 1957. The necessary and sufficient conditions of therapeutic personality change. *Journal of Consulting Psychology* 21:95–103.

Roland, A. 1982–83. The therapeutic relationship and resistance-analysis in Japan, India and America: A cross-cultural psychoanalytic perspective. *Hiroshima Forum for Psychology* 9:35–39.

Roll, S., Millen, L., and Martinez, R. 1980. Common errors in psychotherapy with Chicanos: Extrapolations from research and clinical experience. *Psychotherapy: Theory, Research and Practice* 17:158–168. Reprint 1981. In R. H. Dana (ed.), *Human services for cultural minorities*. Baltimore: University Park Press.

Rosenzweig, S. 1936. Some implicit common factors in diverse methods of psychotherapy. *American Journal of Orthopsychiatry* 6:412–415.

Salan, R., and Maretzki, T. 1983. Mental health services and traditional healers in Indonesia: Are the roles compatible? *Culture, Medicine and Psychiatry* 7 (4): 377–412.

Schumacher, H. E., and Guthrie, A. M. 1984. Culture and counseling in the Philippines. *International Journal of Intercultural Relations* 8:241–253.

Singer, K. 1976. Cross-cultural dynamics in psychotherapy. In J. Masserman (ed.), *Social psychiatry*. Vol. 2, *The range of normal in human behavior*. New York: Grune and Stratton.

Strunkard, A. 1961. Motivation for treatment: Antecedents of the therapeutic process in different cultural settings. *Comprehensive Psychiatry* 2:140–148.

Strupp, H. H. 1973a. Toward a reformulation of the psychotherapeutic influence. *International Journal of Psychiatry* 11:263–327.

———. 1973b. On the basic ingredients of psychotherapy. *Journal of Consulting and Clinical Psychology* 41:1–8.

———. 1982. The outcome problem in psychotherapy: Contemporary perspectives. In J. H. Harvey and M. M. Parks (eds.), *The master lecture series*. Vol. 1, *Psychotherapy research and behavior change*. Washington, DC: American Psychological Association.

Sullivan, H. S. 1954. *The psychiatric interview*. New York: Norton.

Thomas, A. 1962. Pseudo-transference reactions due to cultural stereotyping. *American Journal of Orthopsychiatry* 32:894–900.

Tobin, J. J. 1986. (Counter) transference and failure in intercultural therapy. *Ethos* 14:120–143.

Torrey, E. F. 1986. *Witchdoctors and psychiatrists: The common roots of psychotherapy and its future*. New York: Harper and Row.

Tseng, W. 1978. Traditional and modern psychiatric care in Taiwan. In A. Kleinman, P. Kunstadter, E. R. Alexander, and J. L. Gate (eds.), *Culture and healing in Asian societies*. Cambridge, MA: Schenkman.

Tseng, W., and McDermott, J. F. 1975. Psychotherapy: Historical roots, universal elements and cultural variations. *American Journal of Psychiatry* 132:378–384.

Tung, M. 1984. Life values, psychotherapy and East-West integration. *Psychiatry* 47:285–292.

Tung, T. M. 1985. Psychiatric care for Southeast Asians: How different is different? In T. C. Owan (ed.), *Southeast Asian mental health: Treatment, prevention, services, training, and research.* Washington, DC: National Institute of Mental Health.

Useem, J., and Useem, R. H. 1967. The interface of a binational third culture. *Journal of Social Issues* 23:130–143.

Useem, J., Useem, R. H., and Donaghue, J. 1963. Men in the middle of the third culture: The roles of American and non-Western people in cross-cultural administration. *Human Organization* 22:169–179.

Vassiliou, G., and Vassiliou, V. G. 1973. Subjective culture and psychotherapy. *American Journal of Psychotherapy* 27:42–51.

Wessels, W. H. 1985. The traditional healer and psychiatry. *Australian and New Zealand Journal of Psychiatry* 19 (3): 283–286.

White, G. M., and Marsella, A. J. 1982. Introduction: Cultural conceptions in mental health research and practice. In A. J. Marsella and G. M. White (eds.), *Cultural conceptions of mental health and therapy.* Dordrecht, Holland: D. Reidel Publishing.

Wintrob, R. M., and Harvey, Y. K. 1981. The self-awareness factor in intercultural psychotherapy: Some personal reflections. In P. B. Pedersen, J. G. Draguns, W. J. Lonner, and J. E. Trimble (eds.), *Counseling across cultures.* Rev. ed. Honolulu: University of Hawaii Press.

Wittkower, E. D., and Warnes, H. 1974. Cultural aspects of psychotherapy. *American Journal of Psychotherapy* 28:566–573.

Wohl, J. 1976. Intercultural psychotherapy: Issues, questions, and reflections. In P. B. Pedersen, W. J. Lonner, and J. G. Draguns (eds.), *Counseling across cultures.* Honolulu: University of Hawaii Press.

———. 1978. Counseling and guidance in Asia: Impressions of a developing profession. *International Journal for the Advancement of Counseling* 1:209–223.

———. 1983. White psychotherapists and black patients: Advice from the experts, 1950–1983. Paper presented at the Arkansas Psychological Association Meeting, Hot Springs, Arkansas.

Yamamoto, J., and Acosta, F. 1982. Treatment of Asian Americans and Hispanic Americans: Similarities and differences. *Journal of the American Academy of Psychoanalysis* 10:585–607.

5

Ethics in
Multicultural Counseling

TERESA D. LAFROMBOISE
SANDRA L. FOSTER

Over the past 20 years a number of articles on the role of cultural pluralism in psychology have appeared in response to the criticisms of the
profession as elitist and racist (Zwerlig 1976) or ethnocentric and culturally encapsulated (Wrenn 1962, 1985; Zuniga 1975). These articles
contend that if organized psychology carries out its stated mandates,
that is, uses and applies a specific body of knowledge, adheres to a code
of ethics, commits to service and community interest over financial
gain, and maintains autonomous, economic self-regulation (Campbell
1982), then the profession must continuously examine its regulation
systems in a number of areas. This chapter reviews the current status of
regulation systems employed by the profession in the areas of cross-cultural research, multicultural counseling, and graduate-level training.
The limitations of the American Psychological Association's Ethical
Principles for guiding decisions over multicultural dilemmas are deli-
neated. The need to consider a care perspective emerging in the context
of dialogue with the community in the ethical reasoning of multicultural
dilemmas is underscored.

Issues in Professional Self-Regulation

The specification of ethical principles for psychologists in practice is the
work of members of the American Psychological Association (APA).
The most recent enumeration of these rules of conduct and specialty
guidelines was published in 1981. These principles are organized into
10 categories: responsibility, competence, moral and legal standards,
public statements, confidentiality, welfare of the consumer, professional
relationships, assessment techniques, research with human subjects,
and guidelines for the use of animals in research.

These guidelines are the collective view of persons representing the
profession of psychology and the result of their efforts to define prescrip-

tives for proper professional conduct. Ethical principles must be broadly stated to include the moral behavior of psychologists in private practice; in public agencies; in academic settings, which offer training, scholarship, and research; and at industrial and other business sites. The enormity of the task to include a comprehensive set of guidelines is difficult to imagine.

It is important to note that the APA Principles (American Psychological Association 1981a, 1981b) reflect the prevailing individualistic orientation (based on majority culture values) to which most psychologists have been exposed during their training (Bellah et al. 1985). The perceptions of the majority culture fail to take into account the rich diversity of worldviews held by those who are members of non-white cultures, or who do not have the economic resources to be termed "middle class," or who are female, either white or of color.

A debate has been growing for several years concerning the limitations of the APA ethical guidelines. On the one hand are those in specialized areas of psychology, for example, consultants, who suggest that the guidelines lack specificity and clarity in stating how practitioners in their particular domain should behave. Apart from the call for greater specificity of the principles is the position of an increasing number of psychologists who say that the principles do not adequately reflect the diversity of race, culture, economic status, or even the gender differences encountered by all psychologists. The domain of ethical decision making, as it pertains to counseling persons whose lifestyle is different from the white majority culture, is relatively unexplored and in need of serious attention.

The major impetus for the examination of ethics as they pertain to race and culture in counseling is the 1973 Vail Conference resolution that states that it is unethical to serve clients from culturally defined backgrounds when a counselor is not competent to work with that cultural group. But this resolution further declares that it is "equally unethical to deny such persons professional services because the present staff is inadequately prepared" (Korman 1974, 305). The Vail resolution equates the importance of multicultural competence with proficiency in other specialized therapeutic skills areas. Therefore, it is the obligation of all counseling agencies and their training programs to provide consultation or education for counselors to meet the service delivery needs of the multicultural populations they serve. As a result, training and supervision in multicultural counseling should be given equal intensity along with that given to training in other counseling competencies.

Momentum to render psychological ethics more multiculturally appropriate has been building since the gains of the Civil Rights movement, affirmative action legislation, the population growth of minority groups, the burgeoning dependence by agencies on minority clients, and other social movements that insist on a new level of public morality (Casas, Ponterotto, and Gutierrez 1986). Pedersen and Marsella (1982) were the first to describe the ethical crisis in cross-cultural counseling practice. Their article attacked the continued exportation of mental health assumptions and interventions developed within the majority cultural context to clients from totally different cultures without empirical support for doing so.

A number of articles reiterate concern over this crisis and advocate that psychology render its training, research, and practice more ethically conscientious when issues of cultural diversity are present (Casas, Ponterotto, and Gutierrez 1986; Cayleff 1986; Ibrahim & Arredondo 1986; Pedersen & Marsella 1982; Tapp et al. 1974). This concern may embrace the thoughts, attitudes, and feelings of an increasing number of psychologists. Riegal (1977) criticizes the field of psychology for fostering a sterile view of human behavior, a view that fails to reflect its developmental and cultural-historical underpinnings. Levine (1982) reminds us that behavior associated with the white middle and upper middle classes is considered by most psychologists to be the standard for normal adult human behavior and the yardstick against which culturally different others are measured and then diagnosed. As a consequence, "women, ethnic/racial minority persons, poor persons, and old people who by definition fail the 'normal adult behavior test' are considered deviant" (Levine 1982, 139).

The aforementioned authors maintain that the relationship of psychologist to consumer (be it client, student intern, or business consultee) must necessarily reflect the social, cultural, and economic fabric of our society. The social stratification, inequities of opportunity, and other forms of prejudice that exist within U.S. society can unfortunately be replicated on a smaller scale between consumer and psychologist. These same authors insist that the APA Ethical Principles must reflect cultural diversity. At present, the principles do not do so. A better goal for rewriting the Ethical Principle might be the incorporation of a view that Triandis (1976) has termed "positive multiculturalism"—that differences are perceived as beneficial to society as a whole.

Casas (1986, 2) recently noted the "lack of professional interest and concern for minority groups" evident in the Ethical Principles. He found only three references to individual differences in the principles (Principles 1a, 2d, and 3b). Principle 1a appears under the heading *Responsibility* and prescribes guidelines for carrying out research. It reads as follows: "As scientists, psychologists accept responsibility for the selection of their research topics and the methods used in investigation, analysis, and reporting. They plan their research in ways to minimize the possibility that their findings will be misleading. They provide thorough discussion of the limitations of their data, especially where their work touches on social policy or might be construed to the detriment of persons in specific age, race, ethnic, socioeconomic, or other social groups. In publishing reports of their work, they never suppress disconfirming data, and they acknowledge the existence of alternative hypotheses and explanations of their findings. Psychologists take credit only for work they have actually done."

Principle 2d appears under the heading *Competence*. It reads as follows: "Psychologists recognize differences among people, such as those that be associated with age, sex, socioeconomic, and ethnic backgrounds. When necessary, they obtain training, experience, or counsel to assure competent service or research relating to such persons."

The third principle in which some reference is made to human diversity is 3b. This principle appears under the heading *Moral and Legal Obligations* and states: "As employees or employers, psychologists do not engage in or condone practices that are inhumane or that result in illegal or unjustifiable actions. Such practices include, but are not limited to, those based on considerations of race, handicap, age, gender, sexual preference, religion, or national origin in hiring, promotion, or training." In Pedersen's view (1986), the intent of Principle 3b has yet to be realized.

Kitchener (1984, 45) notes the shortcoming of decision making based upon ethical rules. ". . . ethical codes were developed historically to protect professions from outside regulation. . . . As a consequence, ethical codes are frequently more protective of the profession itself than of the consumer and omit many issues of ethical concern." The APA principles reflect the concerns of the writing committee, which, in turn, voices the opinions of the majority. The "issues of ethical concern" that are not included reflect the voices of the minority, namely those professionals who are not white and male. (There is only one ethnic minority member on the APA ethics committee now, and the committee is revising the APA principles.)

Casas (1986) points out a major problem inherent in the guidelines even as they currently appear: that of the profession of psychology assuming that its practitioners can automatically extrapolate from these principles to respond sensitively to ethnic minority groups. He notes the lack of specific guidelines describing how a practitioner might step beyond a personal worldview to behave in a manner that was beneficial for a client, employee, or trainee from another culture. Casas explains a second problem in applying the principles in their current form. This latter dilemma is the assumption that training curricula apply equally well to all served groups when, in reality, the premises of counseling interventions are based only on normative data from the white middle class.

Pedersen (1986) also addresses the issue of "cultural encapsulation" of the Ethical Principles. He observes that Principle 1a directs psychologists to assume responsibility for incorporating into their work the diversity of clients' cultural mores and values. Pedersen says that the intent of Principle 1a is to promote an *unbiased* perspective but cites evidence that institutional racism, sexism, and ageism exist and that scientific gatekeepers continue to deter publication of studies providing disconfirming data. These forms of discrimination are likely to persist in the face of ethical principles that are themselves culturally encapsulated. Principle 2d states that *when necessary* psychologists obtain training in a client's culture. Pedersen would argue that it is *always* necessary to seek training with culturally unique clients. In reviewing Principle 3b, Pedersen calls attention to abundant data documenting the disproportionately small numbers of minority members, women and other special groups as faculty in the field of psychology, as well as the limited services currently available to bilingual and bicultural students. Although there are remedies in civil law that attempt to ensure nondiscriminatory labor practices, Pedersen (1986) further states that the Ethical Principles fall short of suggesting how psychologists might incorporate cultural variables in their daily work.

To this end, Pedersen and Ivey suggest the following rewording of the Preamble for the Principles: "Psychologists respect the dignity and worth of the individual's fundamental human rights. To protect, preserve, and promote these fundamental rights requires the psychologist to recognize that each individual lives in a socio-cultural and historical context. The application of these fundamental human rights in practice, research, and writing requires the consideration of ethnographic, demographic, status, and affiliations of the socio-cultural and historical context. It is the responsibility of every psychologist to be informed about the presence of cultural factors in his or her own conduct and perspectives, and in the areas of psychological endeavor in which he or she represents himself or herself as qualified to function" (Pedersen and Ivey 1987, 37). They further assert that the implications of this responsibility need to be incorporated in all policy statements and related guidelines of the APA.

Pedersen and Ivey (1987) have recently recommended specific changes in each principle to the APA Ethics Committee that is currently charged with the responsibility for revising the Ethical Principles. Their proposed modifications, now under consideration by the APA Ethics Committee, incorporate the earlier report by Tapp and her working group (1974) and Ibrahim (1986). The revisions coming out of that committee are not expected to be decided upon until fall of 1989.

Other writers have made significant statements promoting inclusion of cross-cultural concerns in the profession's ethical code. Axelson's brief review (1985) of ethical guidelines of the APA, American Association for Counseling and Development (AACD formerly the American Personnel and Guidance Association [APGA]), and American School Counselor Association is the first to appear in a multicultural counseling compilation text. Goodyear and Sinnett's (1984) article on current and emerging ethical issues for counseling psychologists includes a position on cultural discrimination arising from computerized vocational assessment. Kitchener (1984) distinguishes between cultural relativism and tolerance and calls for increased cultural awareness, improvements in training, and development of unbiased services. The most recent APA general guidelines for providers of psychological services include a mandate for competent and available services that are sensitive to factors related to life in a pluralistic society (American Psychological Association 1987). Should the APA Ethics Committee reviewing the principles look carefully at the foregoing recommendations, the principles would better reflect cross-cultural factors in ethical decision making.

Ethical Issues in Research

A similar concern for ethics in cross-cultural research emerged during a time of widespread expansion in international research. Campbell (1969) challenged scientists in the United States and other nations conducting research to use experimental approaches to solve social problems. This touched off an intense debate within the profession over the relevance of social science research. The debate focused on the fact that even critical and disciplined research does not exist in a moral vacuum and that the process of studying a culture may, in fact, simultaneously change that culture. Critics of the social role of research further argued that social scientists are obliged to communicate what they know about social problems but are under no obligation to solve the problems they encounter (Miller 1969; Robinson 1982). Obviously, these disparate positions on the role of social science research yield correspondingly different ethical interpretations. The uniqueness of each research project and the increased complexity of collaboration among culturally different investigators and host communities present even further difficulties in judging ethical problems by any simplistic formula (Warwick 1980; Wax 1982).

The complexities of these issues were addressed by the APA Committee on International Relations in Psychology appointed to design a set of guidelines for the conduct of cross-cultural research and training in this methodology. The Tapp subgroup (Tapp et al. 1974) conducted a series of exchanges at international psychological meetings over a five-year period. This extensive dialogue produced a set of 16 guidelines for cross-cultural research collaboration that, according to Tapp, have been almost entirely ignored since by APA. To date the Tapp subgroup's guidelines remain the most thorough attempt to address multicultural ethics for psychological researchers. Moreover, cross-cultural researchers gained an awareness of the need to consider seriously how their research would enrich rather than harm the host country.

Warwick (1980) emphasizes the inseparability of political from ethical issues when working with a multicultural clientele. Ethical controversies are most intense over fieldwork that deals with ethnic or minority groups who are dominated or exploited by the majority (Munroe and Munroe 1986). Kelman (1972) suggests that there are legitimate ethical concerns regarding the self-determination of minority groups and that there is the need for greater equity in power relationships between the researcher and the minorities involved in the research. Zuniga (1975) most poignantly criticizes American psychological training as ethnocentric and negligent in preparing professionals for the demands of crosscultural work. By his account, ethnocentrism remains benign until the researcher is transferred to an unfamiliar cultural context. Then, "what was a localized deficiency becomes a universalistic ideology and an unconscious (or guilt-ridden) advocacy of a cultural intrusion that is often extremely naive. It often isolates the psychologists from other social scientists with disciplines in which competing centers of production make comparative and critical modes of thought necessary" (Zuniga 1975, 105).

Ethical Issues in Counseling

Many ethical issues in cross-cultural research are germane to issues in multicultural counseling. Conflicts arise in multicultural counseling that involve diametrically opposed moral views of proper behavior. For example, a counselor who asks politically sensitive questions of a client recently immigrated from a country with a repressive dictatorship (and who could possibly have been a torture victim) might be seen by some as causing harm to that client. The need to benefit clients must be extended to all and especially to vulnerable groups that Loo (1982, 108) defines as: "Persons who, relative to the majority society, have less power, opportunity, or freedom to determine outcomes in their lives or to make decisions that affect their situation because of their age, physical or mental condition, race, economic or political position, or captive status." Practitioners must work cautiously with populations who temporarily or continuously experience oppression, discomfort, harm, or danger.

Clients have a right to psychological treatment that benefits them and, therefore, protects them from harm or denial of services based on race, creed, color, natural origin, or sex (Cayleff 1986). Clients also have the right to competent services, respect for their integrity, and to be extended reasonable financial arrangements for payment (Hare-Mustin et al. 1979). In a study by the President's Commission on Mental Health (1978), the responsibilities of therapists to protect the rights of bicultural and bilingual minority clients were found to be inadequately executed. The Human Rights Committee of the Association for Counselor Education and Supervision (ACES) recently joined the ranks of professional organizations that have identified ethnic minorities among those groups that are typically underserved in the United States (Association for Counselor Education and Supervision 1982; Ibrahim et al. 1986). In the case of American Indians, for example, there is only one psychology service provider "broadly defined" for every 8,000 Indian people compared to a ratio of one service provider for every 2,000 people in the general population (LaFromboise 1988).

It is true that ethnic minorities significantly underutilize mental health services. Sue, Allen, and Conaway (1978) found that approximately half of the ethnic minority clients seeking help from 17 Seattle community mental health facilities failed to return after the first session, compared to 30% of the whites not continuing treatment. A number of reasons have been posited for the tendency of ethnic minorities to refuse or underutilize counseling services. Among them is the minority consumer's perception that counseling services are insensitive to their needs and unable to contribute to their health and welfare. They also fear that counselors will try to impose the values of the dominant culture upon them. Help seeking for them is a threat to their self-determination.

Goodyear and Sinnett (1984, 89) identified a number of areas involving client welfare where ethical issues arise: "(1) misunderstanding about who the client is; (2) lack of knowledge or skills necessary for working with special populations; (3) the intrusion of prejudicial (though perhaps well-intentioned) attitudes and values into the assessment and treatment of special populations; (4) failure to provide clients with information about the consequences of undergoing certain assessment and/or treatment procedures; (5) failure to assume an activist stance when necessary to protect client populations in the face of abuses of the authority wielded by others."

Each of these areas has been problematic in multicultural counseling. Services delivered to an ethnic minority person are often delivered under the contract of another professional (e.g., an attorney) or institution (e.g., a public health service provider). Counselors, of course, are supposed to consider the client to be their primary responsibility. The identified client is often vulnerable, however, because those who are remunerating the services are frequently in positions of influence over the counselor and service delivery agency itself.

Client rights are endangered when counselors lack the knowledge and skills necessary to work with a specific population. Counselors often fail to consider a client's unique frame of reference and psychosocial history before deciding whether or not to work with that particular client. A list of attitudinal, cognitive, and behavioral competencies for cross-cultural counseling have been identified by Division 17 (Counseling Psychology) of the APA (Sue et al. 1982). The concept of cross-cultural competence has been applied to the various stages of counselor training for identification of facilitative learning environments and approaches by writers Carney and Kahn (1984). Cross-cultural competence is now being assessed in the national licensing examination for psychologists. However, much work lies ahead in delineating specific professional qualifications for competence in multicultural counseling (Pedersen and Marsella 1982).

The most famous example of harm caused by misdiagnosis and biased attitudes in the treatment of a culturally unique client is the Larry P. v. Riles case in California (Lambert 1981). In this well-known decision a San Francisco federal district court judge ruled that the IQ testing of Larry P., a black student in the Oakland public schools, was unlawful. The testing and subsequent placement in a special education class for the mentally retarded deprived Larry P. of his right to unbiased assessment and stigmatized him, possibly for life. The court's decision forbade the use of IQ tests for diagnosis of the educably mentally retarded. One outcome of the Larry P. decision was an attempt to discover assessment instruments that were less culturally biased, such as the Adaptive Behavior Scale (ABS; American Association on Mental Deficiency 1974) and the System of Multicultural Pluralistic Assessment (SOMPA; Mercer 1979). This case also focused attention on the power of diagnostic criteria in general and the potential harm imposed upon an individual once labeled.

Client rights are not respected when counselors fail to provide the necessary information for a client to make informed choices about entering, continuing, or terminating therapy. Hare-Mustin et al. (1979) specify that clients, particularly those who are unfamiliar with the counseling process, should be told explicitly about the procedures and goals of counseling. From the outset counselors should call attention to their qualifications for working with members of the client's cultural group. Clients should not only be informed of the treatment plan but also be alerted to possible alternative intervention methods available (e.g., support groups, traditional healers, or self-help groups). The potential outcomes of treatment for the client, the client's family, and the client's community should also be explored. Outcomes should include consensus between counselor and familial/community judgment of client's status, improvement in the client's role competence, and self-enhancement rather than mere symptom reduction (Acosta et al. 1987).

Counselors are obliged to make clients aware of the various avenues open to them for expressing grievances that cannot be resolved within the counseling context. Many ethnic minority clients who have historically been denied power are unaccustomed to defending their rights. They become resigned to having their rights denied and their complaints go unheeded. It is clear from the recent report of the APA Ethics Committee that minority clients rarely use their right to redress of grievances. Of the 174 ethics complaints filed in 1982, only two cases concerned discrimination in therapy on the basis of age, race, or sex. In 1986, there were only three discrimination cases out of a total of 203 complaints (Ethics Committee of the American Psychological Association 1987). Most graduate training programs do not emphasize the rights of clients or the limits of therapists' power (Liss-Levinson et al. 1980). It is, however, the counselor's responsibility to inform all clients of the channels for redress of grievances, redress that extends beyond the termination of counseling.

Counselors are also obligated to be alert to possible abuses of authority directed toward clients. Culturally different clients are often vulnerable to human rights abuses despite numerous laws and regulations prohibiting discrimination against minority groups (Atkinson 1981). Most training programs focus primarily on the clients' own contributions to their problems, thereby minimizing the impact of external social forces that influence client behavior. APA's Ethical Principles (1981a) state that scientist and practitioner alike should be concerned with the "legal and quasi-legal regulations (that) at best serve the public interest." Seldom do we hear of grievances filed against majority psychologists even though institutional racism exists within governmental and organizational bodies (Pedersen and Marsella 1982). Mindful of such discrimination, Sobel and Russo (1981) specify nonclinical areas of advocacy and public policy advising for psychologists. Lopez and Cheek (1977) also suggest ways in which psychologists can work to help eliminate institutional racism. These efforts are directed at decreasing client dependency and enhancing client efficacy that will eventually lead to more satisfying and equitable helping relationships.

Ethical Issues in Training

Many of those advocating the careful monitoring of the American Psychological Association's (1986) Accreditation Criterion II, "cultural and individual differences," realize that ethical infractions will persist until cultural pluralism is both reflected in the composition of the faculty who provide training and programmatically infused into the content of the graduate-level curriculum.

Demographic parity requires a profession to be composed of socioculturally diverse members representing the composition of the society served by its members. Based on the 1980 census, ethnic minorities compose 20% of the U.S. population. The massive influx of immigrants from Asia, South and Central America, the Middle East, and the Caribbean cannot be ignored. By the year 2000, ethnic minorities are expected to form 26% of the U.S. population (U.S. Bureau of the Census 1980).

Representation of ethnic minorities in psychology has gradually declined following a peak in the 1970s (Boxley and Wagner 1971; Padilla 1977; Sue 1983). Doctoral graduates from ethnically diverse backgrounds have decreased from a disproportionately small 8% in 1981 to 5% in 1983 (Russo et al. 1981; Stapp, Tucker, and VanderBos 1985). Kagehiro, Mejia, and Garcia (1985) contend that the dearth of psychological theorists and researchers from socioculturally diverse backgrounds limits the range of assumptions and values considered during psychological theory building and hypothesis development. This restricted sampling of professional expertise has implications for all phases of development in counseling and research. Although nonminorities can and some do possess the prerequisite multicultural sensitivity and motivation to counsel ethnic minorities effectively, a number of benefits could be realized by increasing the number of ethnic minority psychologists. Service delivery approaches could become more relevant if they were influenced by individuals who themselves have experienced oppression. The societal forces of misrepresentation and stereotyping could thus be counterbalanced. However, more ethnic minority graduates need to be in teaching and administrative positions to increase the number of relevant role models (Smith 1982). Unfortunately, the strategies for increasing the numbers of ethnic minority graduate students, faculty, and practitioners continue to be seriously overlooked despite detailed and effective recommendations put forth by a number of advocates in this area (Atkinson 1981; Ridley 1985; Russo et al. 1981; Suinn and Witt 1982).

Surveys of the curriculum in APA-approved programs (Bernal and Padilla 1982; Parham and Moreland 1981; Wyatt and Parham 1985), school counseling programs (Ibrahim and Thompson 1982), and community counselor education programs (Conyne 1980; Stadler and Stahl 1979) amply document the reluctance of graduate programs to train students in cross-cultural factors. Many programs are still reluctant to offer even one seminar in which culturally sensitive training material is comprehensively covered. Moreover, seldom do instructors incorporate

multicultural examples in their curriculum materials, missing an opportunity to expand the training model beyond the premises of the majority
culture. Many programs do, however, attempt to satisfy Accreditation
Criterion II by providing practicum experiences with ethnically diverse
clients. Unfortunately, practicum students are seldom afforded the
opportunity to be supervised by ethnic minority supervisors.

Numerous writers have designed models and methods for including
multicultural information to improve the psychology curriculum. Recently, an approach whereby cultural and human rights issues are integrated into every course and clinical experience of graduate training has
been recommended over the separate course, area of concentration, or
interdisciplinary course models (Copeland 1982). Advocates of the curriculum integration model who have suggested extensive inclusion of
cross-cultural materials include Atkinson (1981); Chunn, Dunston, and
Ross-Sheriff (1983); Irving et al. (1984); LaFromboise and Foster
(1987); and Ridley (1985), among others. Casas (1984), in favor of the
curriculum integration model, believes that until integrated curricular
reform takes place, ethical violations will prevail in counseling and will
include cultural bias and cultural homogeneity disregard for within-
group differences and a tendency to overlook the effect of intrapersonal
styles and oppressive extrapersonal life circumstances. The gap between idealistic policy statements laden with multicultural platitudes
and the reality of training is wide.

The quality of ethics training in psychology, despite the APA accreditation mandates, is questionable. Welfel and Lipsitz (1984a, 37) report
that ethics education is defined by many programs as "familiarity with
the ethical codes." These programs indicate that they offer exposure to
ethical issues as these issues emerge in supervised training sessions
(Newmark and Hutchins 1981). In psychology departments, faculty
and mentors are considered the principal source of education regarding
research ethics, yet few of these faculty teach courses dealing specifically
with ethical dilemmas in research (Stanley, Sieber, and Melton 1987).

Abeles (1980) encourages departure from teaching professional codes
of ethics as a static body of knowledge by analyzing critical incidents
depicting ethical dilemmas in psychotherapy research and practice. He
encourages as highly influential discussions of conflicts in professional
values with personal and contemporary societal values and the values
implicit in the APA Ethical Principles. This process regards difference
as a starting point for reflection and action. Controversial topics include
conflicting cultural values inherent in concepts of morality and major
theories of personality (Abeles, personal communication, May 11,
1988). Pelsmas and Borgers (1986) suggest a model for encouraging students to arrive at their own ethical decisions, thereby risking disagree-

ment with stated ethical codes. Ehrlich (1987) argues for an interdisciplinary approach to ethics training. He suggests that professionals identify common ethical dilemmas facing those who serve clients in various ways (e.g., counselors, attorneys, doctors) and systematically study ethical dilemmas that are troublesome to professionals across service-oriented disciplines: confidentiality, conflicts of interest, and informal consent.

Studies investigating the impact of formal ethics training on trainees found that instruction in ethics had a positive influence on later professional conduct. However, the lack of rigorous design in these studies leads one to question the purported impact of such training (Welfel and Lipsitz 1984b). In their own investigation, Welfel and Lipsitz conclude that the ethical concerns of counselors are significantly correlated with their education in the fundamentals of moral reasoning, with their counseling experience, and with their involvement in professional and social action organizations. They criticize the design of studies on ethics education for overlooking the influence of training on actual counselor responses with clients.

A major barrier to multicultural ethics training is the paucity of text material on cultural manifestations of morality. Most ethics casebooks present ethical dilemmas from a culturally neutral perspective. A review of 10 frequently used ethics counseling casebooks yielded only five pages of attention to ethnic minority issues (Biggs and Blocher 1987; Corey, Corey, and Callanan, 1979; Keith-Spiegel and Koocher 1985; Rosenbaum 1982). Keith-Spiegel and Koocher (1985), in recommending their approach to ethical decision making, do suggest that decision-making strategies be broadened to include cross-cultural perspectives. The annual casebook presentations prepared by the APA Committee on Professional Standards and published in the *American Psychologist* have only included two cases on ethnic minority issues since 1981 (Committee on Professional Standards 1981, 1985, 1987).

A number of uncommon situations also need to be included in ethics training materials to help prepare trainees for ethical dilemmas often encountered when working in multicultural settings. For example, accepting goods for payment, attending a client's special event, accepting services in lieu of a fee, accepting client gifts, asking for favors from clients, and lending money to a client are behaviors that might be considered unethical in one context (Hall and Hare-Mustin 1983) yet culturally appropriate in another context. Specific examples illustrating these behaviors in various settings could help trainees develop a greater sensitivity to the details of the situation and an appreciation for divergent client belief systems (Pope, Tabachnick, and Keith-Speigel 1987). Critical incidents using culturally relative examples could then be compared to culture-general analyses of critical incidents (Brislin et al. 1986) to assess the impact of various ethics training approaches on multicultural competence (Barrow 1986).

Future Directions in Multicultural Ethics

The number of investigators studying the manner in which moral understanding is tacitly communicated culturally is increasing (Edwards 1987; Harding 1987; Hwang 1984; Nisan 1987; Shweder, Mahapatra, and Miller 1987). Freedom, rights, and justice are principled moral standards and guilt a major moral emotion in cultures that celebrate the unconnected individual. In cultures where the individual's loyalty and interdependence on the group is primary, respect for social role and status and, in communal cultures, anxiety over the disapproval of others is the primary moral emotion (Shweder, Mahapatra, and Miller 1987).

Hillerbrand (1987), in noting that psychologists are not trained as moral philosophers, suggests that psychologists refrain from trying to resolve ethical dilemmas by reasoning through principles alone. He proposes a popular feminist approach that urges the field of psychology to take a stance of relation to the community and seek resolution of ethical dilemmas in the context of dialogue with the community. He asserts that "psychology's understanding of its social role emerges from a dramatic balancing of facts and values" (1987, 117). Ivey (1987) also suggests that it is time for a more relational view of ethics where we move from a discourse of power of the majority to a new form of dialectical inquiry. He suggests that serious dialectics with those individuals embedded in the community (but often not in power) must occur as the APA Ethical Principles are revised (Hofstede 1980; Horowitz 1982; Kagan and Lamb 1987; Spence 1985). According to Ivey (1987), opportunities for consideration of co-constructed ethics that overcome inequality and detachment can be more readily accommodated.

Gilligan (1982) made an important contribution to the literature with her delineation of "the female view" of the theory of good as distinct from "the male view" of the supremacy of the theory of rights. In a similar vein Noddings (1984, 1986) describes the ethic of caring as feminine and maintains that women are less involved in the ordering of their priorities in accordance with rights. Instead, women concern themselves with the maintenance of relationships, rather than adherence to abstractions in the form of ethical rules.

We, the authors of this chapter, speculate that the ethic of caring and responsibility (Gilligan 1982, 1987; Noddings 1984, 1986) is a promising dialectic that could be considered in resolving ethical dilemmas across cultures. The justice perspective substantiated by John Lock, Immanual Kant, John Rawls, to a certain extent John Stuart Mill, and Lawrence Kohlberg is committed to personal liberty, the ideal of autonomy, and use of a social contract model wherein a group of people consent to a set of mutually acceptable principles to justify a social role. In place of the hierarchical ordering of values characteristic of the justice perspective (Kitchener 1984), a care perspective espoused by philosophers Hume, Aristotle, McIntyre, Williams, and Gilligan emphasizes the importance of virtue rather than justice in moral life. This perspective views detachment as the moral problem. Moral problems are embedded in a contextual frame that eludes abstract, deductive reasoning and are reliant upon a web of relationships that is sustained by the process of communicating perceptions and interpreting events (Kittay and Meyers 1987).

In complex multicultural ethical dilemmas, moral systems are subject to constraints of culture, history, and economy. Harding (1987) cites a number of parallels between feminism and African worldviews and associates the ethic of caring with the altruism of African culture and the shared experience with women of oppression. She suggests that a justice perspective may be an ideology open only to the dominant class.

We encourage consideration of both a care perspective and a justice perspective in multicultural ethical decision making. Gilligan's (1987) recent work suggests that people can view moral problems in more than one way; they can even alternate perspectives with different permutations of justice and care reasoning without blending or reducing them. A reasoned process of ethical relativism that takes into account both the autonomous and relational aspects of the situation and considers factors such as worldview, intergroup differences, political ramifications, and the impact of an individual's actions on the group before advancing analysis of personal liberty or rights is recommended. This process is arduous for the counselor—no simplistic technique or rigid application of principles will suffice.

The following case example is provided to illustrate the different focus and strategies that emerge from the care perspective and the justice perspective. An American Indian client was referred to a counselor by the personnel office of an engineering firm. The referral said that the client, Ms. Daisy Yellow Horse, was having serious problems with her supervisor. The client was a somewhat reticent young woman who had recently completed her engineering degree. She reported that she was routinely subjected to sexual innuendos and ostracism from her male colleagues. She begged the counselor to help her qualify for medical leave with pay so that she could look for another job. She wanted the counselor to concur with her statements that she was emotionally impaired by the harassment and isolation she experienced on the job due to sexism and possibly racism. The counselor thought that the client's story was true but felt that the client needed treatment for problems not directly related to the sexual harassment.

A counselor operating from a care perspective might urge the client to examine her relationships with her coworkers and interactions among a number of people. An understanding of the corporate culture might be encouraged, so that the client might examine any possibility that her behavior is an antecedent to her coworkers' responses. The counselor might encourage the client to seek a support group to better represent herself in a larger social context, particularly in the workplace. The issue of addressing the sexual harassment itself might be discussed from an interpersonal perspective: that responding to it might first take the form of discussions with the offending coworker(s), then his (their) supervisor(s). Then, in the absence of satisfactory results, the client could discuss the matter with the personnel department. A last resort might be seeking outside legal counsel and the filing of a grievance or civil suit.

If the counselor were operating from a Kohlbergian rights perspective (Kohlberg 1981), she or he might well urge the client to file a grievance citing sexual harassment as having a deleterious effect on her working conditions. The counselor might encourage the client to seek training in assertiveness and management of social anxiety so that she might better stand up for herself and her rights.

A competent multicultural counselor would hopefully consider both perspectives before suggesting intervention. The counselor would recognize that sexual harassment constitutes a violation of the client's rights but that more subtle forms of racism as well as sexism might well be occurring in this client's case. The counselor would take into consideration the client's cultural upbringing that discouraged assertive behavior. Perceiving the client's distress as social anxiety and proposing assertive training without considering the client's worldview and cultural reinforcements would be a disservice to the client. In her view, she may not be atypically quiet or reticent.

The counselor would discuss fully the impact on the client of attempting to talk with the offending coworkers. Could she, the counselor would want to know, cope with the outcome of pursuing this strategy? The counselor would also be concerned about the even greater impact on the client of addressing her coworkers' supervisors on the matter or taking her concerns to the personnel department. Although the counselor would want the client to know that she had ways to redress the violation of her rights through a grievance or suit, the counselor would understand how difficult these options might be for the client, not only for herself but for her family and community. The counselor would reassure her that a medical leave might be a very appealing and understandable response to the problem, a face-saving means of stopping what is happening. Nevertheless, the counselor would want the client to think through the impact of this decision because it reinforces the client's avoidance of the situation and role as a victim.

To practice and thus internalize moral reasoning skills, exposure to a professional in the field is helpful. This experience could be gained during an internship. Struggling with difficult questions in a real-life setting would help trainees refine their ethical decision-making skills. In sum, comprehensive training for multicultural counselors requires the development of culturally sensitive moral reasoning, modeling of culturally sensitive ethical decision making in their workplace by practitioners, thorough academic instruction, and involvement in community and professional organizations. Once the insights of vulnerable populations are ascertained through a caring perspective and once justice comes to be understood as respect for people in their own terms, the ethical decision making of multicultural counselors will be much improved.

References

Abeles, N. 1980. Teaching ethical principles by means of value confrontation. *Psychotherapy: Theory, Research, and Practice* 17:384–391.

Acosta, F., Baron, A., Bestman, E., LaFromboise, T., Liu, W., Marsella, A., Padilla, A., and Takeuchi, D. 1987. Outcome of mental health services delivery. In F. Cheung (ed.), *Minority mental health services research conference proceedings,* 48–54. Rockville, MD: National Institute of Mental Health.

American Association on Mental Deficiency. 1974. *Adaptive behavior scale: Manual.* Washington, DC: the Association.

American Psychological Association. 1981a. Ethical principles of psychologists. Rev. ed. *American Psychologist* 36:633–638.

―――. 1981b. Specialty guidelines for the delivery of services by counseling psychologists. *American Psychologist* 36:652–663.

―――. 1986. *Accreditation handbook.* Washington, DC: Committee on Accreditation and Accreditation Office.

―――. 1987. General guidelines for providers of psychological services. *American Psychologist* 42:712–723.

Association for Counselor Education and Supervision. 1982. *Human rights training manual.* Alexandria, VA: AACD Press.

Atkinson, D. R. 1981. Selection and training for human rights training. *Counselor Education and Supervision* 21:101–108.

Axelson, J. A. 1985. *Counseling and development in a multicultural society.* Monterey, CA: Brooks-Cole.

Barrow, R. 1986. Socrates was a human being: A plea for transcultural moral education. *Journal of Moral Education* 15:50–57.

Bellah, R. N., Madsen, R., Sullivan, W. M., Swidler, A., and Tipton, S. M. 1985. *Habits of the heart.* Berkeley: University of California Press.

Bernal, M. E., and Padilla, A. M. 1982. Status of minority curricula and training in clinical psychology. *American Psychologist* 37:780–787.

Biggs, D., and Blocher, D. 1987. *Foundations of ethical counseling.* New York: Springer Publishing.

Boxley, R., and Wagner, N. N. 1971. Clinical psychology training programs and minority groups: A survey. *Professional Psychology* 2:75–81.

Brislin, R. W., Cushner, K., Cherrie, C., and Yong, M. 1986. *Intercultural interactions.* Beverly Hills, CA: Sage.

Campbell, D. M. 1982. *Doctors, lawyers, ministers: Christian ethics in professional practice.* Nashville: Abingdon Press.

Campbell, D. T. 1969. Reforms as experiments. *American Psychologist* 24:409–429.

Carney, C. G., and Kahn, K. B. 1984. Building competencies for effective cross-cultural counseling: A developmental view. *Counseling Psychologist* 12:111–119.

Casas, J. M. 1984. Policy, training, and research in counseling psychology: The racial/ethnic minority perspective. In S. D. Brown and R. W. Lent (eds.), *Handbook of counseling psychology,* 785–831. New York: John Wiley and Sons.

———. 1986. Falling short of meeting the counseling needs of racial/ethnic minorities and the status of ethical accreditation guidelines. Paper presented at the annual meeting of the American Psychological Association, Washington, DC.

Casas, J. M., Ponterotto, J. G., and Gutierrez, J. M. 1986. An ethical indictment of counseling research and training: The cross-cultural perspective. *Journal of Counseling and Development* 64:347–349.

Cayleff, S. E. 1986. Ethical issues in counseling gender, race, and culturally distinct groups. *Journal of Counseling and Development* 64:345–347.

Chunn, J., Dunston, P., and Ross-Sheriff, F., eds. 1983. *Mental health and people of color: Curriculum development and change.* Washington, DC: Howard University Press.

Committee on Professional Standards. 1981. Casebook for providers of psychological services. *American Psychologist* 36:682–685.

———. 1985. Casebook for providers of psychological services. *American Psychologist* 40:678–680.

———. 1987. Casebook for providers of psychological services. *American Psychologist* 42:704–706.

Conyne, R. K. 1980. The "community" in community counseling: Results of a national survey. *Counselor Education and Supervision* 20:22–28.

Copeland, E. J. 1982. Minority populations and traditional counseling programs: Some alternatives. *Counselor Education and Supervision* 21:187–193.

Corey, G., Corey, M. S., and Callanan, P. 1979. *Professional and ethical issues in counseling and psychotherapy.* Monterey, CA: Brooks-Cole.

Edwards, C. P. 1987. Culture and the construction of moral values: A comparative ethnography of moral encounters in two cultural settings. In J. Kagan and S. Lamb (eds.), *The emergence of morality in young children,* 123–151. Chicago: University of Chicago Press.

Ehrlich, T. 1987. Common issues of professional responsibility. *Georgetown Journal of Legal Ethics* 1:3–14.

Ethics Committee of the American Psychological Association. 1987. Report of the ethics committee: 1986. *American Psychologist* 42:730–734.

Gilligan, C. 1982. *In a different voice.* Cambridge: Harvard University Press.

———. 1987. Moral orientation and moral development. In E. F. Kittay and D. T. Meyers (eds.), *Women and moral theory,* 19–33. Totowa, NJ: Rowman and Littlefield.

Goodyear, R. K., and Sinnett, E. R. 1984. Current and emerging ethical issues for counseling psychology. *Counseling Psychologist* 12:87–98.

Hall, J. E., and Hare-Mustin, R. T. 1983. Sanctions and the diversity of ethical complaints against psychologists. *American Psychologist* 38:714–729.

Harding, S. 1987. The curious coincidence of feminine and African moralities: Challenges for feminist theory. In E. F. Kittay and D. T. Meyers (eds.), *Women and moral theory,* 296–315. Totowa, NJ: Rowman and Littlefield.

Hare-Mustin, R. T., Maracek, J., Kaplan, A. G., and Liss-Levinson, N. 1979. Rights of clients, responsibilities of therapists. *American Psychologist* 34:3–16.

Hillerbrand, E. 1987. Philosophical tensions influencing psychology and social action. *American Psychologist* 42:111–118.

Hofstede, G. 1980. *Culture's consequence: International differences in work-related values.* Beverly Hills, CA: Sage.

Horowitz, A. V. 1982. *The social control of mental illness.* New York: Academic Press.

Hwang, K. 1984. A psychological perspective of Chinese interpersonal morality. Unpublished manuscript. National Taiwan University, Taipei, Taiwan.

Ibrahim, F. A. 1986. Reflections on the cultural encapsulation of the APA ethical principles: Recommendations for revisions. Paper presented at the annual meeting of the American Psychological Association, Washington, DC.

Ibrahim, F. A., and Arredondo, P. M. 1986. Ethical standards for cross-cultural counseling: Counselor preparation, practice, assessment, and research. *Journal of Counseling and Development* 64:349–352.

Ibrahim, F. A., Stadler, H. A., Arrendondo, P. M., and McFadden, J. 1986. *Status of human rights issues in counselor preparation: A national survey.* Paper presented at the annual meeting of the American Association of Counseling and Development, Los Angeles.

Ibrahim, F. A., and Thompson, D. L. 1982. Preparation of secondary school counselors: A national survey. *Counselor Education and Supervision* 22:113–120.

Irving, J., Perl, H., Trickett, E. J., and Watts, R. 1984. Minority curricula or a curriculum of cultural diversity? Differences that make a difference. *American Psychologist* 39:320–321.

Ivey, A. E. 1987. The multicultural practice of therapy: Ethics, empathy, and dialectics. *Journal of Social and Clinical Psychology* 5:195–204.

Kagan, J., and Lamb, S., eds. 1987. *The emergence of morality in young children.* Chicago: University of Chicago Press.

Kagehiro, D. K., Mejia, J. A., and Garcia, J. E. 1985. Value of cultural pluralism to the generalizability of psychological theories: A reexamination. *Professional Psychology* 16:481–494.

Keith-Spiegel, P., and Koocher, G. P. 1985. *Ethics in psychology.* New York: Random House.

Kelman, H. C. 1972. The rights of the subject in social research: An analysis in terms of relative power and legitimacy. *American Psychologist* 27:989–1016.

Kitchener, K. S. 1984. Intuition, critical evaluation and ethical principles in counseling psychology. *Counseling Psychologist* 12:43–55.

Kittay, E. F., and Meyers, D. T., eds. 1987. *Women and moral theory.* Totowa, NJ: Rowman and Littlefield.

Kohlberg, L. 1981. *The philosophy of moral development.* San Francisco: Harper and Row.

Korman, M. 1974. National conference on levels and patterns of professional training in psychology: Major themes. *American Psychologist* 29:301–313.

LaFromboise, T. D. 1988. American Indian mental health policy. *American Psychologist* 43:388–397.

LaFromboise, T. D., and Foster, S. L. 1987. *Cross-cultural training: Model and methods.* Paper presented at the Division 17 National Conference for Counseling Psychology: Planning the Future, Atlanta.

Lambert, N. M. 1981. Psychological evidence in *Larry P. v. Wilson Riles. American Psychologist* 36:937–952.

Levine, E. K. 1982. Old people are not all alike: Social class, ethnicity/race, and sex are bases for important differences. In J. E. Sieber (ed.), *The ethics of social research: Surveys and experiments,* 127–143. New York: Spring-Verlag New York.

Liss-Levinson, N., Hare-Mustin, R. T., Marecek, J., and Kaplan, A. G. 1980. The therapist's role in assuring client rights. *Advocacy Now* 2:16–20.

Loo, C. M. 1982. Vulnerable populations: Case studies in crowding research. In J. E. Sieber (ed.), *The ethics of social research: Surveys and experiments,* 105–126. New York: Spring-Verlag New York.

Lopez, R. F., and Cheek, D. 1977. The prevention of institutional racism: Training, counseling psychologists as agents of change. *Counseling Psychologist* 1:64–69.

Mercer, J. R. 1979. *Technical manual, System of Multicultural Pluralistic Assessment.* New York: Psychological Corporation.

Miller, G. 1969. Psychology as a means of promoting human welfare. *American Psychologist* 12:1063–1075

Munroe, R. L., and Munroe, R. H. 1986. Field work in cross-cultural psychology. In W. J. Lonner and J. W. Berry (eds.), *Field methods in cross-cultural research,* 111–136. Beverly Hills, CA: Sage.

Newmark, C. S., and Hutchins, T. C. 1981. Survey of professional education in ethics in clinical psychology internship programs. *Journal of Clinical Psychology* 37:681–683.

Nisan, M. 1987. Moral norms and social conventions: A cross-cultural comparison. *Developmental Psychology* 23:719–725.

Noddings, N. 1984. *Caring: A feminine approach to ethics and moral education.* Berkeley: University of California Press.

————. 1986. Fidelity in teaching, teacher education, and research for teaching. *Harvard Educational Review* 56:496–510.

Padilla, E. R. 1977. Hispanics in clinical psychology: 1970–1976. In E. L. Olmedo and S. Lopez (eds.), *Hispanic mental health professionals* (Monograph No. 5). Los Angeles: Spanish Speaking Mental Health Research Center, University of California.

Parham, W., and Moreland, J. R. 1981. Non-White students in counseling psychology: A closer look. *Professional Psychology* 12:499–507.

Pedersen, P. 1986. Are the APA ethical principles culturally encapsulated? Paper prepared for the Committee on International Relations in Psychology Roundtable at the annual meeting of the American Psychological Association, Washington, DC.

Pedersen, P., and Ivey, A. 1987. Draft recommendations for changes in the APA Ethical Principles. *Internationally Speaking* 12:37–38.

Pedersen, P. B., and Marsella, A. J. 1982. The ethical crisis for cross-cultural counseling and therapy. *Professional Psychology* 13:492–500.

Pelsmas, D. M., and Borgers, S. B. 1986. Experienced-based ethics: A developmental model of learning ethical reasoning. *Journal of Counseling and Development* 64:311–314.

Pope, K. S., Tabachnick, B. G., and Keith-Spiegel, P. 1987. Ethics of practice: The beliefs and behaviors of psychologists as therapists. *American Psychologist* 42:993–1006.

President's Commission on Mental Health. 1978. *Task panel report to the President* (Vols. 1–4). Washington, DC: Government Printing Office.

Ridley, C. R. 1985. Imperatives for ethnic and cultural relevance in psychology training programs. *Professional Psychology* 16:611–622.

Riegel, K. F. 1977. History of gerentological psychology. In J. E. Birren & K. W. Schaie (eds.), *Handbook of the psychology of aging*, 70–102. New York: Van Nostrand Reinhold.

Robinson, D. N. 1982. Ethics and advocacy. *American Psychologist* 39:787–793.

Rosenbaum, M. 1982. *Ethics and values in psychotherapy.* New York: Free Press.

Russo, N. F., Olmedo, E. L., Stapp, J., and Fulcher, R. 1981. Women and minorities in psychology. *American Psychologist* 36:1315–1363.

Shweder, R. A., Mahapatra, M., and Miller, J. G. 1987. Culture and moral development. In J. Kagan and S. Lamb (eds.), *The emergence of morality in young children*, 1–83. Chicago: University of Chicago Press.

Smith, E. J. 1982. Counseling psychology in the marketplace: The status of ethnic minorities. *Counseling Psychologist* 10:61–68.

Sobel, S. B., and Russo, N. F. 1981. Equality, public policy, and professional psychology. *Professional Psychology* 12:180–189.

Spence, J. T. 1985. Achievement American style. *American Psychologist* 12:1285–1295.

Stadler, H. A., and Stahl, E. 1979. Trends in community counselor training. *Counselor Education and Supervision* 19:42–48.

Stanley, B., Sieber, J., and Melton, G. B. 1987. Empirical studies of ethical issues in research: A research agenda. *American Psychologist* 42:735–741.

Stapp, J., Tucker, A. M., and VanderBos, G. R. 1985. Census of psychological personnel: 1983. *American Psychologist* 40:1317–1351.

Sue, D. W., Bernier, J. E., Durran, A., Feinberg, L., Pedersen, P., Smith,

E. J., and Vasquez-Nuttall, E. 1982. Position paper: Cross-cultural counseling competencies. *Counseling Psychologist* 10 (2): 45–52.

Sue, S. 1983. Ethnic minority issues in psychology: A reexamination. *American Psychologist* 38:583–592.

Sue, S., Allen, D. B., and Conaway, L. 1978. The responsiveness and equality of mental health care to Chicanos and Native Americans. *American Journal of Community Psychology* 6:137–146.

Suinn, R. M., and Witt, J. C. 1982. Survey on ethnic minority faculty recruitment and retention. *American Psychologist* 37:1239–1244.

Tapp, J. L., Kelman, H. C., Triandis, H. C., Wrightsman, L. S., and Coelho, G. V. 1974. Continuing concerns in cross-cultural ethics: A report. *International Journal of Psychology* 9:231–249.

Triandis, H. C. 1976. The future of pluralism. *Journal of Social Issues* 32:179–208.

U.S. Bureau of the Census. 1980. *Characteristics of the population.* Washington, DC: Government Printing Office.

Warwick, D. P. 1980. The politics and ethics of cross-cultural research. In H. C. Triandis and W. W. Lambert (eds.), *Handbook of cross-cultural psychology.* Vol. 1, *Perspectives,* 319–371. Boston: Allyn and Bacon.

Wax, M. L. 1982. Research reciprocity rather than informed consent in fieldwork. In J. E. Sieber (ed.), *The ethics of social research: Surveys and experiments,* 33–48. New York: Spring-Verlag New York.

Welfel, E. R., and Lipsitz, N. E. 1984a. The ethical behavior of professional psychologists: A critical analysis of the research. *Counseling Psychologist,* 12:31–42.

———. 1984b. Ethical orientation of counselors: Its relationship to moral reasoning and level of training. *Counselor Education and Supervision* 23:35–45.

Wrenn, C. G. 1962. The culturally encapsulated counselor. *Harvard Educational Review* 32:444–449.

———. 1985. Afterword: The culturally encapsulated counselor revisited. In P. Pedersen (ed.), *Handbook of cross-cultural counseling and therapy,* 323–329. Westport, CT: Greenwood Press.

Wyatt, G., and Parham, W. 1985. The inclusion of culturally sensitive course materials in graduate school and training programs. *Psychotherapy* 22:461–468.

Zuniga, R. B. 1975. The experimenting society and radical social reform: The role of the social scientist in Chile's Unidad Popular experience. *American Psychologist* 30:99–115.

Zwerlig, I., ed. 1976. *Racism, elitism, professionalism: Barriers to community mental health.* New York: Jason Aronson.

PART THREE

Ethnic and Cultural Considerations

There is no single right answer or method for multicultural counseling, although all of us might wish such a simple solution existed. There are alternative models and approaches that can be modified and adapted to each complex and dynamic combination of culturally different clients in counseling. This section is a discussion of several such alternative models.

Harry H. L. Kitano describes a model that combines elements of traditional Japanese culture with elements of traditional American culture in a unique combination suitable for the Japanese-American client. Other Asian-American clients will find some of the combinations Kitano discusses familiar as well. Kitano presents a uniquely suitable approach for multicultural counseling in which the Japanese-American cultural background of the client becomes an illustrative case.

J. Manual Casas and Melba J. T. Vasquez describe the importance of a bilingual and bicultural approach for working with Hispanic clients. The importance of bilingualism and biculturalism extends beyond the boundaries of any single group. The reader will be able to apply principles of this case example on Hispanics to a wide variety of populations.

Joseph E. Trimble and Candace M. Fleming describe a model for working with American Indians that summarizes a great variety of other alternative approaches. Trimble and Fleming's approach combines the complexity of a highly diversified American Indian culture with the dynamics of constant change in response to social, economic, and political forces. This chapter will help the reader be more informed on the whole range of counseling-related issues of American Indian society.

Kay Thomas and Gary Althen provide practical guidelines for counseling foreign students in a theoretical context. The diversity of international students makes generalized counseling guidelines difficult. This chapter provides important starting points to enable persons working with international students to begin asking the right questions.

6

A Model for Counseling Asian Americans

HARRY H. L. KITANO

There have been changes in the Asian-American community since the appearance of the revised edition of *Counseling across Cultures* (1981), just as there have been changes in the field of counseling dealing with Asian Americans. For example, recent publications on Southeast Asians (Owan 1985) and on problems in service delivery to minority populations (Miranda and Kitano 1986) show an increasing awareness of some of the problems related to differences in culture. Part of the sensitivity is no doubt related to the influx of new immigrants, especially from Asia, and the awareness that models based on the experiences of European immigrants of acculturation, assimilation, and integration may not be as relevant as other models that emphasize a bicultural or pluralistic perspective.

But Asian Americans remain an "invisible group" since many still do not use counseling services. There also remains an assimilationist bias in American society as the following case illustrates. In a conference on Chinese health problems in America reported in *East-West News* (1986), there was discussion of a case of a middle-aged Chinese female immigrant who had sought psychiatric treatment for depression. She was reported to have recovered through her becoming more assertive with her husband and getting more in tune with the Western model of wife and mother. From a cross-cultural perspective we might ask, Was this a successful resolution? What happened to the family? Does the solution take into account cultural differences? And, where does the counselor stand in relation to the outcome?

Increased cultural sensitivity, however, can also lead a counselor to err on the side of an unrestrained cultural determinism. For example, we have heard of cases in which wife beating has been dismissed as being an integral part of a culture or of counselors tolerating bizarre behavior that would have been inappropriate in almost any setting. The question for the counselor is whether he or she feels more comfortable in reinforcing an assimilationist or an ethnic perspective. How does the counselor feel about dealing with people who do not wish to participate in the American mainstream? The purpose of this paper is to present a model of counseling that takes into account the variations among Asian Americans.

Review of the Literature

Current generalizations concerning counseling and Asian Americans are consistent with past studies. Leong, Sasao, and Uomoto (1983) note the lack of research, training, funding, and service delivery concerning Asian Americans. More indirect services and the use of broader models of health and psychology are needed.

Tong (1983) also mentions the need for further research, especially in relation to the diagnostic and treatment models of Asian Americans. An expanded role for the "insider," defined as those of Asian-American background, experience, and activity in ethnic community life, will be important.

Kim (1983), in discussing Asian-American children in the public schools sees their lack of use of counseling services. Factors inhibiting use include shyness and hesitancy on the part of the children, stereotypes of Asians held by teachers, and the referral policies of the schools. Other factors include the general invisibility of Asian-American children and the limited availability of bilingual, bicultural counselors.

Atkinson (1983) notes the lack of representation of Asians, as well as blacks and Hispanics, in the student and faculty ranks in counselor education. Minorities are less likely to be students in full-time and doctoral degree programs, and at the faculty level they are more likely to hold more nonacademic, nontenured, and part-time appointments than their nonminority peers.

A study by Yamamoto, Machizawa, and Steinberg (1986) assessed the effects of wartime internment on Japanese Americans. The authors concluded that the experiences of prejudice and fear that occurred over 40 years ago were related to current physical complaints and quality of life.

Chen and Yang (1986) measured the self-image of Chinese-American adolescents. They concluded that attitudes toward dating and sex became more similar to American norms with acculturation. Although Confucian values of loyalty, conformity, and respect for elders still remained, Chinese-American adolescents in the United States were virtually identical to a white sample, but very different from a Chinese sample, in their attitudes and perceptions of themselves.

Uomoto and Gorsuch (1984) in a study of mental health referrals among Japanese Americans found that the use of mental health resources would occur only when extreme symptoms of psychopathology were present.

In sum, the literature indicates that (1) Asian Americans remain outside of the mainstream in terms of their knowledge and use of counseling services; (2) acculturation brings Asian Americans closer to American norms; and (3) counselors need to develop different models for treating Asian Americans.

Changes in the Asian-American Population

The significant change in the Asian-American community has been the influx of new immigrants. In 1970 the Japanese were the most numerous group, but by 1980 they had been replaced by the Chinese and Filipinos (see table 1). Future estimates indicate a rising number of Koreans, so that by the end of the 20th century the demographic picture of Asians in America will be again drastically different.

The change is primarily because of the Immigration Act of 1965, which abolished nationality quotas, and refugee legislation that affected immigration from Southeast Asia. Prior to the 1965 act Asian immigration was severely restricted: the 1924 immigration legislation was basically anti-Asian and excluded Asian immigration; the McCarran-Walter Act of 1952 opened the door a little but still retained many of the anti-Asian aspects of previous legislation. The 1965 act was designed to encourage the flow of immigrants from Southern and Eastern Europe, but because it also gave priority to the unification of families and assigned priority to those with skills deemed necessary to the United States, the flow of Asians also resulted. Immigration legislation passed in 1986 seems more relevant to Hispanic, rather than Asian, immigration (Kitano and Daniels 1988).

The major point of interest, however, deals with the nature of immi-

Table 1. Asians and Pacific Islanders in the United States

	1980	1970
Chinese	806,027	435,062
Filipino	774,640	343,060
Japanese	700,747	591,290
Asian Indian	361,544	—
Korean	354,529	69,130
Vietnamese	261,714	—
Hawaiian	167,253	—
Samoan	42,050	—
Guamanian	32,132	—

Source: U.S. Dept. of Commerce 1980, PC 80-51-3, pp. 7, 13.

gration since 1970. Prior to that year most immigrants were Europeans; from 1970 on they have been Latinos and Asians. For example, the increase in immigration of Asians from 6% in 1950 to 36% in 1980 is the steepest for any group.

The large number of different Asian groups currently in the United States makes it unrealistic to present them all. For example, in a study of refugees from Southeast Asia the following were identified: Blue, White, and Striped Hmong; Chinese, Krom, and Mi Khmer Cambodians; Chinese, Mien, Thai Dam, and Khmer Laotians; and Lowlander and Highlander Vietnamese (State Department of Mental Health 1986). Basically, there are many Asian-American groups, each with their own history and culture, and there are further stratifications within each group. Counselors need to become acquainted with the general history and culture of the various Asian Americans.

Their background experiences cover a wide range. For example, a Cambodian refugee remembers the following when he was 10 years old: "I was in a labor camp. My father and my brothers had been soldiers. They were killed by the Khmer Rouge." He continues his story of starvation, murder, and lack of schooling (Nidorf 1985, 400). A Japanese American might have grown up in a World War II concentration camp. Others, however, may have more "normal" backgrounds.

The error is to assume that no matter what the background of the client, there is a standard approach in therapy. For example, there is evidence that a directive approach is appropriate for Asian-American clients. But what if the client is a fifth-generation Asian American with little ethnic identification and almost totally Americanized? Yet, a directive style might be effective with a newly arrived immigrant who has grown up in a vertically structured society and who has had minimal contact with the American culture.

✗ The Counseling Model: Assimilation and Ethnic Identity

The two variables that appear most critical when dealing with Asian Americans are assimilation and ethnic identity. Assimilation involves the processes of acculturation and becoming "Americanized"; ethnic identity refers to the retention of customs, attitudes, and beliefs of the culture of origin. The interaction of these two variables makes up the basic framework of our model.

Assimilation, which includes acculturation, integration, and amalgamation, is a variation of straight line theory (Sandberg 1986). This theory predicts the lessening of ethnic identity with length of time in America. Over the course of generations there is a "straight line" from a strong ethnic identification to a much weaker one. The model has

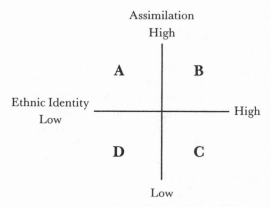

Figure 1. Assimilation and Ethnic Identity

been criticized by Gans (1985); there is the so-called Hansen (1938) effect, whereby the third generation tries to remember what the second generation has forgotten. Nevertheless, it is a model that predicts the experiences of immigrant groups in the United States.

Ethnic identity is correlated with assimilation, but we have conceptualized it as a separate variable (see figure 1). Immigrants constantly struggle with these two dimensions—how American can or should they become and how much of their ethnic culture can or should they retain? In our model of assimilation and ethnic identity there are two further questions. One asks where immigrants actually are, and the second, where they would like to be along the two dimensions. For example, an individual may be strongly ethnic today but expects and desires to become assimilated in the future.

From this model we are able to identify four types; Type A, high in assimilation and low in ethnic identity; Type B, high in assimilation, high in ethnic identity; Type C, high in ethnic identity, low in assimilation; and Type D, low in ethnic identity, low in assimilation. We believe that each of these types will exhibit different problems and require different counseling procedures. It should be emphasized that these are "ideal types"; few individuals will fit neatly into the categories.

Type A: high assimilation, low ethnic identity. Individuals in this category are for all intents and purposes "American." Lifestyles, values, language, and culture are typically mainstream. Clothes and entertainment, especially during adolescence, show little influence of an ethnic background. Close friends may still be Asian, however. This adaptation is what sociologists call structural pluralism; for example, clubs and voluntary organizations remain ethnic, even though their practices and actions may closely resemble American groups. Some individuals may integrate almost totally into the majority group.

Generation and length of time in America are the most important factors influencing this category. By the third generation, there generally is a high degree of assimilation (i.e., the "straight line"), and a counselor is dealing with an "American," but one with an Asian face. Counseling techniques based on prescriptions drawn from traditional Asian cultures would probably be inappropriate; most of the individuals in this category have little knowledge of their ancestral heritage and are unfamiliar with the language of their grandparents. There may be high rates of interracial marriage (Kitano 1985). The self-image may lie close to American norms, and generally counseling with individuals in this category may not be that different from majority group populations. The reality of looking different in a society in which role models are primarily Caucasian, however, precludes complete absorption into the mainstream. Counseling that ignores this factor may foster unrealistic expectations and a barrier to credibility.

Sue and Sue (1972), in working with college students during the Civil Rights era, mentioned variations in the assimilationist perspective. A militant stance meant emphasizing one's own cultural heritage and developing ethnic pride and self-identity. Counseling was often perceived as irrelevant since problems were viewed as stemming from the sociopolitical and economic arrangements in the society. Counselors were thus agents of the establishment with the goal of adjusting clients to the status quo, and therapy was viewed with suspicion and hostility. Direct challenges to counselors were common; it was difficult for students to see problems as arising from individual emotional and personal difficulties. Counselors often found themselves engaging in debates and adopting defensive stances.

Generally, individuals in this category will have problems that are similar to majority group members. Job opportunities, advancement, mobility, dating, marriage, child care, and child guidance as well as personality and intrapsychic problems will be issues. Interpersonal relationships, the need for creative expression, and assertiveness training are other common problems.

Low ethnic identity does not necessarily mean the total absence of an ethnic consciousness. The factor of visibility cannot be avoided; Asian Americans, even of the fourth and fifth generations are often mistaken for newcomers, and the question "But where did you learn to speak English so well?" is a reminder that the individual is perceived by many members of the majority group as an Asian.

Gans (1985) writes of a "symbolic ethnicity"; the individual may partake of ethnic foods, attend an occasional ethnic movie, and participate in an ethnic festival. But if identification means a total commitment—learning the language, immersing oneself in the history and the culture, and actively participating in the ethnic community, then the individual might reconsider the commitment.

Type B: high assimilation, high ethnic identity. This category is essentially bicultural; the individual feels comfortable and knowledgeable about both cultures, has friends in each, and belongs to organizations spanning the cultures. Few people at present fall into this category—intellectuals and businesspeople who have to deal with both cultures are examples. But this category might well be the wave of the future since there is much discussion among Asian intellectuals about the desirability of the bicultural perspective. Counselors who are unicultural may have difficulty with individuals in this category since their clientele possesses knowledge and insights drawn from more than one culture.

Type C: high ethnic identity, low assimilation. Type C identifies those who retain a high degree of their ethnic ways with little tendency to assimilate. This category includes most newly arrived immigrants and old-timers who have spent most of their lives in ethnic communities. Tung (1985) offers some insight and advice to counselors working with Southeast Asian refugees:

1. Expect understatement. Grief and depression may be expressed with little emotion. Anger may be exhibited obliquely and indirectly; severe outbursts may indicate a serious degree of personality disorganization. Females may be allowed a greater degree of emotional expression than males.

2. Modesty, discretion, and self-deprecation are not necessarily related to poor self-concept. Clients may not voluntarily offer details about themselves: they may not want to seem boastful, or they may fear that something they say might reflect upon their family or community.

3. Family matters may be cause for even more discretion. Family dynamics, especially those concerning parents and elders, may be difficult to discuss.

4. Expect difficulty in obtaining sexual information. Female patients may be especially uncomfortable in discussing sexual matters with a male therapist.

5. Physical symptoms and bodily discomfort are more acceptable topics for discussion. Bizarre sounding symptoms, such as a "hot liver," do not necessarily indicate pathology.

6. All symptoms should be examined for cultural relevance. Talking with a dead spouse does not necessarily indicate a flight from reality.

There are a number of other generalizations by Tung (1985), Carlin and Sokoloff (1985), Kinzie (1985), Bliatout et al. (1985), Nidorf (1985), and Westermeyer (1985) that, although focused on Southeast Asian refugees, have relevance to other Asian Americans. For example, therapeutic and counseling sessions are better if they are short—the idea of "imposing" on strangers, rather than on friends and relatives, is difficult to overcome. Toupin (1980, 9) presents the case of an Asian-American student in therapy three times a week, who left to spend a month at home during the Christmas break. At the final session before the holidays, the therapist said, "Call me if you need to see me." The patient, feeling ashamed to impose himself on the therapist's time, spent four weeks at home unable to discuss his problems with anyone and was eventually hospitalized.

There is also a preference for short-term, goal-directed treatment; the cessation of symptoms is important, and therapists are expected to be active, to take charge, and to be directive. Group and family sessions may be difficult; interaction in traditional families may be stilted and ineffective. Sessions that may have the best potential are those in which the groups are relatively homogeneous in terms of sex, background, profession, and social class. Goal-oriented sessions may be more productive than free-floating, process-oriented ones; there is a tendency to look for mature, firm leadership and a clear structure. In addition, participants may need or prefer to speak in their native tongues, in which case translators may need to be present.

Asians come from cultures that are not primarily psychologically oriented. Discussions of feelings or of psychological motives for behavior and analyzing behavior from a psychological frame of reference are not common in most Asian-American homes, even those of the second and third generations. Disturbed behavior is often viewed as the result of a lack of will, supernatural causes, or physical illness. We are acquainted with cases of school failure in which the common parental complaint is that children are lazy and lack character: the solution then lies in stricter parental restrictions, more homework, and other negative sanctions that are believed to foster character development. Hard work, effort, and developing character are presumed to be the best "cure" for most disturbances. The problem is especially acute for Asian-American children with limited abilities.

They also come from cultures that have few mental health professionals. Elders and grandparents—and even departed ancestors—are consulted for advice and guidance. Families may refuse treatment, especially if it consists of "talking out." It should be emphasized that "treatment" takes place in a cultural context; our verbally-oriented models may be inappropriate for most Type C's.

It is difficult to accurately assess the role and use of indigenous healers. If they are being used, the most likely clientele will be drawn from the newly arrived, less acculturated groups. Bliatout et al. (1985) list some traditional healers in Southeast Asia. For the Hmong there are herbalists and shamans; for the Khmer and Lao, Buddhist monks; and for the Vietnamese, ethnic health practitioners, Taoist teachers, and sorcerers. Counselors should see indigenous healers as another possible resource rather than discount them. But it should also be added that not all Type C immigrants believe strongly in the efficacy of traditional forms of healing.

Few Type C's will voluntarily show up for our Western-style counseling services. But, it is also sobering to note that the great majority of Asians are new immigrants, and the resources available to them are scarce. Their thoughts and feelings may remain unverbalized, but their conflicts and struggles are no doubt enormous. They face life in a new land as total strangers; they have to make a living with education and skills that may be irrelevant or disregarded; there is the reality of downward mobility, of questions of dependence, of vulnerability, and of changing roles. It may be helpful to think of the counseling role as that of education and orientation rather than that of therapy.

Type D: low assimilation, low ethnic identity. This category includes "dropouts," those alienated from both the ethnic and the American communities. It also includes the mentally ill and those with severe problems based on their inability to accept either the ethnic role or their role in the dominant society.

A Japanese-American alcoholic, currently in Alcoholics Anonymous, discussed his problem of being an Asian (a role that he did not want) in an all-white world. Everything became all right, however, when he could buy everyone a drink in a high-class bar. He enjoyed the first-name recognition when he set up drinks; his Asianness disappeared temporarily under the influence of alcohol. He thought that Japanese Americans were too uptight, yet he felt uncomfortable in the white world, except when he could drink (Kitano et al. 1985).

A common problem drawn from our model deals with conflict within families, in which often parents are in one category and the children in another. The term "culture conflict" is most appropriate, as in the case of Mr. B, a second generation Korean high school student. He had difficulty getting along with his immigrant parents, who violently objected to his long hair. He later withdrew from treatment without having successfully resolved his conflict with his parents (Ho 1976, 198).

Chen (1987) describes the conflict of children of recently arrived Asian immigrants. They are caught between negotiating between their parents' culture and school, which represents the dominant culture, with little power to influence or change either. Immigrant children also serve as unofficial translators, are called upon to perform a variety of clerical actions, such as filling out forms, applications, and licenses, and may also have to babysit siblings and other relatives; many do not have the "luxury" of having a childhood.

Many traditional Asian parents have little understanding of the American peer-oriented teenage culture. Clothing, appearance, and peer approval can create difficult situations even for American parents;

for the immigrant the chasms appear enormous. Many parents also view nonacademic courses as frivolous; extracurricular activities for their children are often discouraged.

Counseling Techniques

Yamamoto and Yap (1984) discussed the need for developing appropriate counseling procedures for populations that do not fit the classical psychotherapeutic modes. Most of his Asian clients were Type C's, high ethnic identity, low assimilation. Their values were different from American ones—they did not value self-actualization, the fostering of egalitarian principles, and open expressions of feelings. Instead, there was an emphasis on familism (the family as the more important unit than the individual), on hierarchy (the therapist as the authority), and on brief, rather than long-term, treatment.

Nakao and Lum (1977) found that Asian-American counselors used more formal techniques and less confrontation when dealing with Asian clients.

Sue and Zane (1986) write that counselor credibility cuts across all facets. Status is one part of credibility—ascribed status, such as sex and age, governs many traditional Asian interactions. Achieved status is closely related to therapeutic skills, empathic understanding, and an accurate assessment of client needs and problems. Ascribed and achieved credibility are related; the lack of ascribed credibility (i.e., assignment of nonethnic counselors of inappropriate age and sex) may be one reason for the underutilization of therapy, while the lack of achieved credibility (i.e., no quick symptom relief) may explain premature termination.

Kitano and Matsushima (1981) described several therapeutic techniques from Japan. Morita therapy was group-centered, ritualistic, and behavioristic in contrast to the more talk-centered Western therapies. The concentration was on the here and now, on behavior over moods and feelings, and on the interdependence among individuals.

Naikan therapy focused on the important influences in the client's life, especially the mother. The goal was for the individual to gain a better understanding of his or her relationships with significant others and to acknowledge the indebtedness to them. In the process the client becomes more sympathetic to the views of others, including the trouble and problems that he or she has created for them.

Okonogi (1978) wrote about the Ajase complex, developed by the Japanese psychoanalyst Kosawa (1897–1968) and based on Buddhist scriptures. The basic concept is that of strong mother-child ties, especially mother to son, and the consequences of these bonds. There are strong feelings of love and hostility, with the theme of forgiveness as the child returns to the mother.

Okonogi contrasts the Japanese view of forgiveness with the more punitive orientation of Western psychology. Japanese are much more apt to forgive transgressions upon return to the fold than are Europeans. He also comments that the Ajase complex may be a more fundamental explanation of facets of the Japanese culture than Freud's more widely known Oedipus complex.

Summary

The family is central for Asian Americans, and many individual problems arise from family conflict. Nowhere is this conflict more clearly demonstrated than in immigrant families, in which parents reflect "old values" and the children are exposed to another way of life.

Our model, contrasting the four "types," illustrates the problem. Learning about the dominant society and teaching their children the old country ways have always been a part of American immigrant life. Although conflict was common—the term culture conflict has become a part of our vocabulary—the conflict was thought to be resolved through the processes of acculturation and assimilation. But our model also indicates that not all groups are involved in these processes—many individuals remain ethnic throughout their lives. As of now we have little access to them, and even if we did we may not have the skills to be of much assistance.

Creative counseling can be helpful. Counselors can clarify relevant norms and values of the new culture as well as discuss the alternatives and consequences of selected paths of action. Questions of identity remain paramount—is the client Asian, American, or a combination of the two? Which cultural insights and values will aid the client in solving problems? Perhaps the ideal occurs when the client comes to terms with both the Asianness and Americanness of his or her identity.

The same questions are relevant for the counselor. Where does he or she stand in relation to assimilation and ethnic identity? Which values and lifestyles fit most comfortably in the counselor's view of the world? Understanding where clients are is a good first step, but it should be emphasized that the direction of change is a value choice.

Our model can help ascertain where various Asian-American groups are in terms of assimilation and ethnic identity. Each of the typologies describes differences within the population, and culture conflicts can be clearly seen. We hope that appropriate diagnostic and therapeutic tools will be developed to serve the various types of Asian Americans.

References

Atkinson, D. R. 1983. Ethnic minority representation in counselor education. *Counselor Education and Supervision* 23 (1): 7–19.

Bliatout, B. T., Rath, B., Vinh, T. D., Kham, O. K., Bliatout, H. Y., and Lee, D. T. 1985. Mental health and prevention activities targeted to Southeast Asian refugees. In T. Owan (ed.), *Southeast Asian mental health: Treatment, prevention, services, training, and research*, 183–207. Washington, DC: National Institute of Mental Health.

Carlin, J., and Sokoloff, B. 1985. Mental health treatment issues for Southeast Asian refugee children. In T. Owan (ed.), *Southeast Asian mental health: Treatment, prevention, services, training, and research*, 91–112. Washington, DC: National Institute of Mental Health.

Chen, C., and Yang, D. 1986. The self-image of Chinese American adolescents. *Pacific Asian American Mental Health Research Center Review* (3/4): 27–29.

Chen, S. 1987. Suicide and depression identified as serious problems for Asian youth. *East-West News* 9 April: 6.

East-West News. 13 November 1986. Vol. 20 (47): 12.

Gans, H. 1985. Symbolic ethnicity: The future of ethnic groups. In N. Yetman (ed.), *Majority and minority*, 429–442. Boston: Allyn and Bacon.

Hansen, M. 1938. *The problems of the third generation.* Rock Island, IL: Augustana Historical Society.

Ho, M. K. 1976. Social work with Asian Americans. *Social Casework* March: 195–201.

Kim, Y. J. 1983. Problems in the delivery of school-based psycho-educational services to Asian immigrant children. *Journal of Children in Contemporary Society* 15 (3): 81–89.

Kinzie, J. D. 1985. Overview of clinical issues in the treatment of Southeast Asian refugees. In T. Owan (ed.), *Southeast Asian mental health: Treatment, prevention, services, training, and research*, 113–135. Washington, DC: National Institute of Mental Health.

Kitano, H. 1985. *Race relations.* Englewood Cliffs, NJ: Prentice-Hall.

Kitano, H., and Daniels, R. 1988. *Asian Americans.* Englewood Cliffs, NJ: Prentice-Hall.

Kitano, H., Hatanaka, H., Yeung, W. T., and Sue, S. 1985. Japanese American drinking patterns. In L. Bennett and G. Ames (eds.), *The American experience with alcohol*, 335–359. New York: Plenum Press.

Kitano, H., and Matsushima, N. 1981. Counseling Asian Americans. In P. B. Pedersen, J. G. Draguns, W. J. Lonner, and J. E. Trimble (eds.), *Counseling across cultures*, 163–180. Honolulu: University of Hawaii Press.

Leong, C. A., Sasao, T., and Uomoto, J. M. 1983. Selected mental health issues for Asian American psychologists in the eighties. *Asian American Psychological Association Journal* 8 (1): 1–13.

Miranda, M., and Kitano, H. 1986. *Mental health research and practice in minority communities.* Rockville, MD: National Institute of Mental Health.

Nakao, S., and Lum, C. 1977. Yellow is not white and white is not right:

Counseling techniques for Japanese and Chinese clients. Master's thesis, University of California, Los Angeles.

Nidorf, J. F. 1985. Mental health and refugee youths: A model for diagnostic training. In T. Owan (ed.), *Southeast Asian mental health: Treatment, prevention, services, training, and research,* 391–429. Washington, DC: National Institute of Mental Health.

Okonogi, K. 1978. The Ajase complex of Japanese. *Japan Echo* 5 (4): 88–105.

Owan, T., ed. 1985. *Southeast Asian mental health: Treatment, prevention, services, training, and research.* Washington, DC: National Institute of Mental Health.

Sandberg, N. 1986. *Jewish life in Los Angeles.* Lanham, MD: University Press of America.

State Dept. of Mental Health Refugee Project. 1986. Oakland, CA: Asian Community Mental Health Services.

Sue, D. W., and Sue, S. 1972. Counseling Chinese Americans. *Personnel and Guidance Journal* 50 (8): 637–644.

Sue, S., and McKinney, H. 1975. Asian American in the community mental health care system. *American Journal of Orthopsychiatry* 45 (1): 111–118.

Sue, S., and Zane, N. 1986. Therapists credibility and giving: Implications for practice and training in Asian-American communities. In M. Miranda and H. Kitano (eds.), *Mental health research and practice in minority communities,* 157–175. Rockville, MD: National Institute of Mental Health.

Tong, B. 1983. Challenges before the AAPA: The 1980's. *Asian American Psychological Association Journal* 8 (1): 14–18.

Toupin, E. 1980. Counseling Asians. *American Journal of Orthopsychiatry* 50 (1): 76–86.

Tung, T. M. 1985. Psychiatric care for Southeast Asians: How different is different? In T. Owan (ed.), *Southeast Asian mental health: Treatment, prevention, services, training, and research,* 5–40. Washington, DC: National Institute of Mental Health.

Uomoto, J., and Gorsuch, R. 1984. Japanese American response to psychological disorder: Referral patterns, attitudes, and subjective norms. *American Journal of Community Psychology* 12 (5): 537–550.

U.S. Department of Commerce, Bureau of Census. 1980. Census of the population, supplementary reports, race of the population by states. PC 80-51-3. Washington, DC: Government Printing Office.

Westermeyer, J. 1985. Mental health of Southeast Asians over two decades from Laos and the United States. In T. Owan (ed.), *Southeast Asian mental health: Treatment, prevention, services, training, and research,* 65–89. Washington, DC: National Institute of Mental Health.

Yamamoto, J., Machizawa, S., and Steinberg, A. 1986. The Japanese American relocation camp experience. *Pacific Asian American Mental Health Research Center Review* 5 (3/4): 17–20.

Yamamoto, J., and Yap, J. 1984. Group therapy for Asian Americans and Pacific Islanders. *Pacific Asian American Mental Health Research Center Review* 3 (1): 1–3.

7

Counseling the Hispanic Client:
A Theoretical and Applied Perspective

J. MANUEL CASAS
MELBA J. T. VASQUEZ

Recent years have witnessed an increasing interest in culture and the role multicultural awareness plays in counseling. Cultural diversity is a reality in the United States—ethnic minority persons are 20% of the population—and counselors and therapists are confronted with the very real possibility of counseling persons who are different from themselves. We will focus on key issues involved in providing effective and ethical mental health services to Hispanic populations.

Fortunately, we have also witnessed an increase in the number of mental health–related journal articles, chapters, and books focusing on Hispanic Americans. In reviewing these works, it quickly becomes apparent that a major impetus for this increase relates to specific demographic characteristics that have had or are destined to have direct and major implications for the provision of counseling, educational, and other social services to the Hispanic populace. The characteristics most frequently mentioned include population statistics, including size, age, and birth rate, and access to key resources in society, such as education, professions, and economic status.

With respect to population, Hispanics are a sizable and rapidly growing ethnic minority in the United States. Estimates from the 1985 advance census conservatively suggest that Hispanics number 16.9 million, or 7.2% of the population (this figure is conservative because most undocumented Hispanics are not included in the census) (U.S. Bureau of the Census 1985). Comparing these figures with those reported in the 1970s reveals that Hispanics are the fastest growing ethnic group in the United States with a 6.1% annual rate of growth, compared to 1.8% for blacks and 0.06% for whites.

The Hispanic population is young. The median age for all U.S. residents combined is 30; for whites it is 31.3; for persons of Spanish origin

The authors would like to acknowledge the editorial support of Jacqueline Masters and Mary Lou Lumpe.

it is 23.2. Even more dramatic, almost one-third of all Hispanics are under the age of 15. That Hispanics generally, and Mexican Americans and Puerto Ricans specifically, maintain high fertility rates partially explains this phenomenon. Mexican-American females can be expected to average close to three births each, compared to 2.4 births for blacks and 1.7 for whites. Given its youthfulness, prevailing fertility rates, and strong and continuous immigration from Latin America, demographers can safely predict that the Hispanic population will continue to increase at an accelerated rate, especially in large metropolitan areas.

Occupational, economic, and educational levels are symbols of status and power in this country. The levels attained by Hispanics are relevant here and to many social scientists because the possession or lack of power and status can affect an individual's or a group's well-being, image, and identity in positive or in negative ways (Sherif 1982). We draw attention to the absence of an increase in educational and socio-economic attainment concomitant with the increasing number of Hispanics in the general population. For instance, 83.9% of the Anglo population aged 18–24 received high school diplomas, whereas only 55.5% of the Hispanic population of similar ages did so (Duran 1983). Although academic achievement seems to be improving for the general population, a 1976 survey demonstrated that the highest level of education attained by Hispanics averaged approximately 2.6 years less than that of the Anglo population (Ford Foundation Report 1984). More alarming are educators' figures of 50% to 80% Hispanic dropout rates in the larger U.S. cities (National Commission on Secondary Schooling for Hispanics 1984).

Because education in the United States is considered the most important step toward economic stability (Carter and Segura 1979), it is not astonishing to find the Hispanic group, with its poor academic profile, represented at the lower scale of professional status and income (Ford Foundation Report 1984). Economically, the Hispanic population maintains a lower income and is more likely to fall below poverty level than its Anglo counterpart.

Using these demographic characteristics as impetus for their work, most authors in mental health literature have directed their writing and research toward specific topical areas considered requisite for relevant and effective counseling, educational, and social service delivery to Hispanics. The myriad topics generally fall into one of the following broad categories: client variables, counselor variables, and counseling process variables.

The largest amount of published work on Hispanics focuses on client variables. This category includes such topics as client sociocultural characteristics (i.e., family dynamics, socialization practices, cognitive styles, gender roles); psychopathology and presenting problems, that is, the prevalence of specific problems—depression, somatic complaints, stress; utilization patterns (the major theme in most of these works has been a tendency by Hispanics in general to underutilize certain services or to overuse others); counselor preference and effectiveness in relation to race and ethnicity; preference for types of help (e.g., counselor, parents, friends, relatives, clergy); and client expectations of treatment (i.e., what kind of help do Hispanics expect [directive, nurturing, practical, problem solving, advice giving]). Most literature in this category seeks to provide information to improve the understanding of Hispanics and in turn the services provided to them.

Counselor expectations and attitudes predominate in the counselor variables category of literature. This concentration presupposes the counseling profession's belief that attitudes and expectations of the counselor play an extremely important role in the counseling process. As we will note later, a positive and realistically oriented predilection may work to the client's benefit; a negative and prejudicial one may work to the client's detriment.

The third category concerns counseling process variables (i.e., counseling approaches and techniques, according to Casas 1984) and presents two lines of inquiry relative to counseling Hispanics. First are works that identify, from a theoretical perspective, counseling/service models and techniques assumed culturally appropriate and effective for use with all Hispanics. Second are those that are empirically based and actually demonstrate positive counseling outcomes from specific approaches and techniques in the counseling process. Unfortunately for practitioners, the theoretically based articles far outnumber the empirically based.

The increase in the literature as a response to changing demographics denotes an important step toward improving counseling services provided to Hispanics. Inherent in this increase, however, is the potential for using these works to the detriment of the Hispanic client. The potential for such use-misuse is especially high for individuals having limited contact with and knowledge of Hispanics or minimal training in counseling.

Various researchers (e.g., Casas 1984; Sundberg 1981) express concern about the significant number of empirically based works plagued with methodological flaws. The more descriptive studies too frequently provide subjective perspectives on Hispanics that reinforce the negative characteristics and stereotypes attributed to Hispanics in general.

Most writers address their focal topic without benefit of a theoretical framework into which their work can be placed and subsequently understood and evaluated. Thus, while one individual underscores the importance of understanding the family structure of the Hispanics, another enthusiastically identifies an effective technique to use with

Hispanics in general. Such information may have value, but greater value would accrue if a framework existed that enabled the reader to determine the relative importance of the information vis-à-vis the total and dynamic counseling process. Lacking such a framework, much of the information available in the literature has been inappropriately understood and evaluated and, in turn, used ineffectively with the Hispanic client. The purpose of this section is to provide such a framework.

A Counseling Framework

The proposed framework presents categorical variables along a continuum, starting with those more covert and distal to the counseling process and progressing toward those ever more integral. As evident in figure 1 the first category enumerates selected personal and professional attitudes and beliefs inherent to the counselor and strongly affecting Hispanic counseling. The second category identifies individual, sociocultural, and environmental variables that must be accurately understood and appropriately addressed in counseling. Finally, the third category lists approaches to the counseling process, an innovation that provides a more comprehensive and directional perspective of benefit to counseling Hispanic clients and to minority counseling in general.

The Counselor

To understand Hispanic clients, counselors must first become aware of the professional and personal influences, assumptions, and biases that determine and direct their own interactions with clients from diverse backgrounds. Counselors frequently espouse the notion that theirs is an impartial helping profession relating to the essential humanity in each client (Korchin 1980). Actually, the counseling profession is anything *but* impartial. A fundamental set of cultural values forms its core—values that reflect the majority culture: a white, middle-class culture. Unaware of this basic bias, the counselor may ascribe universal value and importance to such factors as rugged individualism, competition, action orientation, the Protestant work ethic, progress and future orientation, the scientific method of inquiry, the nuclear family structure, and rigid timetables.

Giving value and importance to any and all of these factors is, of itself, neither good nor bad. Blind and unquestioning adherence to the importance of these values, however, can become problematic to a counselor working with a client who strongly identifies with traditional Hispanic culture. As will be made evident later, the Hispanic culture

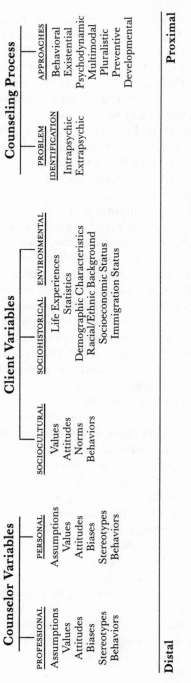

Counselor Variables

PROFESSIONAL
Assumptions
Values
Attitudes
Biases
Stereotypes
Behaviors

PERSONAL
Assumptions
Values
Attitudes
Biases
Stereotypes
Behaviors

Client Variables

SOCIOCULTURAL
Values
Attitudes
Norms
Behaviors

SOCIOHISTORICAL
Life Experiences
Statistics
Demographic Characteristics
Racial/Ethnic Background
Socioeconomic Status
Immigration Status

ENVIRONMENTAL

Counseling Process

PROBLEM
IDENTIFICATION
Intrapsychic
Extrapsychic

APPROACHES
Behavioral
Existential
Psychodynamic
Multimodal
Pluralistic
Preventive
Developmental

Distal   **Proximal**

Figure 1. A Framework for Counseling the Hispanic Client

does *not* assign high value to many of these factors. In fact, many values predicate to traditional Hispanic culture conflict with those of the Anglo culture. The interpretation of behavior in terms of the counselor's values rather than those of the client can result in erroneous assessment and diagnosis and potentially ineffective or destructive intervention.

Real complications arise when Anglo values are used to underscore and validate basic assumptions of the counseling profession. Pedersen (1987) recently identified several culturally biased assumptions that frequently emerge in the literature of multicultural counseling within international contexts. They are relevant also to counseling racial and ethnic minorities in the United States, and the effective cross-cultural counselor needs to examine each of them.

A primary, all-pervasive assumption is that a more or less universal definition of "normal" behavior exists regardless of social, cultural, economic, or political backgrounds and that consequently all people share this common measure of normalcy. This assumption can lead counselors to presume that describing a person's behavior as "normal" is meaningful and implies a particular pattern of behaviors by the normal person. According to Pedersen, "if the label *normal* is challenged in a particular instance, the variation can frequently be explained as a deviation from otherwise normal behavior because of socio-cultural differences from the norms of society" (1987, 17). Interestingly enough, the need to explain variations in normality in a manner that protects the status quo of normality is so ingrained that very creative and elaborate rationalization often results (Pedersen 1987).

In fact, there *is* no universal measure of normality, and this is extremely difficult to accept. Perhaps it would help to examine the term itself. It is easy to see that the root word is norm; after that the extensive dictionary entries reflect rather than resolve our conflictual reactions to the designation "normal." After stating the word's origin as a measure of construction (perpendicular from a tangent; literally, a carpenter's square), Webster's listing continues: "2. Not deviating from a norm, rule, or principle; 3. Occurring naturally; 4. Relating to or characterized by average intelligence or development, *free from mental disorder*" (emphasis added) (Woolf 1980). There are more definitions, but the sequence is clear. What began as one type of measurement became recognized as a general measure of conformity to a specific set of rules or principles; then comes the connotation that this conformity is "natural"; and finally, that failure to follow this particular measurement, by definition, indicates below average intelligence and the presence of mental disorder! What was specific has become universal, and those who do not share or recognize this are not "normal." This illustrates a natural—and potentially dangerous—progression of assumptions. It is one thing to believe in the existence of universal values but quite another thing entirely to define *your* values as the one universal truth.

What is considered normal behavior must be evaluated and understood according to the situation, the cultural background(s) of the person or persons demonstrating the behavior, and the time during which the behavior is being displayed and observed. When a counselor applies a definition of normal behavior based in one culture to a culturally diverse population, and disregards such variables, diagnostic errors result. This section will describe just how such errors occur.

The basic assumption that individuals are the building blocks of a society inheres in a culture valuing rugged individualism. Counselors who share that assumption work from the premise that counseling's primary goal is the development of the individual rather than units of individuals or groups, such as the family, organization, or society (Pedersen 1987). This cultural bias works to the detriment of persons from cultures that put family or another designated social unit above the individual. In traditional Hispanic culture the family unit (including the extended family) is given great importance; consequently, in that cultural context it is "normal" to deal with the reality and necessity of valuing the welfare of the family higher than one's individual welfare. To speak of an individual's health and welfare independent of the health and welfare of the family unit simply does not make good sense within traditional Hispanic culture (Pedersen 1987).

Complementing the high valuation of individualism is the assumption that independence has value and dependence does not. Once again, it is necessary to note that other cultures, the traditional Hispanic among them, view interdependencies as both healthy and necessary. This perspective must be incorporated by the counselor who assesses the appropriateness of relationships among and between Hispanic clients, including the healthy function that their reliance on others serves. Anglo counselors must challenge their personal, culturally conditioned notions and presumptions of pathology regarding interdependence and learn to reframe such constructs. The value of connecting, supporting, and cooperating within a group is easily understood and observable from a different context than that of rugged individualism.

Cultural differences also pertain to evaluating acceptable patterns of client behavior during counseling sessions. A premise prevalent among professional counselors equates cooperativeness in counseling with the client's willingness to be verbally open and direct. In fact, many if not most of the world's cultures view revelations to a stranger of intimate personal and family details as highly unacceptable. The acceptable pattern of behavior for the traditional Hispanic is to handle one's problems discreetly, from within the family or other natural support systems, and, once again, cultural expectations conflict with the counselor's professional expectations.

There exists in this nation's majority culture the assumption that individuals depend on linear thinking—wherein each cause has an effect and each effect a cause—in order to understand the world around them. Not all cultures ascribe to this philosophical orientation. According to Pedersen (1987), some cultures routinely describe an event independent of its relationship to surrounding, preceding, or consequent events.

The next three premises of the counseling process are extremely important to the Hispanic client, and although only briefly touched on in this section, they are addressed in greater detail later in the chapter. The first premise is that the role of the counselor is to change individuals to fit society rather than change society to fit the individuals. Psychology is the study of human behavior; thus, counseling interventions from a psychological perspective tend to focus on the individual and how the individual should change, regardless of the possibility that the environment may be the problem. Hispanics in the United States experience second-class citizenship, oppression, and discrimination to varying degrees. Given this sociohistorical reality, the effective counselor will know how to facilitate the Hispanic client's empowerment in that environment (focusing on skills of assertion, stress management, but especially supporting the attitude that the Hispanic client is entitled to work toward changing the environmental factors that deter one's goals) as opposed to colluding with the unhealthy dynamics of oppression and "blaming the victim." The effective counselor may become directly involved in taking an active role in the community to change the oppressive elements.

Second, past history has little relevance to the presenting problem. "Counselors are more likely to focus on the immediate events that created a crisis, and if clients begin talking about their own history or the history of their 'people,' the counselor is likely to stop listening and wait for clients to 'catch up' to current events, which the counselor considers more salient than past history" (Pedersen 1987). The past and the present interrelate so complexly for most Hispanics that without an understanding and appreciation of their sociohistorical reality it is impossible to understand the total individual.

The third premise is that counselors are aware of the assumptions inherent in their profession and, concomitantly, that they already possess all information and skills necessary for dealing with them effectively. Such is not the case. The assumptions and the values that generate them are so implicit, so interwoven into the fabric of the majority culture, that they go unchallenged even by broad-minded and insightful psychologists, and unfortunately, "the consequences of these unexamined assumptions are institutionalized racism, ageism, sexism, and other forms of cultural bias" (Pedersen 1987, 16). Until examination of these culturally learned assumptions becomes an integral part of the training curriculum for counselors, the profession is poorly prepared to deal with a diversified society.

According to Katz (1985), the counseling profession's failure to recognize its own implicit cultural milieu results in counselors, and all mental health professionals, being identified as agents of the status quo (Halleck 1971) and—more seriously—as perpetuators of cultural oppression (Sue 1981). Members of minority groups often view counselors not as benign helpers but as social agents whose primary function is to assure the client's adaptation and conformance to the majority culture's values (Szasz 1974).

An awareness of the profession's cultural encapsulation (Wrenn 1962) and the negative effect such encapsulation has on the credibility and effectiveness of counselors with minority group clients should serve as adequate impetus to self-examination by individual counselors and by the profession. Counselors must realize that the beliefs, attitudes, and values on which their patterns of behavior are based have evolved from their own cultural biases. At this time, most counselors in this nation—like the tenets of the profession they have created—are products of a white, middle-class, male value system, and there is a high probability that the system's beliefs, attitudes, stereotypes, and biases relative to Hispanics and all other value systems are firmly and invisibly imbedded in both theory and practice.

A study investigating the attitudes of practicing psychotherapists toward blacks, Chinese Americans, Japanese Americans, Jews, and Mexican Americans found that of all the responses provided by the therapists, 79.2% indicated the presence of subtle stereotypic attitudes, and 22.6% demonstrated highly blatant stereotypic attitudes. The stereotypes most frequently ascribed to Hispanics tend to be negative (lazy, dumb, dirty, overemotional) or, when different from the majority (passive, cooperative, present-time oriented), negatively perceived. Wampold, Casas, and Atkinson (1981) conducted a study that provided evidence that prevailing stereotypes preclude counselors' accurately processing information relative to their minority clients and thereby impede their ability to provide those clients with the most appropriate help and services.

Worse yet is the research evidence that strongly suggests prevailing stereotypes are affecting clinical diagnoses and judgments. For example, Cole and Pilisuk (1976) found that blacks and Chicanos were provided psychotherapy less often than whites. Furthermore, they reported that persons from these groups were more likely to be diagnosed as psychotic or having serious illnesses than whites. Finally, they found that

white counselors frequently viewed cultural differences in clients'
behavior as pathological even when different responses may have been
realistic and adaptive to the situation.

These biased approaches to the assessment of Hispanics probably
account for the early psychiatric epidemiological studies revealing incidence of psychotic diagnoses substantially higher among ethnic minorities, especially Hispanics, compared to nonminority populations
(Gross, Knatterud, and Donner 1969 as cited by Malgady, Rogler, and
Costantino 1987). These studies failed to mention various factors that
may have contributed to the discrepant representation of psychoses,
including subject variables such as economic status.

At this time, given the availability of research, the question is no
longer *whether* counselors are personally and professionally encapsulated
and biased but *to what degree and in what ways*. Each and every human—
including professional counselors—is encapsulated by the values and
beliefs of the society and ethnicity that nurtured that individual. Once
we accept that axiom, we can turn our attention to generating and
implementing professional training and developing mechanisms that
free us from both personal and professional prejudice.

The Client

This section examines external sociocultural, sociohistorical, and environmental factors identified as highly important in the psychosocial
development of Hispanic clients. A Hispanic individual's culture, history, and experience with oppression causes variations in human behavior. Visible behavior may not mean the same to the client as it does to
the counselor in his or her worldview or perspective. Thus, this section
will look at those variables, rather than the innate variables, that influence all basic human behaviors. We do acknowledge that the accumula-
tion of evidence strongly suggests that an individual's genetic makeup,
for example, may determine a propensity to certain psychological disorders (e.g., depression, anxiety, alcoholism). We acknowledge the
genetic component in the counseling process and urge every professional to continue and extend diagnostic and evaluative attention to all
innate individual variables. This section, however, concerns the sociocultural, sociohistorical, and environmental factors that overlay the
innate individual factors influencing human behavior.

As with all clients, counselors must develop the ability to see individual Hispanic clients as products of their unique life experiences and
maintain a valid and realistic perspective on the differences between the
counselors' and the clients' cultural environments and the learning and
conditioning that result from the cultural contexts. Unfortunately, the

development of such a perspective requires an effort, since the majority of counselors have had little or no generic or specific training relative to cross-cultural counseling of racial and ethnic minorities. Without such training many counselors fail to appreciate the role culture plays in psychological development and functioning and are apt to focus solely on the presenting problem, totally failing to evaluate it within an appropriate sociocultural context.

In addition to lack of training few counselors have extensive personal and professional contact with Hispanics, and most lack timely, valid, and realistic sociocultural information about this group. The lack of awareness, training, and information often leads counselors to use stereotypical and static perspectives, resulting in the distortions and misinformation we have previously discussed.

The Hispanic client frequently does not have the opportunity to be accurately understood and effectively counseled. If the profession is to counteract this unfortunate state of affairs, counselors must seek statistical and empirically based information, interpersonal training with Hispanics, and personal experiences that provide direct and extensive contact with diverse segments of the Hispanic culture. From such a basis they can finally distinguish between stereotype and truth, bias and health, effective counseling and cultural oppression.

It is impossible to adequately address here all socioculturally relevant variables of the Hispanic; the following topics are merely representative of the multitude of factors at work in cross-cultural experiences.

Who is Hispanic? As noted earlier, statistically and demographically, the generic term *Hispanic* refers to a very large, young, rapidly growing, highly diverse and dynamic group of people. Race and ethnicity are important in the diversity among Hispanics. Depending on geographical origin (Argentina, Mexico, Puerto Rico, Venezuela, and so on), Hispanics can be Caucasian, Mongoloid, Negroid, or various combinations of these races. While Hispanics have much in common, including history, ancestry, language, and traditions, each of the numerous ethnic subgroups—Costa Ricans, Cubans, Peruvians, and others—adheres to unique and distinguishing social and cultural practices.

As is true for all races and ethnicities, further diversification results from time of immigration, whether immigration was from an urban or rural society, educational level, socioeconomic level, and region of residency within the United States. Some of these factors correlate significantly with distinct Hispanic subgroups. For example, although Hispanics generally fare quite poorly in both the economic and educational realms, Cubans and South and Central Americans are consistently higher achievers in these areas. Consequently, members of those subgroups attain higher occupational status than other Hispanics; Dominicans, Puerto Ricans, and Mexicans, conversely, are reportedly lower in these areas. Knowledge of this diversity within the Hispanic ethnic group makes obvious the errors that can result from faulty and stereotypical interpretations of a Hispanic client's socioeconomic status and educational level. Intragroup differences in socioeconomic status among Hispanics may be best understood by examining immigration and migration factors as well as the sociopolitical history of each subgroup.

Acculturation contributes to the dynamic, ever-changing aspect of the Hispanic populace. In its original and still quite acceptable definition, acculturation is a process of "those phenomena which result when groups of individuals having different cultures come into continuous firsthand contact, with subsequent changes in the original pattern of either or both groups" (Redfield, Linton, and Herskovitz 1936). Although originally perceived from the perspective of the group, acculturation occurs in both groups and individuals.

Recent studies identify facets of acculturation. It is not simple and unidirectional; its direction can be reversed; its rate can be halted, slowed, or accelerated. Viewed in the framework of the much talked about bicultural phenomenon, Malgady, Rogler, and Costantino (1987, 233) underscore this aspect of acculturation: "It is also not uncommon for acculturation to be situation specific in the sense that one may act Anglo American and speak English at work, for example, but maintain a traditional Hispanic life-style and speak Spanish at home."

A variety of factors determine the direction and rate of acculturation. Among them are changes in the racial or ethnic demographics of a community or geographical region; proximity or availability of inexpensive means of travel to the native homeland (a significant factor for Hispanics along our southern borders, for example); prevailing sociopolitical attitudes and policies (segregation policies, for example); economic conditions and practices (the means and opportunities for improving employment and economic status); and access to high-quality, advanced education. According to Szapocznik and Kurtines (1980), differentially available opportunities and the continued prevalence of traditionally prescribed gender roles cause the acculturation rate to vary by generation and gender. The rate is faster for the younger generations, and men acculturate more quickly than women.

Three major dimensions reflect acculturation: (1) language proficiency, preference, and use; (2) socioeconomic status; and (3) culture-specific attitudes and value orientations (Olmedo 1979). Although the less acculturated Hispanic may speak both Spanish and English, gain lower socioeconomic status, and adhere to attitudes and values that include a strong family orientation, personalism, idealism, and informality (characterized as a more passive and humanistic orientation toward life), the more acculturated Hispanic may no longer speak Spanish, may attain middle- or upper-class status, and may strongly adhere to majority- culture values, including individualism, pragmatism, effectiveness, efficiency, and a strong orientation toward achievement (characterized as the Protestant work ethic).

When acculturation occurs in an environment lacking relevant support networks from among family, teachers, friends, and counselors, it can and often does create conflict, stress, and loss of self-esteem as the individual struggles with an inevitable clash of values. Furthermore, acculturation, as a direct affront to ethnic identification, often affects an individual's mental health. According to Tumin and Plotch (1976), the choice to maintain important aspects of his or her sociocultural background can create a "healthy aware" individual. In contrast, Fitzpatrick (1971, 80) presents a somewhat extreme description of what a Hispanic undergoes during acculturation without support: "Frustrated and not fully accepted by the broader social world he wishes to enter, ambivalent in his attitude toward the more restricted social world to which he has ancestral rights, and beset by conflicting social standards, he develops, according to the classic conception, personality traits of insecurity, moodiness, hypersensitivity, excessive self-consciousness and nervous strain."

Acculturation contributes tremendously to the increasing diversity prevalent among Hispanic groups. Individual Hispanics can be found at different levels of the acculturative process, and the process may be more or less evident in different areas of the same individual's life, as illustrated by the apparently acculturated Hispanic in the workplace who returns to traditional values and attitudes at home. Ruiz (1981) points out that Hispanics can range from "completely Hispanic" to "completely Anglo" but most fall somewhere in between on the continuum of acculturation; consequently, it is necessary to assess the degree to which an individual Hispanic ascribes to the traditional sociocultural attributes assigned to the "typical" Hispanic. Even while acknowledging the role acculturation plays in bringing about change within the Hispanic populace, we must understand that Anglo-Americans and a significant number of Hispanics have and will continue to have different sociocultural dimensions into the foreseeable future.

Hispanics often display a great concern for immediacy and the "here and now" (as opposed to a more teleological orientation in Anglo-American culture); Hispanics frequently attribute control to an external locus (causality replaced by luck, supernatural powers, and acts of God); Hispanics favor an extended family support system (rather than a basic adherence to the nuclear family); Hispanics often take a concrete, tangible approach to life (rather than an abstract, long-term outlook); with authority figures Hispanics may practice a unilateral communication pattern that uses avoidance of eye contact, deference, and silence as signs of respect (as opposed to more self-assertive patterns); and Hispanics may develop multilingual communication skills, using English, Spanish, and "Spanglish," a hybrid of the two. Counselors must be aware of these culturally dictated traits just as they must avoid broad, all-encompassing generalizations.

Hispanic clients are not solely products of their sociocultural background, nor are they mere reflections or extrapolations of the statistically derived "average" Hispanic found in the literature. Just as there are specific sociohistorical factors that distinguish Hispanic subgroups, there are also unique sociohistorical life factors that differentiate Hispanics regardless of subgroup. These life factors play major roles in the psychosocial development and adjustment of each and every Hispanic as they do for the general populace. Such life factors can be as mundane and "normal" as family size, birth order, childhood illnesses, family mobility, family deaths, authoritarian parenting, and family overprotectiveness; they can also be as dramatic and sociopolitically generated as racism, segregation, unequal opportunities for education, unequal accessibility to health and social services, unfair employment (or unemployment) practices, and political disenfranchisement.

Through training or lack of training, counselors tend to be more or less adept at understanding and addressing mundane sociohistorical life factors. Culturally encapsulated and ignorant of the sociopolitical system of the United States in regard to its treatment of minorities and women (Sue et al. 1982), too many counselors ignore or deny the existence of the more dramatic factors listed above. Given the times and the urgency of the issues, the helping professions cannot afford this ignorance and denial. If we are to fulfill our stated purpose of providing effective and ethical services to Hispanic and other clients, we must acknowledge, learn, and understand the external stresses that unequal power, voice, and opportunity exert on members of society that are casually designated as "minorities." There is no way to understand and counsel a Hispanic client, or any client, without assessing cultural factors as well as the individual's experience of oppression.

The Counseling Process

Sociocultural, sociohistorical, and environmental factors affect the counseling process itself. The literature representative of the counseling process variables (counseling approaches and techniques) relative to counseling Hispanics presents two lines of inquiry: empirical and theoretical. Little empirically based work on counseling Hispanics has been conducted. A review of the literature of cross-cultural (pluralistic) counseling reflects the following two trends: (1) attempts to identify the particular approach, theory, or philosophy that most effectively facilitates cross-cultural counseling (Ibrahim 1985; Sue and Zane 1987; Casas 1976; Ponterrotto 1987; Suinn 1985); and (2) conceptualizations or modifications of perspectives from which to view the interaction between the individual (personality, strength of ethnic identity) and the environment (culture and race, assimilation, social support systems, etc.) (Katz 1985; Levine and Padilla 1980; Smith 1985; Ivey, Ivey, and Simek-Downing 1986).

Such trends suggest ways that the effective cross-cultural counselor can sharpen and integrate professional skills and knowledge. Ibrahim (1985), for example, identifies existential philosophy as an enhancement of cross-cultural counseling effectiveness because it honors and recognizes cultural differences as it organizes human experience in ways that reflect universal concerns of humankind. The ability and willingness to understand both one's own worldview and that of the client, Ibrahim points out, is key to *all* effective counseling, none more so than when the client and counselor differ in cultural backgrounds.

In a similar vein, Ivey, Ivey, and Simek-Downing (1986) stress the importance of *cultural empathy* to the *intentional* counselor. The authors define the empathic counselor as one who has the capacity to understand many individuals who are vastly different from the couselor and who also has the ability to generate a maximum number of thoughts, words, and behaviors to communicate with a variety of diverse groups inside and outside the counselor's culture.

Casas (1976), Bouletter (1976), Ruiz and Casas (1981) identify the behavioral approach as more appropriate for many ethnic minority groups, including Mexican Americans. The behavioral approach has an environmental focus: most behavioral interventions typically involve activating (empowering) the client's role in the environment as well as changing the environment. These interventions focus on skill building and move away from the "blaming the victim" tone inherent in some insight-oriented therapies.

While acknowledging that the behavioral approach is successful in adapting culturally relevant characteristics, other writers suggest that various theoretical orientations and approaches may be appropriate. The key ingredient to successful cross-cultural counseling, according to this group, is the ability to combine respectful understanding of the cultural differences of behaviors, thoughts, and feelings with an informed understanding of the sociopolitical and economic issues relevant to a particular group.

Suinn (1985), for example, suggests that we think more seriously about how the three traditional major approaches to intervention (psychodynamic, humanistic, and behavioral) relate to cross-cultural considerations. Citing evidence that some existing theories do recognize cultural variables, he proposes the notion of reorienting existing concepts. Some of the concepts he believes need review and revision include:

1. Recognition of general intrapsychic variables as opposed to acceptance of culture as a real variable in the assessment process. This is cited as an agreement with Smith and Vasquez (1985).
2. Role definitions of counselor and client in each major theory and their match or mismatch with the client's cultural system. As examples he cites the possibility that an Asian-American client might be initially reassured by the counselor as expert (psychodynamic approaches), but a black client might be initially resentful of the same approach, seeing it as a superior-inferior interaction.
3. The rationale given by counselors to clients about how change is brought about in the counseling process. Suinn suggests that such process rationales may be in direct conflict with clients' cultural values. The humanistic-existential orientation, with its focus on the individual as essential for progress, could be disruptive rather than supportive for the ethnic minority whose family, community, or tribe comes before the self. Likewise, the psychodynamic orientations that require verbal self-disclosure and expression of feelings and insights may conflict with the values of Asian-American and Hispanic cultures according to other authors.
4. Certain universal meanings given to words, actions, and events by the traditional approaches (especially psychodynamic and behavioral). In the interpretation of dreams, for example, Suinn suggests that a pig would not necessarily have the same symbolic association to both an Occidental and an Asian born in the Year of the Boar. Likewise, the interview behavior of "lack of eye contact" may have different significance for an Anglo student and a Hispanic student. Suinn thus provides examples of needed modifications of the three major approaches for use with Hispanic clients.

Ponterotto (1987) recommends a multimodal approach, suggesting that such a model has the flexibility to be adapted to the tremendous intracultural diversity of Hispanics. He recommends this approach since it is comprehensive, attending to behavior, affect, sensations, images, cognitions, interpersonal relations, and biological (drugs/diet) functioning. This approach, he contends, enhances the probability of behavioral change and can include factors that are external (i.e., social, environmental, institutional) to the Hispanic client's control. He does emphasize the importance of assessing degree of acculturation.

Levine and Padilla (1980) suggest that a therapeutic approach in pluralistic counseling (which recognizes the client's culturally based beliefs, values, and behaviors and which is concerned with the client's adaptation to his or her particular cultural milieu) should focus on the interaction of both individual and cultural dynamics. They stress the importance of a counselor's assumptions about the interaction of culture and the individual, as these affect goal setting in therapy.

In addressing the universality versus cultural aspects of mental health and maladjustment, Levine and Padilla (1980, 10) provide a succinct and helpful statement: "Mental health involves a realistic acceptance of self, a clear perception of the world, open relationships with others, and the ability to handle stress and crisis. The overall processes of mental health and maladjustment are universal attributes of culture. The specific events creating stress and the behavior manifestations of disturbances are culturally defined."

Indeed, the unique life experiences of ethnic minorities have high potential for stressful psychological consequences. Smith (1985) proposes a model of the life stress process for ethnic minorities, identifying the various types of life stresses that ethnic minorities experience, such as out-group status, social isolation, marginal social status, and status inconsistency. She presents several hypotheses to describe the situation of members of ethnic minority groups as well as a model for counseling members of ethnic minority groups.

A theme in the models and approaches described thus far stresses the importance of cultural knowledge and awareness of the sociohistorical and political reality of members of ethnic minority groups. The purpose of cultural and sociopolitical knowledge in counseling is to promote understanding and prevent error in diagnosis. Behavior that may be interpreted in one way may be perceived or interpreted differently if one understands relevant cultural values, norms, and behaviors as well as the unique stresses that ethnic minorities face. Regardless of theoretical orientation, the effective and ethical counselor must assess which aspects of that orientation may result in colluding with the unhealthy dynamics of oppression (such as blaming the victim by presenting certain interpretations of psychodynamic formulations).

Knowledge of the historical status of women and ethnic minorities, especially Hispanics, in the sociopolitical system in the United States is crucial. This implies understanding racism and sexism, including one's own beliefs and attitudes and how those may be problematic. In working with indigent people, we must ask ourselves whether we see behavior as stemming more from unconscious motivation or from elements in the environmental class structure.

In addition to using culturally sensitive or modified approaches to counseling and therapy with Hispanics, counselors must use other frameworks and approaches beyond the traditional one-to-one model.

We propose the incorporation of *preventive* and *developmental* interventions as alternative options in enhancing the quality of life for Hispanic groups.

Preventive interventions may be defined as those that "present or forestall onset of problems or needs through anticipation of the consequence of non-action" (Drum and Lawler, in press). Various theoretical models have been developed incorporating preventive interventions in school psychology, industrial organizational psychology, community psychology, and in counseling psychology. Many aspects of consultation theories (Gallessich 1980) and the environmental adjustment, ecosystems theories and models from the student development field are preventive in nature (Banning 1980; Morrill, Oetting, and Hurst 1974). Preventive environmental interventions to forestall problems for ethnic minorities are many and varied. Examples include development of national, state, and local policy and law that affect the mental health and general well-being of ethnic minority individuals. On college campuses, increasing the number of ethnic minority faculty and staff is an attempt to improve the collegiate environment, and it is also important in recruiting and retaining ethnic minority students.

Preventive interventions are unique in that they help anticipate, forestall, and prevent problems; have an impact before a person needs help; occur more often in stand-alone format; use both active and passive change strategies; have a less complex change methodology; and are more private (Drum and Lawler, in press).

Preventive interventions require some degree of commitment to enhancing the lives of others through management of the milieu. Such a commitment is an aspect of social responsibility that an effective cross-cultural counselor should reaffirm and embrace.

Developmental interventions facilitate "normal development by adding new skills or dimensions or by providing strategies for resolution of critical issues" (Drum and Lawler, in press). Drum and Lawler further describe developmental interventions as similar to preventive in that both are highly preplanned; focus on a single issue; seek to raise consciousness and to educate; and require a high degree of leader expertise. Developmental interventions are different in that they empower through acquisition or enhancement of critical life skills; assist after the need for help arises; occur more often in workshops or group settings; use mostly active change strategies; possess a more complex change methodology; and are less private.

Widick, Knefelkamp, and Parker (1980) identify five clusters of theories to describe development, including psychosocial theories, cognitive development theories, maturity models, typology models, and person-environment models. Most of the applications of developmental theory in counseling psychology focus on the critical issue of career development among university students. The theory, methods, and technology of developmental interventions provide the most room to grow and to contribute to professional practice in a unique manner. Drum and Lawler (in press) contend that most adult problems originate not in serious, underlying pathology but in the far simpler and more common short-circuiting of normal developmental processes. Critical issues such as aging (midlife, geriatric), grief from loss, failure, and relationship problems are common but may lead to crises if individuals do not understand or have the skills to cope with such experiences. Drum and Lawler have developed a detailed, step-by-step guide to designing developmental interventions that provides some techniques to apply to many of those critical life issues.

Ethnic minority populations have problems with many of the same critical issues as does the majority population, but often a given, common problem may have additional complications. Cultural values and norms as well as unique stresses are additional factors to consider in planning and implementing developmental interventions for Hispanic populations.

For example, one would expect most older students who return to school for graduate or other training to experience several adjustments, for example, loss of income, change of status, need for new academic skills. A Hispanic female may experience the additional stresses of conflict about commitment to children, partner, or family of origin. The positive valuation of family and relationships can be a source of guilt and frustration when a rigorous study schedule monopolizes time. Encountering negative and at times discriminatory attitudes from peers and faculty provides additional stress. Well-meaning faculty may express doubts about the Hispanic woman's ability to succeed. A peer may express resentment to the recipient of a minority fellowship or affirmative action policy. Such experiences are (unfortunately) predictable for the older Hispanic woman who chooses to pursue higher education. Workshops, support groups, or materials could be designed to provide direction for confronting such challenges.

Drum and Lawler (in press) define personal development as a subtle process that occurs slowly as individuals acquire new skills, learn to respond more effectively, learn ways to reduce inner conflict, and through all this gain a sense of self. They identify four components of personal development intervention: (1) a deliberate plan for directing self-inquiry; (2) the transmission of accurate and timely information; (3) a problem-solving strategy; and (4) the proper sequencing of these elements into a low resistance-generating treatment plan. Interventions may include informational materials, workshops, and groups.

An example of such an intervention for ethnic minorities is the development of a brochure for ethnic minority students on campus, *Making the Most Out of College* (Minority Student Program Development Committee 1986), designed to provide information about developmental issues faced uniquely by that group. The brochure identifies potential challenges for minority students, such as being among the first members of their family or ethnic community to attend college; seeing few other members of their ethnic or minority group on campus; and wanting to prove themselves worthy of attending school. It also identifies numerous important issues that may "contribute to uncomfortable feelings," such as dating, sexuality, religious and spiritual values, exploring career life plans, political and social action, developing a personal and unique identity, acceptance of diverse people and their values. Suggestions for action are provided, including the challenge to retain and enhance one's ethnic and cultural identity, finding role models and mentors, and using student services and campus resources.

Designing and providing workshops and group experiences for special populations is another means of developmental intervention. An empowerment and entitlement workshop for Hispanic women, for example, could emphasize attitudes and beliefs regarding second-class status and the rights to a quality life; development of assertiveness skills to deal with discriminatory and other difficult attitudes; and provision of social support in handling relationship problems. Development of such an intervention requires knowledge of the technology in developing such an intervention and knowledge of the population, including critical issues addressed in this chapter.

The strength of developmental interventions is their potential to prevent more serious deterioration of individual behavior or coping skills because of the ineffective resolution of everyday challenges. They teach critical skills and can support the acquisition of satisfaction in life.

Summary

The increase in the number of mental health–related journal articles, chapters, and books on Hispanic Americans in response to changing demographics is an important step toward improving counseling services for Hispanics. However, a framework to enable the reader to determine the relative importance of the information vis-à-vis the total dynamic counseling process would enhance the value of the literature. Specifically, the framework should promote better understanding, accurate evaluation, and more effective and appropriate use of the information the literature provides.

This chapter proposed a framework of categorical variables along a continuum from those variables more distal to the counseling process progressing toward those more proximal to the process. The variables include counselor, client, and counseling process. Among the counselor variables attention was selectively directed to professional and personal attitudes and beliefs that strongly affect the counseling of Hispanics. In the client variables category the identification of individual, sociocultural, sociohistorical, and environmental variables that must be understood and considered within the counseling process was emphasized. Finally, in the counseling process category an effort was made to examine the way varied counseling approaches use or misuse the sociocultural, sociohistorical, and environmental milieu that creates the Hispanic client. Within the framework the categories and variables ascribed to each category are nonexhaustive. Other categories representing relevant topics in the literature, such as training and counseling techniques, could fit into the proposed framework. Given time and space limits, however, the authors chose those categories and variables that best serve to sensitize and stimulate thought and promote movement toward improving the quality of counseling for Hispanics.

References

Banning, J. 1980. The campus ecology manager role. In U. Delworth and G. Hanson (eds.), *Student services: A handbook for the profession.* San Francisco: Jossey-Bass.

Boulette, R. R. 1976. Assertive training with low income Mexican-American women. In M. R. Miranda (ed.), *Psychotherapy with the Spanish speaking: Issues in research and service delivery,* 67–71. Los Angeles: Spanish-Speaking Mental Health Research Center.

Carter, T. P., and Segura, R. D. 1979. *Mexican Americans in school: A decade of change.* Princeton, NJ: College Entrance Examination Board.

Casas, J. M. 1976. Applicability of a behavioral model in serving the mental health needs of the Mexican American. In M. R. Miranda (ed.), *Psychotherapy with the Spanish speaking: Issues in research and service delivery,* 61–65. Los Angeles: Spanish-Speaking Mental Health Research Center.

———. 1984. Policy, training, and research in counseling psychology: The racial/ethnic minority perspective. In S. D. Brown and R. W. Lent (eds.), *Handbook of counseling psychology.* New York: John Wiley and Sons.

Cole, J., and Pilisuk, M. 1976. Differences in the provision of mental health services by race. *American Journal of Orthopsychiatry* 46:510–525.

Drum, D. J., and Lawler, A. C. In press. *Developmental interventions: Theories, principles and techniques.* Columbus: Charles Merrill.

Duran, R. P. 1983. *Hispanics' education and background.* New York: College Entrance Examination Board.

Fitzpatrick, J. P. 1971. *Puerto Rican Americans.* Englewood Cliffs, NJ: Prentice-Hall.

Ford Foundation. 1984. *Hispanics: Challenges and opportunities.* New York: Ford Foundation.

Gallessich, J. 1980. Consultation. In U. Delworth and G. Hanson (eds.), *Student services: A handbook for the profession.* San Francisco: Jossey-Bass.

Gross, H., Knatterud, G., and Donner, L. 1969. The effect of race and sex on the variation of diagnosis and disposition in the psychiatric emergency room. *Journal of Nervous and Mental Diseases* 148:638–642.

Halleck, S. L. 1971. Therapy is the handmaiden of the status quo. *Psychology Today* 4:30–34, 98–100.

Ibrahim, F. A. 1985. Effective cross-cultural counseling and psychotherapy: A framework. *Counseling Psychologist* 13 (4): 625–638.

Ivey, A. E., Ivey, M. B., and Simek-Downing, L. 1986. *Counseling and psychotherapy: Integrating skills, theory and practice,* 97–105. Englewood Cliffs, NJ: Prentice-Hall.

Katz, J. H. 1985. The sociopolitical nature of counseling. *Counseling Psychologist* 13:615–624.

Korchin, S. J. 1980. Clinical psychology and minority problems. *American Psychologist* 35:262–269.

Levine, E. S., and Padilla, A. M. 1980. *Crossing cultures in therapy: Pluralistic counseling for the Hispanic.* Monterey, CA: Brooks-Cole.

Malgady, R. G., Rogler, L. H., and Costantino, G. 1987. Ethnocultural and linguistic bias in mental health evaluation of Hispanics. *American Psychologist* 42:228–234.

Minority Student Program Development Committee. 1986. *Making the most out of college: A guide for the minority student.* Counseling Learning and Career Services, University of Texas, Austin.

Morrill, W. H., Oetting, E. P., and Hurst, J. C. 1974. Dimensions of counselor functioning. *Personnel and Guidance Journal* 52 (6).

National Commission on Secondary Schooling for Hispanics. 1984. *Make something happen: Hispanics and urban high school reform.* Vol. 1. Washington, DC: National Commission on Secondary Schooling for Hispanics.

Olmedo, E. L. 1979. Acculturation: A psychometric perspective. *American Psychologist* 34:1061–1070.

Pedersen, P. B. 1987. Ten frequent assumptions of cultural bias in counseling. *Journal of Multicultural Counseling and Development* 15:16–24.

Ponterotto, J. G. 1987. Counseling Mexican Americans: A multi-modal approach. *Journal of Counseling and Development* 65 (6): 308–312.

Redfield, R., Linton, R., and Herskovitz, M. J. 1936. Memorandum for the study of acculturation. *American Anthropologist* 38:149–152.

Ruiz, R. A. 1981. Cultural and historical perspectives in counseling Hispanics. In D. W. Sue (ed.), *Counseling the culturally different: Theory and practice,* 186–215. New York: John Wiley and Sons.

Ruiz, R. A., and Casas, J. M. 1981. Culturally relevant behavioristic counseling for Chicano college students. In P. B. Pedersen, J. G. Draguns, W. J. Lonner, and J. E. Trimble (eds.), *Counseling across cultures,* 181–202. Honolulu: University of Hawaii Press.

Sherif, C. W. 1982. Needed concepts in the study of gender identity. *Psychology of Women Quarterly* 6 (4): 375–398.

Smith, E. M. J. 1985. Ethnic minorities: Life stress, social support, and mental health issues. *Counseling Psychologist* 13 (4): 537–580.

Smith, E. M. J., and Vasquez, M. J. T. 1985. Introduction. *Counseling Psychologist* 13 (4): 531–536.

Sue, D. W. 1981. *Counseling the culturally different: Theory and practice.* New York: John Wiley and Sons.

Sue, D. W., Bernier, J. E., Durran, A., Feinberg, L., Pedersen, P. B., Smith, E. J., and Vasquez-Nuttall, E. 1982. Position papers: Cross-cultural counseling competencies. *Counseling Psychologist* 10 (2): 45–52.

Sue, S., and Zane, N. 1987. The role of culture and cultural techniques in psychotherapy: A critique and reformulation. *American Psychologist* 42 (1): 37–45.

Suinn, R. M. 1985. Research and practice in cross-cultural counseling. *Counseling Psychologist* 13 (4): 673–684.

Sundberg, N. D. 1981. Cross-cultural counseling and psychotherapy: A research overview. In A. J. Marsella and P. B. Pedersen (eds.), *Cross-cultural counseling and psychotherapy: Foundations, evaluation, and cultural considerations.* New York: Pergamon Press.

Szapocznik, J., and Kurtines, W. 1980. Acculturation, biculturalism, and adjustment among Cuban-Americans. In A. M. Padilla (ed.), *Recent advances in acculturation research: Theory, models, and some new findings, 914–931.* Boulder, CO: Westview Press.

Szasz, T. S. 1974. *The myth of mental illness.* New York: Harper and Row.

Tumin, M., and Plotch, W., eds. 1976. *Pluralism in a democratic society.* New York: Praeger.

U.S. Bureau of the Census. 1985. Current population report: Persons of Spanish origin in the United States. Series P-20, No. 403. Washington, DC: Government Printing Office.

Wampold, B. E., Casas, J. M., and Atkinson, D. R. 1981. Ethnic bias in counseling: An information processing approach. *Journal of Counseling Psychology* 28:498–503.

Widick, C., Knefelkamp, L., and Parker, C. A. 1980. Student development. In U. Delworth and G. Hanson (eds.), *Student services: A handbook for the profession.* San Francisco: Jossey-Bass.

Woolf, H. B., ed. 1980. *Webster's new collegiate dictionary.* Springfield, MA: GNC Merriam.

Wrenn, C. G. 1962. The culturally encapsulated counselor. *Harvard Educational Review* 32:444–449.

8

Providing Counseling Services for Native American Indians: Client, Counselor, and Community Characteristics

JOSEPH E. TRIMBLE
AND CANDACE M. FLEMING

It's not a pleasant article to read. In the beginning our curiosity increases as the story about the "psychotic" Navajo male unfolds. The author, Douglas Jewel (1952), takes us through an 11-month ordeal detailing the circumstances leading to an eventual diagnosis of catatonic schizophrenia. Then, without much warning, we discover that the main problem, if indeed there was a "problem," was one of misunderstanding between the clinical staff and the "patient"—no one at the hospital could recognize that the young male Navajo was speaking his indigenous language! As an afterthought Jewel emphasizes the need for practitioners to become more sensitive to the covert personality dynamics of their patients.

The theme is not new. Pioneer anthropologists such as Franz Boas, Bronislaw Malinowski, and William Sumner reminded us of the importance of introducing strict controls to prevent ethnocentric interpretation. The recent development of "discovery procedures" by linguists is a notable example of how we can approach the study of everyday human activities (Werner and Schoepfle 1987). Moreover, ethnographers are ever mindful that "any explanation of behavior which excludes what the actors themselves know, how they define their actions, remains a partial explanation that distorts the human situation" (Spradley 1979, 13).

Distortions of the human situation are frequent enough in everyday interpersonal exchanges, and when we encounter people from unique cultural backgrounds the distortions increase. For many American Indian clients interpersonal and interethnic problems can emerge because a counselor's lack of experience and knowledge, deeply held stereotypes, and preconceived notions can interfere with the counseling relationship and thwart counseling effectiveness. Yet ample evidence is available that a counselor can use to promote trust and improve the

177

counselor-client relationship both in general and with American Indian clients. Matters relating to trust and other counseling considerations form the basis of this chapter and provide information that could stimulate effective cross-cultural counseling contacts with America's indigenous population, the Native American Indian.

Who Are Native American Indians?

To appreciate the complexity of providing counseling services to Indians, it would be instructive to describe the extraordinary diversity that exists among America's native population. Within the past few decades psychiatrists, psychologists, and social workers have devoted considerable attention to psychosocial correlates of the behavior and personality of the first Americans. Kelso and Attneave (1981) compiled 1,360 articles on Indian mental health topics, and Mail and McDonald (1980) list 969 citations dealing exclusively with alcoholism among Indians. A review of the citations from both bibliographic sources reveals that the vast majority refer to Indians in a generic, collective manner and give little attention to the heterogeneity of Indians.

It is difficult to identify the reasoning behind the tendency for social scientists and the public as a whole to view Indians in a collective manner. Certainly a guilty finger could be pointed in the direction of the anthropological school of culture and personality. The school emphasized the effects of cultural lifestyles of a particular indigenous group on the emergence of distinctive personality styles. Information was typically gathered on a tribe's customs and patterns of living and then used to infer the existence of a prevailing collective character. Benedict's research on the Pueblo groups of the southwestern United States and the Kwakiutl of Vancouver Island in the Pacific Northwest are illustrative. Using the Nietzschean concepts Apollonian and Dionysian, Benedict reported, "They (the Kwakiutl) valued all violent experience, all means by which human beings may break through the usual sensory routine, and to all such experiences they attributed the highest value" (1959, 80). Benedict referred to the Indians of the Northwest Coast as Dionysian even though she admits that "they had a culture of no common order" (1959, 173). To an extent the "collective grouping effect" persists especially in comparative research in which we find study after study contrasting Indians with whites, blacks, Hispanics, Asian Americans, and other Indian groups. Descriptions of the respective sample populations are usually stated in global terms without comment on the enormous amount of variability particular to the group in question.

As most scholars know, the term American Indian is an imposed ethnic category with little relevant meaning. At best it is a generalized gloss in the beginning foisted upon the Arawak, a now extinct tribe once indigenous to islands off the southeastern coast of the United States, by a wayward Italian sailor who thought he had reached India. Somehow, and no one is really certain why, the category continued to be used to the extent that almost all indigenous, native people of the Western hemisphere are referred to as Indians. We hear and see everywhere—Canadian Indians, Mexican Indians, Indians of Central America, Brazilian Indians, Indians of the Central Plains. For better or worse the term has become institutionalized and even accepted by the native people themselves.

Within the past decade or so efforts to replace the term "American Indian" with "Native American" were initiated by Indian activist groups and conscientious liberal sympathizers. The effort died rather suddenly when Indian political groups such as the National Congress of American Indians and the National Tribal Chairman's Association recognized that many descendants of early colonists could consider themselves native also since their families had been in America for about 400 years. In the state of Alaska indigenous peoples are referred to as Alaska Natives, and nonindigenous folks are Native Alaskans—the distinction is clear, and most abide by the encompassing categories.

Definitional Criteria

The American Indian and Alaska Native have a unique relationship with the federal government of the United States. The relationship and the social, cultural, and political diversity of the Indian led the U.S. Congress to formulate a legal definition of the indigenous American. The legal definition enabled government agencies, principally the Bureau of Indian Affairs (BIA), to determine if an individual claiming to be Indian in fact is entitled to government services. Basically, the BIA defines an Indian as someone who is (1) an enrolled or registered member of a federally recognized Indian tribe, or (2) at least one-fourth Indian or more in blood quantum and can legally demonstrate that fact to BIA officials.

The legal definition concept was first set forth in the Curtis Act of 1898, through which the BIA had to authorize land allotments to members of the Five Civilized Tribes of Oklahoma. Since then the legal definition has undergone few revisions. Nonetheless, many tribes have established their own blood quantum criteria. Among a few tribes it is whatever can be proved; among certain tribes in the western part of the United States it is more than one-half. Intermarriage has been largely responsible for eroding the question of Indianness. As a consequence it has been estimated that between 10 million and 20 million people in the United States have some Indian blood (Taylor 1984).

Svensson (1973, 9) asserts that "Indianness is a state of being, a cast of mind, a relationship to the Universe. It is undefinable." In a report filed in 1982 to the U.S. Department of Education (DOE), the authors concluded that the "term Indian has no *singular* meaning" (U.S. Dept. of Ed. 1982). Yet despite the agreement on the elusiveness of the definition, the government and the public persist in claiming to know who an Indian is. The BIA and the tribes have their own definitions, and the U.S. Bureau of the Census and the DOE have yet others. The Bureau of the Census definition is self-enumerative; if a person indicates that he or she is an Indian on the census form then the bureau accepts that declaration as sufficient. Consequently, the Bureau of the Census now recognizes more than 500 tribes and 187 Indian languages—far more than recognized by the BIA. The DOE has a slightly more rigid definition that parallels closely the one used by the BIA, but which allows someone to be counted if he or she is a descendant of anyone who was at one time a member of a tribe.

Population counts generated by the various definitions produce such a skewed pattern that the DOE was compelled to investigate Indian enrollment in many of the nation's public schools. As reported in a DOE document, "the Federal government took a number of steps calculated to heighten or validate racial or ethnic self-awareness and our evidence shows there were substantial shifts in the population toward Indian identification" (U.S. Dept. of Ed. 1982, 62).

The American Indian is the *only* ethnic group residing in the United States that has been legally defined. Many Indians and non-Indians, however, simply refuse to accept the criteria. For many non-Indians an Indian must resemble a historical image, one frozen in the past and in archives—the noble, proud warrior worshiping nature's mysteries. For others an Indian is only an Indian if he or she is a full-blood.

Even though a generalized set of definitions exists, there are colloquial efforts to promote further clarification of one's ethnic origins. American Indians constitute an extremely diverse and complicated ethnic group. As stated earlier, according to the 1980 U.S. census there are close to 1.6 million Indians, which is considerably less than 1% of a national population of over 235 million people. There may be many more since many Indians either refuse to participate in the census or do not want to be identified as such for a multitude of personal and social reasons. There are well over 450 identifiable tribal units with some having as few as four or five remaining members.

The diversity is compounded by the fact that greater than 60% are of mixed background, the result of intermarriages among blacks, whites, and Hispanic populations. Many "breeds," or people of mixed marriages, are not considered "ethnically pure" by some Indians and non-Indians alike and hence are not viewed as characteristically Indian in terms of knowledge of traditional mores and folkways. Of course, this assumption is blatantly fallacious as many "breeds" are often much more "native oriented" than many so-called pure Indians—blood quantum is certainly not an accurate gauge of one's ethnic affiliation and knowledge of traditional lifeways.

American Indians represent a range of orientation from fully traditional to fully acculturated. English is a second language for many, but proficiency in English *and* the tribal dialect is also prevalent. Berry, Trimble, and Olmedo (1986) point out that individuals vary in their degree of acculturation and that "not only will groups and individuals vary in their participation and response to acculturative influences, some domains of culture and behavior may become altered without comparable changes in other domains" (1986, 297).

Demographic Patterns

Actual counts of the numbers of natives residing in North America at the time of Columbus' alleged discovery vary. Estimates range from as few as 800,000 to as many as 9,000,000. Josephy (1968) points out that Indians were speaking no less than 2,200 different languages and dialects and in addition some 200 languages were mutually unintelligible. In appearance there were and are some similarities: hair and eye color, dental patterns, amount of body and facial hair, and skin tone are the most distinguishable. There is evidence, however, of a subband of the Mandan-Hidatsa, in which blue eyes, blonde and brown hair, and a light skin tone were prevalent. Today largely because of intermarriage with whites and blacks, the physical characteristics of Indians have changed dramatically.

After Columbus the native population was reduced considerably. Josephy (1968, 278) remarked, "No one will ever know how many Indians or how many tribes were enslaved, tortured, debauched and killed." Diseases unknown to most Indians, such as smallpox, measles, diphtheria, and typhoid fever, led to the deaths of thousands. About 1837 the Mandan tribe of the Dakotas was all but exterminated by a smallpox epidemic; no one knows how many bands from other tribes suffered a similar fate. The devastation and destruction of a 350-year period reduced the Indian population to about 250,000 in 1850. People were talking then about the "vanishing American" and the complete submission of the rebellious "savage."

The Indian population increased slowly to approximately 650,000 in 1960. The growth spurt since then has been quite dramatic as demonstrated in the 1980 figure of slightly over 1.5 million.

Slightly more than half of the present-day Indians reside in urban and metropolitan areas. California has the largest Indian population

(201,000), followed by Oklahoma (170,000), Arizona (153,000), and New Mexico (105,000). The Navajo, who reside on a New Mexico and Arizona reservation comparable in size to West Virginia, is the largest tribe, with over 110,000 members. Numerous tribes have as few as five members, and some may even have only one remaining survivor.

With all of this social, cultural, and psychological diversity, what can a counselor do to provide effective and culturally sensitive mental health services to Indians? Is there a common set of procedures and tactics available that are known to be effective? What does a conventionally trained counselor need to know about facilitating positive relationships with Indian clients? Many counselors have been unsuccessful with Indian clients and not because of their lack of effort and concern. Something was lacking—either the counselor lacked basic knowledge about the client's ethnic background or the counseling style was inappropriate, or a combination of the two interfered, causing the client to decide not to cooperate.

In the past decade a number of Indians and non-Indians have published articles related directly or indirectly to providing counseling services to Indians. Some of the writing is research based; however, most of the content is based on counselors' firsthand experiences with Indian clients. Many of the counselors appear to be providing similar recommendations, which suggests they had some degree of success with their Indian clients. In the following section a summary review of those writings is presented and organized around central counseling-related themes: mental health conditions, the nature of Indian communities, counselor characteristics, client characteristics, values, counseling styles, and the role of the shaman in providing mental health services.

Mental Health Issues

It is important to understand that the indigenous American always had experiences that could well be included under the general category of mental health; depression, feelings of hopelessness and powerlessness, acute and chronic anxiety, hallucinations, chronic and acute phobias are but a few of these likely expressions of thought, emotion, and behavior.

The influx of civilization fostered by colonialism, government control and regulations, forced isolation, and the constant harassment fueled by bigotry and racism enhanced if not accelerated the growth of Indian mental health problems. When the introduction of alcohol and, most recently, psychoactive drugs are added to these factors, we find, not surprisingly, that mental health has become a major concern of most Indian communities.

Indigenous Americans always had formal and informal systems for dealing with mental health problems. Many of those systems persist to this day despite efforts on the part of missionaries and government agents to eliminate them and replace them with supposedly more refined and sophisticated approaches. Manson and Trimble (1982) describe the kinds of mental health services provided to Indians through private agencies and practitioners, county and state agencies, community mental health centers, the Bureau of Indian Affairs, the Indian Health Service, urban Indian health programs, and tribal health departments (cf. McShane 1987). Following their description, the authors present a series of questions intended to stimulate future research and development in Indian mental health.

The mental health services provided through the Indian Health Service extend to about 500,000 Indians. According to Beiser and Attneave, the service seems to be working and "reflects the quip so often encountered . . . 'Mental Health for Indians: they surely need it. It's about time somebody did something' " (1978, 10). Yet counselors working out of community mental health centers are quick to point out that Indians tend to underutilize services, are likely to have a higher dropout rate than other ethnic minorities, and are less likely to respond to treatment than other groups (Sue, Allen, and Conaway 1978). Barter and Barter (1974) argue that many urban Indians sense that the services are not really responsive to their unique needs. Schoenfeld, Lyerly, and Miller (1971) and Manson and Trimble (1982) reason that Indians believe that negatively held images of non-Indian counselors also contribute to underutilization. Fear, mistrust, and counselor insensitivity can also contribute to underuse (Dukepoo 1980; Cooley, Ostendorf, and Bickerton 1979). Differences in value orientations between Indian clients and non-Indian counselors and different beliefs about the etiology of mental health problems also are thought to be part of the problem (Trimble 1981; Trimble et al. 1984; Dinges, Trimble, and Hollenbeck 1981; Red Horse et al. 1978). It would appear that underuse in certain settings is likely to persist. Counselors have to assume a major share of the responsibility in reducing underutilization.

Nature of Indian Communities

If we examine the history of Indian-white relations over the past 400 years, the reasons for the fear and mistrust of mental health practitioners would quickly become evident. Attneave (1985) and Richardson (1981) provide a nice overview of the conditions and policies that have influenced Indian perceptions of mental health settings. A large part of the distrust derives from the many misunderstandings created about a culture that is seemingly ever dependent on the government for services and the providers who are "contracted" to do so. In many cases the

Indian client and local Indian communities have no sense of ownership in the service unit or community center and thus tend to view it as one more enterprise foisted upon them to meet their needs.

Ayres (1977) points out that the geographic isolation of many Indian communities leads to high unemployment, lack of self-confidence, and a distrust of anything that is non-Indian. Access to the welfare system and mental health services is almost prohibitive because many residents prefer to remain on their own lands.

Many writers of the American Indian condition are prone to emphasizing the group and collective orientation as both a strength and a bane to progress. Edwards and Edwards (1984) strongly emphasize the inherent psychosocial differences among Indians, yet despite the differences distinct non-Indian characteristics are evident. For many, ego strength is maintained through identification with the tribe "back home" from which they derive support through customs, values, beliefs, and familial ties. The need for identification may be so strong that a would-be Indian client might refuse help in a non-Indian setting in favor of traveling hundreds of miles to return home just to affiliate with friends and kin who provide help and assistance in an informal, culturally specific manner.

Like many ethnic enclaves Indian communities are fairly intact and operate as quite rigid ecosystems. In describing such communities, Trimble and Hayes (1984) include those elements that reflect the physical and environmental settings, sociocultural characteristics, individual characteristics, and variations in cultural orientations. "Just as every person's life history provides important information for a mental health worker," the authors maintain, "the history of a reservation community provides valuable insights in to past and existing physical and psychosocial conditions" (1984, 307). Knowledge of the nature and history of Indian communities is therefore essential to counseling effectiveness. "The 'newcomer,' 'outsider,' 'stranger,' 'white' who attempted to ask questions without preliminary contacts, agreements, and approvals would find closed doors and, most likely, uncooperative and suspicious persons" (Trimble and Hayes 1984, 307). Knowledge of the community and an understanding of the counselor's role as perceived by the residents may well take a year to unfold. In the course of that development a mutual awareness materializes, and if respected, trust may be a by-product.

Characteristics of Counselors

Certain critics of the counseling process often would want us to believe that a counselor must abandon conventional styles and wisdom to be effective with the culturally different client. Not only is this advice ill conceived, it is foolish. We must be mindful of the fact that in many ways the traditional providers of mental health services—shamans, spirit healers, medicine people, friends, and kin—have personal characteristics that promote healing. Torrey (1986) reminds us that "witch doctors" and psychiatrists have a great deal in common despite differences in their approaches. The similarities have to do with the healer's personal characteristics.

Although there is little empirical evidence to support the following thesis, the traditional providers of helping services in Indian communities most likely exemplify empathy, genuineness, availability, respect, warmth, congruence, and concreteness—characteristics that are likely to be effective in therapeutically treating anyone regardless of theoretical orientation or counseling style. It would be safe to conclude that effective counseling with Indians begins when a counselor carefully attends to these basic characteristics.

A number of counselors have identified other factors that if heeded could improve effectiveness. Building trust and nurturing trustworthiness are highly correlated with client self-disclosure. LaFromboise and Dixon (1981) found that Indian students clearly rated simulated interviews more positively when counselors, regardless of their own ethnicity, enacted trustworthy roles. Trustworthiness appeared to be enhanced when counselors used culturally appropriate communicative styles and trust behaviors. In a similar vein, Bransford (1982) pointed out that the counselor's perceived expertise, attractiveness, and avowed respect for the Indians' culture are likely to improve effectiveness by contributing to rapport building. Trimble and Hayes (1984) echo the findings and place a strong emphasis on the counselor's knowledge and awareness of the Indian's cultural legacy and the historical and present-day influences that could be shaping the client's life.

Bransford (1982), Haviland et al. (1983), and Dauphinais, Dauphinais, and Rowe (1981) are but a few who argue that counselors of Indian ancestry are more likely to be effective than non-Indian counselors. Haviland et al. (1983) added that Indian clients also prefer same sex counselors. Subjects who participated in their study indicated, however, that they would probably pursue counseling even if the counselor was not their first choice.

Other writers disagree with this finding although not completely. Dinges et al. (1981) recognized that counselor-client matching along ethnic lines is important and likely promotes faster rapport. Nonetheless, perceived effectiveness (i.e., warmth, genuineness, respect, empathy, etc.) is more likely to sustain a relationship.

In an interesting line of research Littrell and Littrell (1983) examined nonverbal cues by non-Indian counselors. The authors explored the effect that nonverbal cues, as depicted by a counselor's clothing, had on perceived empathy, warmth, genuineness, and concreteness. Indian subjects rated casual clothing as less indicative of empathy, warmth, and genuineness than did Caucasian subjects. Given the results, the authors suggest that counselors dress and present themselves in a fashion consistent with the values certain Indian groups are likely to hold about authority figures and those in responsible positions. "Dressing down," therefore, could influence the way an Indian client responds to a counselor's attempts to convey a sense of empathy and warmth. The client may interpret the nonverbal cues as expressed in casual clothing styles as indicative of a person who really does not deserve a show of respect.

LaFromboise, Dauphinais, and Rowe (1980) surveyed a number of Oklahoma Indian students on their attitudes toward the characteristics of "helping persons." On the basis of their findings the authors concluded that "it is of overriding importance that a potential helping person be someone who is trusted, . . . (knows) about practical and useful information (and is) willing to meet people outside the office" (1980, 14–15). Trust and flexibility, therefore, appear to be the most important counselor characteristics and suggest that effectiveness depends on a counselor's ability to develop and nurture these important characteristics.

Characteristics of the Client

The degree of cultural and psychological diversity existing among Indian clients is likely to present a multitude of problems for any counselor. Acculturative status, physical appearance, and lifestyle preferences do vary considerably from one client to another. Some clients who come from traditional backgrounds are not likely to maintain direct eye contact, will avoid personalizing and disclosing troubled thoughts, and may seemingly act quite shy in the presence of a counselor (Youngman and Sadongei 1974; Ayres 1977; Trimble and Hayes 1984; and Attneave 1985). Very traditional clients might tell the counselor that their problems have been tended to by Indian doctors and that they have no need for any advice or consultation. Other, more acculturated, clients understand the counseling process and have a good sense for what is expected of them as clients and act accordingly.

Some Indian clients have learned to cope with emotional and stressful conditions in culturally unique ways. Many Siouan-speaking people deal with problems by invoking a form of "cultural time out" (wacinko). Individuals may use wacinko in familial situations in which they believe that they are placing too much of a burden on others (Trimble et al. 1984). Wacinko, usually translated as "pouting," has often been diagnosed as a reactive depressive illness with symptoms ranging from withdrawal to psychomotor retardation. From a traditional Sioux perspective, however, *wacinko* is not pathological and is quite functional and even expected. Older individuals may even reproach a person who has yet to *wacinko* when they recognize the conditions that are likely to prompt the behavior. More than once, Indians who were "pouting" have been referred to counselors and psychiatrists; however, the "would-be clients" knew they were behaving in a culturally specific manner that enabled them to deal with their problems. A counselor might persist in probing for the causes of a client's depressive-like state in hopes of remedying the problem, when, in fact, the "pouting" is the solution and not the cause.

Blue and Blue (1983) point out that many Indians may react to stressful conditions by merely waiting out the circumstances. Since many traditional Indians place an importance on "living with" the environment, they quite naturally expect the environment to eventually offer solutions. Hence, the individual may appear to be depressed and withdrawn, but they are actually waiting for something to happen. In this situation, the authors emphasize, "passivity is not hopelessness but hopefulness" (1983, 20).

Most likely, numerous other tribal-specific normative styles of behavior that people invoke to deal with stressful and problematic life events are yet to be identified. The expressed behaviors may well be similar to what many mental health professionals view as psychopathological symptoms. Clinical and counseling intervention in these instances would be not only disruptive but futile since the seemingly exotic behaviors are actually expressive forms of *self-treatment* and *healing*. Counselors should seek appropriate ways to identify and recognize these often highly stylized forms of self-healing and respect them in their context and the manner in which they are expressed.

Value Differences

Culturally different clients are likely to subscribe to values and beliefs that are distinctly different from those of a counselor. The counseling setting may highlight potential conflicts between client and counselor, introducing sources of misunderstanding, promoting client resistance, and interfering with the process of self-disclosure and the agenda of both parties.

In general terms values are "what is wanted, what is best, what is preferable (and) what ought to be done" (Scheibe 1970, 42). Values reflect one's wishes, desires, goals, passions, or morals and can "define for an individual or for a social unit what ends or means to an end are desirable" (English and English 1958, 576–577).

Indian clients undoubtedly will express values that are inconsistent if not disparate from those of a non-Indian counselor. Variations in valuing styles, of course, could be mediated by clients' acculturative status, the degree to which they identify with "Indianness," and their tribal or village orientation.

Numerous writers have sought to identify the likely value differences between Indians and the dominant culture. Bryde (1971) and Zintz (1963) generated contrasting lists of value preferences for both Sioux and Southwest Pueblo groups. A comparison of the independently derived lists reveals considerable agreement and consensus. Kluckhohn and Strodtbeck (1961) also identified general value categories in which discrepancies among and between many diverse cultural groups may be found. These value perspectives include man-nature orientation (mastery over nature, subjugation to nature, and harmony with nature); time orientation (temporal past, present, and future); and relational orientation (status and power positions along lineal orientations, group consensus, and individualism).

Spang (1965), Burton (1980), Lazarus (1982), and Edwards and Edwards (1984) also emphasize the importance of understanding the value orientations of Indian clients. In slightly different ways but nonetheless writing from a similar perspective they tend to highlight the value orientations expressed by Bryde and Zintz. And each of them concludes that non-Indian counselors must be aware of value differences if only to become aware of their own biases and preferences.

The creation of generalizable contrasting value orientations introduces the tendency to overgeneralize and subsequently categorize clients along one or all of the contrasting dimensions. There is evidence to suggest, however, that Indians' value orientations are more subtle, diverse, and complicated than previously understood. Tefft (1967), for instance, used a slightly modified version of the Kluckhohn value orientations and found more differences between tribal groups than between Indians and Caucasians. Moreover, his Arapaho student sample showed more disagreement over preferred values in contrast to the Shoshone and Caucasian samples combined. Similar but less profound are the findings of Helper and Garfield (1965); using a generalized semantic differential technique, they found "some differences" in value content between Indian and white groups.

Diversification can also result from the degree of contact one group has with another. Often the contact group seeks feedback concerning out-group expectations and attributions. Berreman (1964) found that Aleuts involve themselves in what he calls "evaluation group alienation." They know that Caucasians dislike them. As a consequence, when Aleuts are in the presence of Caucasians, they assume roles that differ markedly from their typical behavior in an effort to compromise. The roles often serve to reinforce the perceived expectations that Caucasians have of them, sometimes reinforcing general Indian stereotypes. Chance (1965), in support of this, found that the St. James Cree act more "Indian" (i.e., as they think Caucasians want them to act) when they are in town than when they are in their own village.

It is often difficult to separate out the differences between role expectations and value orientations, as one is invariably reflected in the other. Behavior can often be construed as representative of what is expected of a person. At the same time, the behavior can be thought of as reflective of a value orientation. Typically, behavior and cognition are combined in many ethnographic studies and subsumed under the general term "ethos." Thus, in the interpretation of indigenous group behavior, the actual meaning is never certain: Is the interpreted value a value or indicative of an expected role? Honigmann (1949) has applied such a perspective in his study of the Kaska in northwestern Canada. His findings suggest that the Kaska ethos of strong emotional constraint, inhibition of emotional expression in interpersonal relations, and apathetic withdrawal from or mistrust of others is related to their low population density, isolation, and general style of life, characterized by hunting and trapping. This may indicate what some would call traditional Kaska values. Alternatively, they may be values that developed as a result of Kaska fear of social contact and acculturation.

Values and traditional personality characteristics tend to persist in spite of the variations in social contact and acculturation (Brown 1969). The return of conservative patterns, unconscious persistency, and generosity have been identified among Cherokees and certain Plains Indians (Meekel 1936; Devereux 1951; Gulick 1960). Schusky noted that differences persisted between Caucasians and Lower Brule Dakotas. He stated that "one readily observes personality differences between Indians and Whites . . . on first acquaintance the young seem excessively quiet. Although this shyness lessens with greater familiarity, children are quite reserved before adults, waiting to be 'spoken to before speaking.' Whites frequently comment on the good behavior of Indian children in this respect" (1970, 115). Freyre (1956) also noted that the practice of and value placed on mercy killing still persist among certain Eskimo groups (who come under the definition of American Indian), despite Caucasians' insistence that such behavior is murder and Eskimos who commit euthanasia should be punished.

Some individual Indians experience a great deal of conflict in attempting to internalize alien values, and the mere presence of a contact group is known to create some value conflicts. In reference to the Teton Dakota, Macgregor related that "in this environment the basic personality has become almost schizophrenic. Individuals were torn between desires to gain status and role outside the reservation and to enjoy warm, stable and positive interrelations by remaining at home.

Through failure to realize either goal, many of the younger generation slipped into a life of apathetic resignation and passivity" (1970, 99).

The same disruption in values apparently can occur when an Indian leaves the reservation even for a short period of time. Vogt (1951) found that many Navajo veterans who had returned to the reservation from a term in the armed forces had modified their value orientation. Some veterans had adopted a concern for the future that went beyond that which the Navajo traditionally value and had taken a position that a person controls nature rather than the other way around. Vogt further indicated that those Navajo males who tended to accept Caucasian values had personal conflicts and feelings of insecurity.

Similar value conflicts emerge for the Indian who leaves the reservation to live in a city or town. Typically, there is a strong tendency for urban Indians to retain their "Indianness," while struggling with the almost daily contact with the dominant culture. In so doing, an urban Indian topology has emerged that emphasizes internalizing values indicative of Indians in general. Invariably, these values are elaborations with modifications of typical tribal values and are characterized more by pan-Indian ideologies. The stretching of tribal values to accommodate Caucasian values had produced what White (1970) has called "the lower class 'culture of excitement.' " In his studies of lower-class Sioux in Rapid City, South Dakota, he found that Indian values may reflect the "reservation ideal," but sometimes the behavior may take on a form particular to Indians living in urban settings. We cannot then infer the value from the role or the role from the value, because the intrinsic value of any behavior is situational. This may well be an explanation for the discrepancies in Tefft's findings on Arapaho-Shoshone values, as well as those of Berreman (1964), Chance (1965), and Honigmann (1949) mentioned earlier.

Ablon (1971) collected data on 50 American Indian and Samoan families who relocated from their native homes to a West Coast city. She found that the Indian family members, but not the Samoans, had difficulty in adjusting to the urban setting. She also noted a "natural reticence" and a tendency to withdraw from encounters. Shyness or "natural reticence," presumably a value preference, was challenged by encounters with other urban residents, especially with those who did not share this orientation. Kemnitzer (1973), in a study of nine "urbanized" Dakota Indians, found dissonance reduction to be a major problem, attributing it to new challenges, forced behavior, and conflicts with cognitively based value preferences.

Conflicts of value orientation are not unavoidable when Indians relocate to urban areas. Affiliation, maintenance of traditional ceremonials, and opportunities to visit native homes may reinforce value retention. "Stayers," those who remain in the cities, can retain tribal-based values if their expectations for goal attainment are realized (Graves and Arsdale 1966). Put another way, if someone voluntarily leaves his or her rural or reservation home of the city and experiences the sense of achieving goals (e.g., finding a suitable home, landing a respectable job and being successful at it), the greater the likelihood that basic values will not change substantially. Presumably, those who stay are more willing to let go of some basic cultural orientations and learn and internalize those that will assist them in adapting to the new lifestyle. To the contrary, "leavers" may recognize that certain culturally rooted lifestyle preferences are not appropriate for city life; rather than change their perspectives, they leave.

Value orientations have staying power and can be resistant to change even when individuals from different cultures mingle in the same environment. Using a 40-item sentence completion instrument, value preferences were assessed among Indians and non-Indians attending the same school in southeastern Oklahoma (Trimble 1981). Based on the response patterns and the use of a step-wise discriminant function analysis, the results produced a significant classification of both groups along distinct cultural lines. The study also revealed a generalized, almost pan-Indian ordering of value preferences for the Indian students. Most, if not all, of the Indian subjects in the study had close interpersonal contacts with the non-Indian students. Yet through all of the interaction, a basic and different value preference had been retained in spite of the influences presented by the dominant culture.

It would be a mistake to assume that Indians (or any other cultural groups) are unvarying in their commitment to basic value preferences. Commitment and subsequent enactment and expression of values certainly vary across individuals and the situations in which they find themselves day by day. Indeed, as discussed earlier, value expressions and preferences can vary among Indians. For many, commitment to tribal values is strong and enduring; for others who may be experiencing identity problems, feelings of marginality could be muddled with uncertainty. Taking this thought a bit further, it could be argued that the strength of a person's value orientation, especially one endorsed by other normal, healthy, functioning individuals, is closely correlated with self-perception. Put into a question, are American Indians with high, positive self-perceptions more likely to express a strong commitment to social values than those with moderate or negative self-perceptions?

To answer this question and a few related ones, Trimble (1981) administered two scales to 791 Indians—a 65-item self-regard scale consisting of six subscales and a social values scale consisting also of six subscales. Based on the responses to the self-regard scale, respondents were placed into two categories—high positive, and moderate to low positive. Results show that the "high" self-perceivers tend to endorse kindness, honesty, self-control, social skills, social responsibility, and reciprocity more significantly than do the "low" self-perceivers. Hence, those Indians who perceive themselves positively do tend to feel more strongly about certain values than those who perceive themselves less positively.

Knowledge of the strength of value convictions can be a useful counseling tool. A client may seek counseling to reduce personal confusion and conflict. Having a negative self-perception can suggest the existence of an unstable value orientation. Consequently, the counselor can aid the client by reviewing the substance of the client's values along his or her valuing process. With some care a counselor can assist the client in examining the existing relationship between the values, the problems, and ways to bring them into perspective.

Through a clarification and analysis of client values, both counselor and client may discover that it is a value that prompts the initial difficulty. A client's perceived inability to acknowledge, respond to, and deal with the value conflict may contribute to feelings of inadequacy and diminished self-worth. Recognition of value differences, therefore, should not be the only concern of counselors of Indians; strength and degree of endorsement of principal value preferences must be considered as well. The association between self-perception and value preferences can be reasonably strong. Clients who tend to have relatively weak or negative value preferences may not perceive themselves in a positive light. By emphasizing the strengthening of value preferences, counselors may assist in improving a client's self-perception and, in the long run, contribute to promoting positive mental health.

Counseling Styles

Given the information and recommendations presented thus far, ultimately we may wonder what counseling styles or theoretical orientations would be most effective and useful with Indian clients. Unfortunately, there is no simple, straightforward recommendation. On the one hand, if a counselor shows evidence of being warm and empathetic, establishes trust and rapport, shows respect for cultural values and beliefs, and expresses flexibility in meeting the client's expectations, then it would make sense that any counseling style would work. Yet a number of writers in the area suggest that certain styles are likely to be more effective than others even though there is at this point little empirical evidence to support their claims.

Youngman and Sadongei (1974) suggest that counselors approach the initial interview slowly to allow the client's confidence level to unfold at his or her own pace. Pacing therefore seems to be important in building up trust levels. Richardson (1981) also suggests that silence, acceptance and acknowledgement of client feelings and thoughts, and careful use of paraphrasing punctuate the counseling sessions. He also recommends that at strategic points counselors summarize the content of counselor-client interactions.

Both Burton (1980) and Richardson (1981) recommend a counseling style that ranges from being directive to nondirective, altering the distinctive approaches according to the client's communication style. Spang (1965); Dauphinais, Dauphinais, and Rowe (1981); and La-Fromboise, Dauphinais, and Rowe (1982) disagree. These researchers strongly recommend the exclusive use of a directive approach. Dauphinais, Dauphinais, and Rowe (1981) and LaFromboise, Dauphinais, and Rowe (1980) present research evidence collected from samples of Indian students that suggests that the directive style is more comfortable for them than the nondirective approach. The latter researchers also stated that "available evidence indicated that the (Rogerian or nondirective style) may be counterproductive for most American ethnic minorities" (1980, 15). This position matches with clinical experience: the directive style seems to be more effective since many Indian clients, especially more culturally traditional ones, are likely to be reticent and taciturn during the early stages of counseling if not throughout the entire course of treatment.

In general, American Indians are very family oriented. Usually, the more traditional families have a tendency to keep their personal problems within the family. Family members connected to a large kinship network assume responsibility for dealing with troubled kin. Counselor intervention in these instances is usually not solicited or considered desirable. Yet there are occasions when family members feel powerless to help their kin. In many cases members will do nothing in the hope that the problem will take care of itself or the kin member will seek advice elsewhere.

Within the past few years counseling and clinical psychologists have been emphasizing that a client's problems are often very situational and contextual. Trimble and Hayes (1984) and Dinges et al. (1981) recommend that counselors of American Indians attempt to understand "the cultural context" in which a client's problem is embedded. Familial patterns, peer group relationships, and community relationships are a few of the "ecological" processes that should be understood and somehow incorporated into one's counseling style (Trimble and LaFromboise 1985).

Family counseling is thus an approach that makes a good deal of sense. Attneave (1969, 1977) and Speck and Attneave (1973) recommend that counselors and therapists account for the social and network characteristics of Indian families and involve kin members in the counseling process. Goldstein (1974) and Shore and Nicholls (1975) used houseparents, parents, and relatives to assist mental health practitioners in working with youth problems in Indian boarding schools. Collaborative relationships between surrogate and natural parents and counselors appear to be a uniquely cultural approach to promote counselor effectiveness (cf. Unger 1977).

The type of problem experienced by the client often requires a counselor to alter the style he or she is likely to use. Grief over the death of someone is an instance in which a counselor needs to understand the meaning of death, funeral and burial customs, and the client's personal wishes (Hanson 1978). Counselors should allow the client to express anger and loss and should assist the client in not owning or showing the guilt associated with a loved one's death. "If we blame the client for feeling angry," Hansen maintains, "we may prolong the grief, shame and guilt, (which could result) in physical and emotional ill-health" (1978, 21).

Indian clients with alcohol- and drug-use problems also may require unique attention (Trimble 1984; Baker 1982). Intervention and treatment that accommodates many of the recommendations made earlier in this chapter may be effective in many cases, but because of the complexity of Indian substance abuse, treatment effectiveness may be compromised.

Summary of Findings

Throughout the writings on the topic of counseling Indians one theme surfaces repeatedly: Counselors of Indian clients must be adaptive and flexible in their personal orientation and use of conventional counseling techniques. Commitment to understanding the cultural context and unique cultural characteristics of clients is also essential. This often requires counselors to extend their efforts beyond what is typically done in a conventional office. Miller (1982) perhaps best captures the essence of this in her outline of the strategies she found most useful in counseling Indians. For example, she found that (1) a counselor's personal identification with the culture of a client is hardly sufficient for a thorough understanding of the impact of a cultural lifestyle on a client; (2) a client's personal history contains information that focuses on certain strengths, and this can be useful in promoting positive counseling expectations; (3) counselors should be aware of their own personal biases and stereotypes about cultural pluralism; (4) counselors should encourage clients to become active in identifying and learning the various thoughts and behaviors that promote positive growth and development; and (5) the most important yet basic counseling approaches involve empathy, caring, and a sense for the importance of the human potential.

Bryde's (1971) sample of Indian students in South Dakota also identified some important characteristics of a counselor of American Indians. The qualities include the following: (1) the counselor should be Indian and be matched with the client on the basis of gender; (2) the counselor should be a friend who is always available for assistance; (3) the counselor should be open-minded; (4) the counselor should be thoroughly knowledgeable about Indian culture and values; (5) the counselor should be patient; and (6) the counselor should have full knowledge of the counseling field and be able to use that knowledge effectively and appropriately.

Acculturative Styles and Counselor Effectiveness

Considering the sociocultural diversity of Native American Indians, the tendency to underutilize mental health services, client reactions to counseling styles, and the existence of variable tribal-specific approaches to mental health problems, how can a conventionally trained counselor expect to know if intervention will be appropriate and effective? Few academic institutions provide training designed to enhance a counselor's sensitivity to the robustness of cultural and ethnic variables; fewer still provide training designed specifically to promote effectiveness with Indian clients (cf. Pedersen 1985; Ponterroto and Casas 1987). Yet ample evidence suggests that many counselors throughout the United States work with Indian clients in some capacity. Many experience the frustrations discussed earlier and are likely puzzled about their lack of effectiveness in rendering assistance.

In addition to internalizing the suggestions discussed earlier, counselors stand a good chance of increasing their effectiveness by learning about an Indian client's acculturative status, preferably during the early intake sessions. Like many clients in general, Indians may not understand the goals and objectives of counseling, their role and responsibilities as clients, and the requirements associated with talking to a stranger about personal problems. A good deal of this lack of knowledge certainly can be attributed to the lack of experience with the counseling process in general. For the potential Indian client much of the ignorance about counseling may also derive from the manner in which he or she was socialized and the extent to which traditional values, beliefs, and customs were instilled by kin and tribal elders.

Although no empirical evidence supports the contention, there is a strong likelihood that Indians raised in a very traditional, native-oriented manner, especially in reservation communities, pueblos, or villages, are not familiar with the conventional counseling process. Consequently, they are not likely to make "good" clients, largely because they are not accustomed to talking out their problems with strangers or, most certainly, non-Indian counselors. Furthermore, the traditional, native-oriented Indian is more likely to receive assistance from kin, friends, and traditional healers or shamans. In contrast, highly acculturated Indians, particularly those raised in urban settings, are more likely to respond to counseling.

An Indian client's responsiveness to counseling is not necessarily a function of where he or she was raised. Rather, it would appear that the acculturation of the client is a potent contributor to a client's receptivity to counseling in a conventional sense. Like many other ethnic minorities and culturally distinctive people in North America, Indians express the full range of acculturation. Many, regardless of age, are traditional and native oriented; others are transitional in the sense that they reflect an understanding and appreciation of tribal-specific folkways yet recognize the value of internalizing the values and beliefs of the dominant, more progressive culture; and others, whether because of geographic isolation from their ancestral homes or personal choice, have fully internalized the folkways of modern society.

To illustrate the responsiveness of Indian clients to counseling, three case studies taken from case records have been condensed and are presented for review. Each of the three clients was judged to fit one of three acculturative styles—the successfully acculturated, the marginally acculturated, and the moderately traditional. Personal information for each client has been changed to prevent identification.

A Successfully Acculturated Client

Mary, an Indian woman in her mid-40s, presented herself at a mental health clinic for support during a time when she and her daughter, age 16, were in extreme conflict. Mary's daughter had been dating an older, non-Indian adolescent who had a reputation for drug abuse. Within the previous year Mary's son, age 18, had been to peer counseling training in the area of chemical dependence prevention, and the entire family had participated in the associated family program. She was proud of her son's growth and grateful for the opportunities the family had had to learn and heal together. Mary was anxious about her daughter's choice of friends and feared that she and her husband would lose the closeness with their daughter that they had had, especially in recent months.

Mary and her non-Indian husband operated a ranch on her reservation allotment, and they enjoyed a comfortable income. Mary also worked in a rest home as an LPN in a nearby town bordering the reservation. Her children attended integrated schools in that town, and they had both done well academically and socially. Over the years, Mary and her husband encouraged their children to participate in tribal and community organizations, such as an Indian dance group and a 4-H club.

Therapeutic issues focused on Mary's own adolescence. She was the eldest of two daughters raised by their widowed mother; Mary's father had been killed in an alcohol-related automobile accident when she was an infant. From that point forward abstinence from alcohol and drugs became a strong family value. Mary and her sister internalized that particular value, but in their teen years conflict with their mother centered around other values. Mary was sent to boarding school when she reached high school age, and her mother was inconsistently emotionally available to her, alternating between rigid limit setting and laissez-faire parenting. This model of parenting had presented much anxiety for Mary, and her therapeutic work was to separate her own unresolved issues from the current issues with her daughter.

A Marginally Acculturated Client

Terry, a 30-year-old American Indian man, was referred to a mental health counselor by his physician because he had not been sleeping well for several weeks. The physician thought that the underlying cause was Terry's unresolved grief for his father who had died a year earlier. Terry reported having a recurring dream about his father and grandfather in which they did chores together around his grandfather's cabin. He would awaken with a sense that the dream had great significance for him and was sad that he couldn't avail himself of the traditional healing ways of his own reservation several states away. Terry had grown up in a native-language-speaking family, and his parents were considered leaders in the teaching of tribal culture. He had gone to a high school boarding school, but he was expelled in his senior year because of substance abuse. His girlfriend from school left with him; they returned to her reservation to stay with her family, and they got married. After several years of labor work Terry earned his Graduate Equivalency Degree and began working for his wife's tribe in the fisheries department. At the time he sought therapy, he was not satisfied with his job, but he was also ambivalent about pursuing further training or formal education. He had some interest in computer technology.

Marital stress was an additional concern to Terry at the time of the referral. Terry's wife was not open to learning the culture of her tribe (a very assimilated group) or his tribe and believed that their daughter needed to learn primarily about non-Indian culture. Terry, in contrast, began renewing the traditional teachings of his grandfather in his own life and wanted to pass that knowledge on to his daughter. Terry and his daughter occasionally attended powwows, but his wife rarely accompanied them. Terry felt at a loss at times about the unique cultural ways his daughter needed to learn from a female perspective and missed the influence of his own mother who had died when he was a teenager.

Terry's wife babysat to earn extra money and enjoyed playing in a women's softball league. Her major social contact outside of her marriage was a sister who also lived in their housing project. Terry was committed to the marriage but felt that he and his wife did not share many common values. She was only minimally open to marriage counseling. He was periodically involved with Alcoholics Anonymous: two or three times a year he engaged in binge drinking at the local "Indian bar," although he had begun to break this pattern during the previous year. He had no significant Indian or non-Indian male friends.

Terry's therapist chose to help him focus on the various losses he had experienced throughout his life and help him affirm his own tribal cultural perspective of those changes. Terry was able to see that his identity crisis was extensive and influenced his relationships with his spouse, child, tribe of origin, significant persons in his past, his current peer group, his vocation, and his future professional and personal development.

A Moderately Traditional Client

Joanne, a 44-year-old American Indian woman from the coastal region of the Pacific Northwest, was taken to an Indian Health Service clinic by her two female cousins after they found her wandering aimlessly on a small beach near the reservation. After what appeared to be a thorough examination, the physician concluded that the woman was severely depressed, acutely undernourished, suffered from hallucinations, and was in desperate need of sleep and relaxation. Although Joanne was reluctant to talk with the physician, she did confide some of her thoughts with one cousin who in turn passed the information along to the physician. From what the cousin could gather, Joanne had not eaten a full meal for about three weeks, had averaged only three to four hours of sleep per night for about one month, and had been absent from work for the week prior to her being discovered on the beach.

Joanne's parents had died in a tragic boating accident when she was four years old. After living with her father's sister for a year, she had moved in with her father's parents, who raised her to adulthood. Joanne's grandparents, by most standards, were very traditional: they spoke their native language in the home and on occasion at social and ceremonial gatherings, gathered and preserved native foods, hunted and fished and smoked their catches, and in general abided by customs of a century or so ago. They were active in Indian religious and ceremonial activities and in every way possible involved Joanne. Joanne followed the traditional ways of her grandparents and passed the knowledge along to her two daughters.

When Joanne was in her mid-20s, she learned that her grandparents were highly regarded shamans, or spirit healers. About the same time, she also learned a good deal about sorcery and about various methods used by those who practiced on the darker side. On a few occasions, partially out of bitterness and dislike for certain tribal members, including her estranged husband, she had made use of sorcery to seek revenge and regress. And her actions had not gone unnoticed.

After the diagnosis and through the insistence of her cousins, Joanne was referred to a local mental health counselor. The counselor's intervention efforts were greeted with great reluctance by Joanne, who seemingly avoided disclosing any of her thoughts and feelings. Concluding that his efforts were in vain, the counselor confided in a highly regarded local spirit healer (shaman), who agreed to work with Joanne. The counselor discussed the matter with her, and Joanne also agreed to the arrangement. She appeared to respond to the healer's efforts, and it seemed that her "problem" had been resolved.

From what the counselor could surmise from his discussions with Joanne's cousin, she apparently had been the target of sorcery instigated in all likelihood by someone who had been victimized by her many years ago. It seemed that Joanne had discovered one evening that someone had sprinkled her personal belongings with a powder made from certain herbs and roots—the sinister mixture was used to capture someone's soul, and Joanne's dysfunctional behavior was typical of people who had lost their souls. If intervention had not occurred through the restoration of her soul, Joanne, like many others who had experienced soul-loss, might have mysteriously died or disappeared.

In each of these cases the counselors had to identify and be sensitive to the client's degree of acculturation, which may or may not have been obvious to the acculturated client. Mary had been raised on a reservation and to an extent had participated in Indian-related ceremonial activities. The influences provided in school and her choice of friends, however, suggested that she was more inclined to respond to counseling than Joanne. Cultural variables were less significant in her case than with Terry and Joanne. Joanne's counselor, for instance, recognized almost immediately that Joanne was reluctant to discuss the problem with him. She, too, knew that he was in no position to assist her. Yet he was helpful in an oblique way as he not only facilitated the arrangement with the local shaman but also affirmed the importance of that helping medium and Joanne's preferred manner of dealing with her personal problems. In a slightly different manner Terry's counselor was also sensitive to Terry's cultural needs and his concern about his identity and attempted to work with him on these matters in the course of the counseling process.

Perhaps the most significant point that can be made about the three cases is that the counselors made substantial adjustments in their counseling styles to accommodate the acculturative status of their clients. In every case the counselor had the foresight to gather culturally related information to assist them in making the adjustments.

An assessment of acculturative status is no small matter and not achievable merely by asking a few questions and gaining inferences from physical appearances. Central to determining acculturative status is the extent to which a particular individual is engaged in acculturation. Is it an active or passive process, voluntary or involuntary, subtle or direct? Equally important is the determination of an attitude toward acculturation. To assess a client's acculturative status, a counselor should develop a line of open-ended questions that generates information about (1) education, (2) wage employment, (3) urbanization, (4) media influence, (5) political participation, (6) religion, (7) language, (8) daily life, and (9) social relations. Berry, Trimble, and Olmedo (1986) discuss useful procedures for obtaining information concerning these variables through the use of measures of contact, adaptation, ownership, and change. Leininger (1984) also not only identifies a list of similar "culturological" topics but also presents a series of useful steps to follow in conducting interviews with culturally different clients. We may conclude that if a counselor obtains information about a client's acculturative status and at the same time affirms the importance and significance of cultural orientation, the counselor will develop greater trust and rapport with a client. In addition, a closer client-counselor bond will be nurtured. Both processes lead to an improvement in client effectiveness and to the promotion of client expectations.

Conclusion

Just as various sections in this chapter provide tenable suggestions for promoting counselor effectiveness, the material also points to the gaps that exist in understanding what works best given the heterogeneity of the population of Native American Indians. The presence of these gaps serves as a reminder for the need for careful documentation of the intervention strategies that appear to be effective for counselors and clinicians who work with Indian clients. These gaps also suggest the need for more carefully controlled research that is inherently sensitive to the cultural orientations of Indians and their respective communities. A blend of the documentation of case studies and empirical findings can only lead to the improvement of the delivery of mental health services to the first American.

References

Ablon, J. 1971. Cultural conflict in urban Indians. *Mental Hygiene* 55 (2): 199–205.

Attneave, C. L. 1969. Therapy in tribal settings and urban network intervention. *Family Process* 8:192–210.

———. 1977. The wasted strength of American Indian families. In S. Unger (ed.), *The destruction of American Indian families*, 29–33. New York: Association on American Indian Affairs.

———. 1985. Practical counseling with American Indian and Alaska Native clients. In P. Pedersen (ed.), *Handbook of cross-cultural counseling and therapy*, 135–140. Westport, CT: Greenwood Press.

Ayres, M. E. 1977. Counseling the American Indians. *Occupational Outlook Quarterly* 21 (1): 22–29.

Baker, J. M. 1982. Alcoholism and the American Indian. In N. Estes and M. E. Heinemann (eds.), *Alcoholism: Development, consequences and interventions*. 2d ed. 239–248. St. Louis: Mosby.

Barter, E. R., and Barter, J. T. 1974. Urban Indians and mental health problems. *Psychiatric Annals* 4 (9): 37–43.

Beiser, M., and Attneave, C. L. 1978. Mental health services for American Indians: Neither feast or famine. *White Cloud Journal* 1 (2): 3–10.

Benedict, R. 1959. *Patterns of culture*. Boston: Houghton Mifflin.

Berreman, G. D. 1964. Alienation, mobility, and acculturation: The Aleut reference group. *American Anthropologist* 66:231–250.

Berry, J., Trimble, J., and Olmedo, E. 1986. Assessment of acculturation. In W. Lonner and J. Berry (eds.), *Field methods in cross-cultural research*, 291–324. Beverly Hills: Sage Publications.

Blue, A., and Blue, M. 1983. The trail of stress. *White Cloud Journal* 3 (1): 15–22.

✕ Bransford, J. 1982. To be or not to be: Counseling with American Indian clients. *Journal of American Indian Education* 21 (3): 18–21.

Brown, J. E. 1969. The persistence of essential values among North American Plains Indians. *Studies in Comparative Religion* 3 (Autumn): 216–225.

Bryde, J. F. 1972. *Indian students and guidance*. Boston: Houghton Mifflin.

Burton, L. 1980. *Counseling Native American high school and college students*. Paper presented at the Annual Conference on Ethnic and Minority Studies, LaCrosse, WI.

Chance, N. A. 1965. Acculturation, self-identification, and personality adjustment. *American Anthropologist* 67:327–393.

Cooley, R. C., Ostendorf, D., and Bickerton, D. 1979. Outreach services for elderly Native Americans. *Social Work* 29:151–153.

Dauphinais, P., Dauphinais, L., and Rowe, W. 1981. Effects of race and communication style on Indian perception of counselor effectiveness. *Counselor Education and Supervision* (September): 72–80.

Devereux, G. 1951. *Reality and dream*. New York: International Universities Press.

Dinges, N., Trimble, J., and Hollenbeck, A. 1981. American Indian adolescent socialization: Review and critique of research. *Journal of Adolescence* 2:259–296.

Dinges, N., Trimble, J., Manson, S., and Pasquale, F. 1981. Counseling and psychotherapy with American Indians and Alaska Natives. In A. Marsella and P. Pedersen (eds.), *Cross-cultural counseling and psychotherapy: Foundations evaluation, and cultural considerations,* 243–276. Elmsford, NY: Pergamon Press.

Dukepoo, F. C. 1980. *The elder American Indian.* San Diego: Campanile Press.

Edwards, E., and Edwards, M. E. 1984. Social group work practice with young American Indians. *Social Work with Groups* 7 (3): 7–21.

English, H. B., and English, A. C. 1958. *A comprehensive dictionary of psychological and psychoanalytical terms: A guide to usage.* New York: McKay.

Freyre, G. 1956. *The masters and the slaves.* New York: Knopf.

Goldstein, G. S. 1974. The model dormitory. *Psychiatric Annals* 4 (11): 85–92.

Graves, T. D., and Arsdale, M. V. 1966. Values, expectations and relocation: The Navajo migrant to Denver. *Human Organization* 25 (Winter): 300–307.

Gulick, J. 1960. *Cherokees at the crossroads.* Chapel Hill: Institute for Research in Social Sciences.

Hanson, W. 1978. Grief counseling with Native Americans. *White Cloud Journal* 1 (2): 19–21.

Haviland, M. G., Horswill, R. K., O'Connell, J. J., and Dynneson, V. V. 1983. Native American college student's preference for counselor or race and sex, and the likelihood of their use of a counseling center. *Journal of Counseling Psychology* 30 (2): 267–270.

Helper, M. M., and Garfield, S. L. 1965. Use of the Semantic Differential to study acculturation in American Indian adolescents. *Journal of Personality and Social Psychology* 2 (6): 817–822.

Honigmann, J. J. 1949. *Culture and ethos of Kaska society.* Yale Publications in Anthropology, No. 40. New Haven: Yale University Press.

Jewell, D. P. 1952. A case of a psychotic Navaho Indian male. *Human Organization* 11 (11): 32–36.

Josephy, A. M. 1968. *The Indian heritage of America.* New York: Knopf.

Kelso, D. R., and Attneave, C. L. 1981. *Bibliography of North American Indian mental health.* Westport, CT: Greenwood Press.

Kemnitzer, L. S. 1973. Adjustment and value conflict in urbanizing Dakota Indians measured by Q-Sort Technique. *American Anthropologist* 75 (3): 687–707.

Kluckhohn, F. R., and Strodtbeck, F. L. 1961. *Variations in value orientation.* New York: Harper and Row.

LaFromboise, T., Dauphinais, P., and Rowe, W. 1980. Indian student's perceptions of positive helper attributes. *Journal of American Indian Education* 19:11–16.

LaFromboise, T., and Dixon, D. 1981. American Indian perceptions of trustworthiness in a counseling interview. *Journal of Counseling Psychology* 28:135–139.

Lazarus, P. J. 1982. Counseling the Native American child: A question of values. *Elementary School Guidance and Counseling* (December): 83–88.

Leininger, M. 1984. Transcultural interviewing and health assessment. In P. Pedersen, N. Sartorius, and A. Marsella (eds.), *Mental health services: The cross-cultural context,* 109–133. Beverly Hills: Sage Publications.

Littrell, M. A., and Littrell, J. M. 1983. Counselor dress cues: Evaluations by American Indians and Caucasians. *Journal of Cross-Cultural Psychology* 14 (1): 109–121.

Macgregor, G. 1970. Changing society: The Teton Dakotas. In E. Nurge (ed.), *The modern Sioux: Social systems and reservation culture,* 92–106. Lincoln: University of Nebraska Press.

Mail, P. D., and McDonald, D. R. 1980. *Tulapai to Tokay: A bibliography of alcohol use and abuse among Native Americans of North America.* New Haven: Human Relations Area Files.

Manson, S., and Trimble, J. 1982. American Indian and Alaska Native communities: Past efforts, future inquiries. In L. Snowden (ed.), *Reaching the underserved: Mental health needs of neglected populations,* 143–163. Beverly Hills: Sage Publications.

McShane, D. A. 1987. Mental health and North American Indian and Native communities: Cultural transactions, education and regulation. *American Journal of Community Psychology* 15 (1): 95–117.

Meekel, H. S. 1936. *The economy of a modern Teton Dakota community.* New Haven: Yale University Press.

Miller, N. B. 1982. Social work services to urban Indians. In J. W. Green (ed.), *Cultural awareness in the human services,* 157–183. Englewood Cliffs, NJ: Prentice-Hall.

Pedersen, P., ed. 1985. *Handbook on cross-cultural counseling and therapy.* Westport, CT: Greenwood Press.

Ponterotto, J. G., and Casas, J. M. 1987. In search of multicultural competence within counselor education programs. *Journal of Counseling and Development* 65:430–434.

Red Horse, J. G., Lewis, R. L., Feit, M., and Decker, J. 1978. Family behavior of urban American Indians. *Social Casework* 59:67–72.

Richardson, E. H. 1981. Cultural and historical perspectives in counseling American Indians. In D. W. Sue (ed.), *Counseling the culturally different: Theory and practice,* 216–255. New York: John Wiley and Sons.

Scheibe, K. E. 1970. *Beliefs and values.* New York: Holt, Rinehart and Winston.

Schoenfeld, L. S., Lyerly, R. J., and Miller, S. I. 1971. We like us. *Mental Hygiene* 55 (2): 171–173.

Schusky, E. L. 1970. Culture change and continuity in the Lower Brule community. In E. Nurge (ed.), *The modern Sioux: Social systems and reservation culture,* 107–122. Lincoln: University of Nebraska Press.

Shore, J. H., and Nicholls, W. W. 1975. Indian children and tribal group homes: New interpretations of the whipper man. *American Journal of Psychiatry* 132 (4): 454–456.

Spang, A. 1965. Counseling the Indian. *Journal of American Indian Education* 5 (1): 10–15.

Speck, R., and Attneave, C. 1973. *Family process.* New York: Pantheon.

Spradley, J. P. 1979. *The ethnographic interview.* New York: Holt, Rinehart and Winston.

Sue, S., Allen, D. B., and Conaway, L. 1978. The responsiveness and equality of mental health care to Chicanos and Native Americans. *American Journal of Community Psychology* 6 (2): 137–146.

Svensson, F. 1973. *The ethnics in American politics: American Indians.* Minneapolis: Burgess.

Taylor, T. W. 1984. *The Bureau of Indian Affairs.* Boulder, CO: Westview.

Tefft, S. K. 1967. Anomy, values and culture change among teen-age Indians: An exploratory study. *Sociology of Education* 40 (2): 145–157.

Torrey, E. F. 1986. *Witch doctors and psychiatrists: The common roots of psychotherapy and its future.* New York: Harper and Row.

Trimble, J. E. 1981. Value differentials and their importance in counseling American Indians. In P. B. Pedersen, J. G. Draguns, W. J. Lonner, and J. E. Trimble (eds.), *Counseling across cultures,* rev. ed. 203–226. Honolulu: University of Hawaii Press.

―――. 1984. Drug abuse prevention research needs among American Indians and Alaska Natives. *White Cloud Journal* 3 (3): 22–34.

Trimble, J. E., and Hayes, S. A. 1984. Mental health intervention in the psychological contexts of American Indian communities. In W. A. O'Conner and B. Lubin (eds.), *Ecological models: Applications to clinical and community mental health,* 293–321. New York: John Wiley and Sons.

Trimble, J. E., and LaFromboise, T. 1985. American Indians and the counseling process: Culture, adaptation, and style. In P. Pedersen (ed.), *Handbook of cross-cultural counseling and therapy,* 127–134. Westport, CT: Greenwood Press.

Trimble, J. E., Manson, S., Dinges, N., and Medicine, B. 1984. American Indian concepts of mental health: Reflections and directions. In P. Pedersen, N. Sartorius, and A. Marsella (eds.), *Mental health services: The cross-cultural context,* 199–220. Beverly Hills: Sage Publications.

Unger, S., ed. 1977. *The destruction of American Indian families.* New York: Association on American Indian Affairs.

United States Department of Education. 1982. *A study of alternative definitions and measures relating to eligibility and service under Part A of the Indian Education Act.* Unpublished report, United States Department of Education, Washington, DC.

Vogt, E. Z. 1951. Navajo veterans: A study of changing values. *Papers of the Peabody Museum of American Archeology and Ethnology* 41 (1, Reports of the Rimrock Project Values Series), 1–223.

Werner, O., and Schoepfle, G. M. 1987. *Systematic fieldwork: Foundations of ethnography.* Newbury Park, CA: Sage Publications.

White, R. A. 1970. The lower-class "culture of excitement" among the contemporary Sioux. In E. Nurge (ed.), *The modern Sioux: Social systems and reservation culture,* 175–197. Lincoln: University of Nebraska Press.

Youngman, G., and Sadongei, M. 1974. Counseling the American Indian child. *Elementary School Guidance and Counseling* 8:273–277.

Zintz, M. V. 1963. *Education across cultures.* Dubuque, IA: William C. Brown.

9

Counseling Foreign Students

KAY THOMAS
GARY ALTHEN

"I'll have to talk to my brother," the female Pakistani graduate student told the female American counselor. "I can't decide what to do until I talk to him." She was married, and her husband was abusing her. He hit her, reviled her, and on at least one occasion burned her with his cigarette. Friends had encouraged her to see the counselor. Her older brother was a post-doctoral researcher at an Ivy League institution. It was his guidance she said she needed.

The counselor saw the problem right away. Here was a woman unable to make up her own mind. She needed to assert herself. It was her life, not her brother's. The counselor explained that the Pakistani woman needed to take responsibility for her own decisions. The Pakistani woman left the counseling session and never saw the counselor again.

After some discussion with people familiar with Pakistani culture, the counselor in this case realized she had made a mistake. A mistake, at least, if she wanted to earn the woman's confidence and have any possibility of helping her. She had (quite naturally) taken the individual-centered view that is the hallmark of most Western cultures. She had supposed that the Pakistani woman was immature (and perhaps even a bit defective) in believing she needed her brother's guidance before she could make an important decision about the course of her life. It had not occurred to the counselor that this woman, in her own eyes and those of all important to her, was behaving in a perfectly appropriate way. It was clear to the Indian woman that the counselor simply did not understand.

This brief case study points out two important factors that must be considered in counseling foreign students. The first is that they have a number of unique characteristics that distinguish them from domestic clients. These are largely due to the different cultural values they bring with them and to their status as temporary sojourners in the host country. Most come to get an advanced education. The second is that counselors, to be effective with foreign clients, must learn to adapt their counseling styles and their expectations to accommodate the differing worldviews and cultural value orientations of their foreign clients.

Counselors cannot expect to understand even the main points, let alone the subtleties, of the hundreds of cultures represented by the hundreds of thousands of foreign students now doing post–secondary school education in the United States and other Western countries. In 1986–1987 nearly 350,000 foreign students were studying in the United States (Institute of International Education 1987). Approximately 50% of these students came from South and East Asia. Dealing with students from the more than 150 countries around the world takes years of training. This essay offers an overview that can help the Western-trained counselor to be cognizant of some of the distinctive issues that arise in counseling students from other countries and offers some specific ideas for dealing with common foreign student problems.

What is Distinctive about Foreign Student Clients?

Foreign students are people in transition. Unlike ethnic minorities, refugees, or recent immigrants foreign students are sojourners in the host culture and are therefore considered people in transition, most having come to accomplish an educational goal. They are in a phase of their lives that will presumably end in the fairly near term, and most plan to return to their home countries.

Although domestic students also look forward to completing their education and are also people in transition, generally more transitions are involved for foreign students than for domestic students, and the transitions are more striking. The foreign students have left their home culture and must somehow "adjust" to the host country so they can realize their academic and other objectives. Whether graduation finds them going home or remaining in the host country, they face issues of accommodating themselves to cultural differences that domestic students do not confront. Questions of purpose and identity are more complex for people in transition. Foreign students must decide where they want to be on a continuum between functional adjustment to the host culture—just learning to do what they must do in order to get by—and assimilation—taking as much of the host culture as possible and making it their own.

Foreign students' basic assumptions and values are different. Anthropologists and others have devised a number of ways to try to describe the dimensions along which cultures vary. Widely used formulations are those of Kluckhohn and Strodtbeck (1961) and Hofstede (1984). Stewart (1972) has applied Kluckhohn and Strodtbeck's framework to a particularly useful analysis of American culture. (For a brief introduction to a variety of models for comparing cultures, see Robert Kohls' paper, "Models for comparing and contrasting cultures," in Reid 1988.) Counselors who work with students from other countries can have a better understanding of the dynamics of their counselor-client relationships if they can place their own culture, and those of their clients, into some framework such as the two summarized here.

Kluckhohn and Strodtbeck posit that there are five basic questions or considerations to which a group of people must have shared answers in order to be called a "culture." The first question is, What is the character of innate human nature? The other questions are, What is the relation of humans to nature? What is the time orientation? What is the mode of human activity? What is the mode of social relationships?

Human nature might be seen as basically evil, basically good, as neutral, or as a mixture of good and evil. Whatever their basic nature is conceived to be, human beings might be viewed as changeable, through education, training, or counseling, or as "immutable." North Americans tend to assume that human beings are basically good and also that they can change for the better. In other societies other conceptions of human nature are more common. When foreign students come to campuses in the United States, they will find an array of manifestations of the North American belief in human improvability. Study skills centers, reading laboratories, writing laboratories, workshops on assertive behavior, interviewing skills, overcoming shyness, test taking, relaxation, weight control, and how to make friends—all such things are based on assumptions that many foreign students do not share.

The relationship of humans to nature might be seen to be a matter of people's subjugation by nature, subjugation of nature, or of living (or trying to live) in harmony with the forces around them. Americans, perhaps to an extent exceeding almost all other peoples in the world, generally accept the mastery-over-nature viewpoint. Perhaps the attractiveness of engineering schools and natural and medical science programs in Western countries is testimony to the achievements of people raised with the belief that they can solve virtually any problem.

An aspect of the mastery-over-nature viewpoint that prevails in the United States is the rejection of the notion that "fate"—or some other external, uncontrollable force—determines an individual's destiny. Cross-cultural specialist Kohls (1984) stresses that most of the world's people assign fate a large role in what happens in their lives. Many foreign students have the notion that if they have problems, they have problems. They do not have the notion that they can "solve" their problems by talking with a counselor, attending workshops, reading books, or "practicing new behaviors," as North Americans are likely to believe. Rather, they may suppose that their problems must simply be borne. Counselors working with foreign students, then, might have to begin by convincing their clients that something can be done about their problems, rather than beginning by talking about what is to be done.

With respect to time orientation, a culture might be oriented mainly to the past, the present, or the future. Americans have traditionally focused on the future, on the goals they will attain later through their hard work. Counseling foreign students who are having academic difficulty is sometimes a matter, at least in part, of getting them to appreciate the connections between their current behavior and the final outcome of their academic career. They might not truly realize that their final cumulative grade-point average is closely related to the way they are currently spending their time.

Americans typically embody a "doing" or "action-oriented" response to the question about human activity. Contrasting responses are the "being" response typical of traditional, religious-oriented societies, and the "being-in-becoming" response typical of a society that values inner development more than success as manifested in the acquisition of material goods. One of the things that most frequently saddens foreign students is the difficulty they encounter making friends with domestic students. A common complaint foreign students have about North Americans is that "they are always so busy." They are "dominated by their clocks and their schedules." Latin, European, African, Indonesian, Malay, and Middle Eastern students are all accustomed to spending long hours talking with friends and relatives. To North Americans this is likely to be "just talking," which is deemed a "waste of time." Foreign students often need help in understanding that the North Americans' seemingly impulsive need to be doing something is not a manifestation of dislike for students from other places.

Social relationships might be basically hierarchical, collective, or individualistic. Americans generally have the latter viewpoint, seeing people as individuals who are essentially each other's equals. Many other peoples in the world have another view. Foreign students frequently have trouble adjusting to the "informal" nature of U.S. society, where, as they perceive it, people who presumably hold high-status positions do not routinely act in ways they consider appropriate. To the degree that counselors are older and wiser than the students they treat, foreign students are likely to expect them to do most of the talking in counseling sessions, to express their opinions, and to offer their suggestions. They are not likely to expect counselors to sit and listen most of the time, since such behavior is not concordant with their notions about the way people who are older and wiser—people with such a title as "counselor"—are expected to act.

This discussion of Kluckhohn and Strodtbeck's five dimensions of cultural variation has included examples of ways in which foreign students might misunderstand or have difficulty coping with typical aspects of life. A related and equally important point is that counselors, unless they are quite familiar with their culture, as foreign students might respond to it, can expect to have difficulty understanding and dealing with foreign student clients. Counselors cannot be experts on all the world's cultures, but they can develop a sound understanding of their own cultural values and the way their own culture affects people from elsewhere.

A more recent framework for comparing cultures is reported in Hofstede's 1984 study of organizations operating in countries around the world. Hofstede identified four dimensions along which culture can be said to vary. They are individualism/collectivism, uncertainty avoidance, power distance, and masculinity/femininity. Parallels with the Kluckhohn and Strodtbeck framework are readily apparent.

In a more individualistic culture people identify themselves as separate persons, operating on their own and responsible for themselves. In Hofstede's sample the United States placed very near the individualism end of the individualism-collectivism continuum. In a society with a collectivist orientation, such as that of the Pakistani woman discussed at the opening of this chapter, people see themselves more as members of groups, families, tribes, etc., than as separate individuals. Recent work by Triandis, Brislin, and Hui (1988) has addressed this individualism/ collectivism dimension of cultural variation and suggested ways for people from individualistic cultures to work more effectively with those from collectivist cultures and vice versa. They suggest that individualists who work with collectivists pay attention to people's group memberships to understand their behaviors; build relationships based on trust; criticize carefully, and never when an individual will lose face; and be sensitive to status hierarchies. Collectivists working with individualists need to learn to talk about personal accomplishments; establish short-term relationships; and engage in fewer superordinate and subordinate behaviors depending on the others' status levels.

In a country high on uncertainty avoidance people generally feel uncomfortable in ambiguous situations, and their societies have many devices (for example, much ritual interchange in conversations or systems that encourage lifetime employment with a particular organization) that limit the amount of uncertainty or ambiguity in people's lives. The United States is relatively low on Hofstede's uncertainty avoidance scale. That is, Americans tend to be more tolerant of ambiguous situations than are people from many other countries.

The power distance dimension has to do with the degree to which people accept the notion that power is distributed unevenly among people. Egalitarian Americans rank low on power distance.

In Hofstede's formulation masculine societies emphasize assertiveness and competitiveness, and feminine ones are more attentive to relationships among people, concern for other people, and the general quality of life. Hofstede found the United States to be on the masculine side, but not as much so as a number of traditionally male-dominated countries.

Some of these various assumptions and values are probably more salient to counseling than others, although none could be said to be irrelevant. We have already seen how one counselor's careless assumption that everyone shared her individualist orientation got her into difficulty with a client from a more family- and group-oriented culture. In addition to ideas about the definition of the person as an individual as opposed to being a member of a group, assumptions and values clearly related to the counseling process have to do with the equality-hierarchy dimension (or power distance in Hofstede's formulation) and the presence or absence of a sense that people in general have significant control over their own destinies. Table 1 depicts some counseling-related assumptions and values, comparing common American viewpoints to those more likely to prevail elsewhere. Ideas from this table are elaborated at various points in this chapter.

Foreign students are living in an academic setting. All foreign and domestic students are in a "down" position vis-à-vis faculty and are constantly under pressure and on trial. They have deadlines to meet, and their work is being evaluated. These factors can disadvantage foreign students more than domestic ones because they are confounded by language difficulties and an array of misunderstandings about the way the academic system operates. Furthermore, for many foreign students the academic stakes are higher than they usually are for domestic students. For them, academic failure or dropping out often seems unimaginable. Such events would have lifelong consequences for their reputations and careers.

Foreign students face other pressures that do not afflict domestic students. These include immigration regulations that require them to be enrolled full time in school and, in many cases, restrictions or at least time-consuming procedures related to the transfer of funds from their own countries. These restrictions, coupled with the legal limitations on employment, leave many foreign students under serious financial pressure.

At this point it seems relevant to address the question of the degree of academic prowess foreign students bring. Traditionally, foreign students represented the best-educated segments of their home societies. More often than not they were among the "highborn" of their countries and had enjoyed the best education and upbringing. If not of the highborn, they were quite likely to be among the most intelligent and highly motivated. Now that nearly 350,000 students are in the United

Table 1. Contrasting Assumptions/Values between America and Other Cultures

American assumptions/values	Contrast-American assumptions/values
People (clients, counselors, and everyone else) are isolable individuals.	People are integrally related with other people (in groups such as families).
Personal growth and change are valuable and desirable.	Conforming to time-tested ways of behaving is desirable.
Individuals have control over their own life circumstances.	One's life circumstances are directed by external (political, economic, social, natural) forces.
Personal problems are often soluble, through greater understanding of their origins or through remedial action undertaken by the individual or both.	Problems are fated to occur, and fate may or may not remove them.
"Professional" people can help other people solve their problems.	One's problems are beyond the control of other human beings.
People (counselors) can be genuinely interested in the welfare of strangers.	Only one's close friends and relatives can be trusted.
People (counselors) can be dealt with as occupants of roles.	Other people are dealt with as whole people.
Open discussion of one's problems can be beneficial.	It can be dangerous to reveal oneself to others.
Emotional disturbances have their root in the individual's past.	Emotional disturbances have their root in external forces or situations.
People are (more or less) equal.	There is a hierarchical ranking of people in society.
Males and females are (more or less) equal.	Males are superior.

Note: Adapted from E. C. Stewart (1972), in D. Horner et al. (1981).

States and an estimated 580,000 students are studying abroad in other countries (Institute of International Education 1987), it is clear that foreign students are not necessarily the "cream of the crop" they were once assumed to be. In fact, there are some who are clearly not. Three situations can be briefly mentioned:

1. In some countries the very best post–high school students, as determined by the results of national school-leaving examinations, remain in their own countries and occupy the limited spaces avail-

able in the domestic universities. This is the case in Malaysia (Steadman 1986), for example, and it was the case in pre-Khomeini Iran (Lockyear 1979).

2. In countries that quickly mount large-scale scholarship programs, some of the students who are granted financial support can be expected to be less academically inclined than others. Some students will simply avail themselves of the opportunity for support for studying outside their country even if they have no particular interest in academic success. The scholarship programs established in the late 1970s and early 1980s by the (temporarily, in some cases) oil-rich nations of Nigeria, Venezuela, Kuwait, and Saudi Arabia sent many young students abroad for whom academic achievement was not especially important.

3. More and more countries are, in effect, competing for students from abroad. Students from ex-colonies often prefer to study with their previous colonial masters, if only because the educational systems and languages are likely to be familiar. Many Malaysians, for example, would prefer to study in the United Kingdom or in Australia. Algerian students might have a preference for study in France. Thus, Malaysian and Algerian students who go to Germany or the United States are not likely to be the best students their countries have produced.

Of course, there are still cases in which outstanding students go abroad to study. And a general impression among faculty seems to be that foreign students are often so highly motivated that they will work hard enough to overcome academic or linguistic deficiencies that might otherwise prevent them from realizing their academic goals. Counselors working with foreign students will want to be circumspect about assuming that given students from abroad are either highly adept academically or highly motivated. The traditional notions about foreign student academic ability fit in some cases and not in others.

Foreign students' social support situations are distinctive. Most domestic clients, at least those who are students, have social support networks that are familiar to Western-trained counselors. They have family members, friends, roommates, classmates, and community organizations to which they can turn for help.

Foreign students, however, are quite far from their families and friends. Furthermore, their families and friends at home probably cannot truly appreciate the experiences the students are having. They may or may not have local friends, depending on, among other factors, the presence or absence of co-nationals with whom they feel compatible. They may face unusual difficulties in being assimilated into the local community, or they may have acquaintances who are more than willing to assist them. Thus, although it is not certain how a foreign student's social support situation will differ from that of a domestic client, it is almost certain that it will differ, perhaps in ways a counselor will not readily comprehend.

Foreign students' customary communicative styles are different. In his study of aspects of Japanese versus American nonverbal behaviors, Barnlund (1975) offered the idea of "communicative style" as a way of comparing important cultural differences. Althen (1984) elaborated on American communicative style compared to that likely to be found in various other cultures. Barnlund set forth five aspects of communicative style: (a) the topics people prefer to discuss in different situations, (b) people's favorite or accustomed forms of verbal interaction (for example, argument, repartee, ritual), (c) the depth of involvement people seek from each other, (d) communication channels people tend to rely on (vocal, verbal, physical), and (e) the level of meaning (factual or emotional) to which people are generally attuned.

Once again, although all aspects of communicative style are in play during a counseling session (and anywhere else), some aspects are likely to be more salient than others. Among the more salient ones are ideas about what topics are appropriately discussed with those outside one's circle of trusted people; the degree of directness with which topics are discussed; vocal volume; eye contact; turn taking in conversation; and the sorts of arguments that are persuasive. Even the way the chairs in the counselor's office are arranged can affect the client's response to the interaction.

Foreign students are unlikely to share the counselor's conception of the counselor's role. Counseling, as we know it, is a Western and, even more, an American invention. American counselors can fairly safely assume that people who come to them as clients believe it is possible to get help from a person who is a "professional helper." Clients generally assume that they will be expected to talk openly about their situations and their feelings. The counselor will ask some questions and perhaps offer comments or suggestions. Together, the counselor and the client will achieve an improved understanding of the genesis of the client's problem and will devise a way to gain improvements.

Foreign students are unlikely to share all these assumptions. If they do visit a counselor about a problem, and often they will not, they need some explanation of the counseling process, the counselor's role, the client's responsibilities, and the manner in which the two people interact in a counseling relationship.

Foreign students face unique problems and issues of adjustment. All new college and university students face the need to "adjust" to their new setting, whether they are foreign or domestic students. Foreign students face some adjustments that domestic students do not, however, and some of the adjustments foreign students must make are unique to students from abroad. Some of the major adjustment problems are discussed below.

1. Initial adjustment to the new culture, including language problems, loneliness, culture shock, and status shock. The literature overflows with discussions and analyses of "culture shock" and "adjustment." Writers differ in how they view this process, with some referring to it as "adjustment," others as "acculturation," and others as "accommodation." Many of these notions will be discussed later in this chapter. However one views this process, there is general agreement that new foreign students need a period of time to learn all the things they must learn in order to manage their daily lives in their new settings and to realize their academic objectives. Unhappy new foreign students may not be aware, or may not want to acknowledge, that their lethargy, hostility, or gastrointestinal problems are the result of a natural adjustment process. "I have decided to go home," a recently arrived and obviously unhappy foreign student might say. Or, "I have decided to transfer to a school that is closer to my cousin." The student is likely to cite particular problems (such as a professor who is difficult to understand or a housing situation that is less pleasant than had been hoped for) that have led to the decision to leave—or at least to serious thoughts about leaving.

Faced with recently arrived and unhappy students, counselors can often help by making clear to the student that nearly all new foreigners confront feelings of unhappiness and frustration that will pass with time. It is quite common to suppose that new foreign students need at least one semester, if not longer, before they can expect to feel generally comfortable and competent in their new environment.

2. Academic difficulty stemming from the novelty of the academic system. Addressing himself to an audience of foreign students, Barnes (1984) describes the U.S. higher education system in terms that compare it to systems that prevail elsewhere. Since the system differs from others, the expectations of students differ, as do the study skills needed for success. Foreign students who have been successful in their own countries can be expected to suppose that they can succeed in U.S. colleges and universities if they follow the same practices that brought them success at home. Often that does not prove to be the case. Aspects of the U.S. system that traditionally cause problems for foreign students include objective-type (as opposed to essay) examinations; the need to do assignments and take examinations throughout each semester, rather than just at the end of the term, the year, or even a two-to-four-year period of studies; and the need to cover a large amount of material and then analyze and synthesize the information.

3. Political, religious, and social conflicts that arise among their fellow nationals in their local community (if there are any). Concerns

among Taiwanese students about "spies" in their midst made the headlines in the mid-1980s, when a Taiwanese who had been a visiting faculty member at an American university, and who had publicly opposed the regime then in power, met an unexplained death while visiting his own country. The Taiwanese community on U.S. campuses is not unique in being divided into factions. Communities of students from Chile, Iran, South Korea, Libya, Malaysia, the People's Republic of China, and South Africa are among those that have been divided by political, social, or religious differences. Some students allow these differences to become the focal points of their lives to the detriment of their studies. Counselors of foreign students ought to guard against the assumption that all the students from a particular client's country are known to and are on good terms with each other.

4. The impact of developments in their home countries—wars, radical changes in government, economic difficulties, and so on. Althen and Riahinejad (1982) used the term "political depression" to describe the state of mind of Iranian students, who, consumed with concern about "the revolution" in their country, could not apply themselves to the task of leading normal daily lives, let alone studying effectively. Counselors of foreign students are better situated to understand their clients if they have even a general idea of what is taking place in the students' countries.

5. Cross-cultural male-female relationships. Whether in daily interactions, romantic relationships, or within marriages, cultural differences in ideas about the proper behavior of males and of females can produce serious misunderstandings. For example, foreign males may find their attentions spurned when they employ their customary means of signaling their interest in a particular female. They may be seen as "too forward," or at the other extreme they may find that their efforts to show interest are so subtle that they are not noticed. Many societies are more male dominated than United States society is (Condon and Yousef 1975) and many other scholars of cross-cultural relations comment on this point, and much disharmony results when male foreign students treat North American females in openly domineering ways.

6. Social isolation, depression, and paranoia (the most common mental disturbance among foreigners). Later in this chapter we discuss these common features of the process of adjusting to a new social and cultural environment.

7. Financial difficulties. As was suggested above, foreign students sometimes face financial diffculties that, compared to the financial difficulties facing domestic students, can seem unresolvable. Laws and regulations of most host countries render foreign students ineligible for most federal financial aid programs. Immigration regulations in most countries also restrict employment opportunities for nonresidents. So

when they do encounter financial problems, foreign students have far fewer options than domestic students have. And unlike domestic students, they cannot, except in certain cases where they can find employment that gives them practical experience in their field of study, interrupt their studies to work, save, and return to school.

8. Anxiety brought on by fear of immigration authorities. It is not unusual to find foreign students who live with noticeable anxiety that their transgressions of the immigration regulations might result in overnight deportation. Foreign students might not understand, as counselors who work with them will want to, that the deportation process in the United States entails a series of time-consuming steps during which the alleged violator has opportunity to present a defense or to leave the country voluntarily.

9. Stressful relationships with particular Americans, especially academic advisers, roommates, and landlords. Brislin et al. (1986) provide a set of cross-cultural "critical incidents" designed to help learners to understand the ways in which culturally based assumptions and values can complicate interactions among people from different cultures. Misunderstandings commonly arise when participants in a situation do not share a common set of assumptions about the behavior that is appropriate to the roles in which they find themselves. Foreign students cannot be assumed to share these understandings with the individuals with whom they relate as academic advisers, roommates, and landlords. The latter are important people in the lives of new students, and if their relationships are troubled the foreign students can be expected to be anxious and upset.

10. Dealing with new-found freedom. Any young college or university student who is living away from home for the first time experiences a sense of liberation from the restraints of parental control. For foreign students the sense of liberation might be even more marked. Anthropologist Edward Hall (1959) uses the terms "high context" and "low context" to distinguish types of cultures in which there are more rather than fewer situations in which proper behavior is culturally prescribed. The United States, Hall says, represents a relatively low-context culture, meaning that there are relatively few situations in which all parties in a situation agree on the sort of behavior that is appropriate. Social restraints are less numerous in a low-context than in a high-context culture. New foreign students, especially ones from a high-context culture, might find themselves almost completely lacking in guidance when they are first apart not just from their parents but from a social order in which such matters as student-teacher relationships, male-female relationships, and young person–older person relationships are structured by socially agreed-upon guidelines. The students may or may not welcome all this freedom.

11. Dealing with disappointed expectations (the student's own and those of family). Althen and Stott (1983) address some of the issues counselors confront when dealing with foreign students who have unrealistic academic expectations. Such students can be particularly difficult to help when they perceive themselves as being under pressure from family members, who themselves are likely to be ignorant of the operations of the U.S. academic system, to achieve outstanding academic records.

12. Dealing with the death of family or friends in the home country and being unable to return home. Relatives or friends of some foreign students may die while those students are away, and sometimes the students are not in a position to return home and participate in the ceremonies that normally take place to show respect for the deceased. Counselors may be called upon to help students in these situations, and those counselors are unlikely to be aware of the customary ways grief is dealt with in the student's own society.

13. Deciding where to live after graduation. No data are available concerning the numbers of foreign students who remain in the United States rather than return to their own countries after they complete their studies. Some students express the intention to remain as soon as they arrive, but many others experience long periods of stressful indecision as they consider the advantages and the disadvantages of staying and of going.

14. Anxieties about returning home. Goodwin and Nacht's (1984) study of Brazilian alumni of U.S. colleges and universities points out the professional and personal difficulties foreign students can experience upon their return home. While many foreign students do not anticipate that they will have particular problems readjusting to their own cultures, some do anticipate the problems, and counselors might encounter students who seem to need assistance in dealing with their fears.

Some Issues in Counseling Foreign Students

The distinctive aspects of foreign students as clients, taken together with the type of training Western counselors receive and the sorts of clients they normally see, give rise to at least four different issues that counselors confront when faced with a client from another country.

1. The general problem of cultural stereotyping. People naturally generalize about other groups of people with whom they have only limited and superficial experience. Most counselors have limited experience with students from other countries. As counselor training pays more attention to the existence and the effects of ethnic and other differ-

ences among clients, the problem of counselor stereotypes gets more attention, and counselors in training presumably become more sensitive to their own stereotypic notions about other categories of people.

Stereotypes can be positive as well as negative, and many Western stereotypes about foreign students are indeed positive. Foreign students are often deemed highly intelligent, highly motivated, courteous, polite, and conscientious. There also may be negative stereotypes about foreign students who do not speak English well, appear clannish, manipulative, and perhaps less than honest. Some particular groups of foreign students are probably subject to more negative stereotyping than others. In any case, counselors must deal with their own stereotypes of students from abroad and look for ways to recognize and overcome them in their counseling with foreign students.

2. The plethora of factors affecting foreign students' situations. Although it may be tempting and sometimes even useful to talk about *the* foreign student, the fact is that any given student's situation is a function not just of his or her cultural background and personality makeup but of a number of other factors as well. Among these factors are the following: country of origin; number of fellow nationals enrolled at the same school or living in the same community and the nature of the relationships among those people; the community's receptivity to foreign students; age; social status at home; English-language proficiency; availability of suitable housing, foods, and opportunities to engage in customary religious practices; goals for the stay in the host country; financial situation; for married students, the situation of dependents (whether they are with the student or back home) duration of anticipated stay; amount of time in the host country; and previous international experience.

3. The difficulty in identifying the source of problems. Many factors can contribute to a client's problems in coping with daily life. Skilled counselors can often isolate the main cause or a few main causes of a client's difficulty. In cross-cultural counseling situations, however, diagnosis can be far more problematic, and consideration must be given to cultural factors that might be having an impact on the client. For example, a foreign student's academic difficulties might stem from limited English proficiency, inappropriate academic background, low intelligence, low motivation, loneliness or other forms of personal unhappiness or preoccupation, some inherited mental illness, a learning disability, difficulty in interacting appropriately with teachers and fellow students, financial strain, concern over the political or family situation at home, or any of a number of other factors. It is unlikely that norms exist for most of the traditional objective diagnostic measures one might employ in diagnosing American clients. The challenge becomes that of assessing how much of a client's problem is because of intercultural problems, interpersonal problems, or pathological disorders.

How, then, can one tell what is behind the problem? It is not easy. And counselors can be *too* "culturally sensitive" or relativistic. Some research by Riahinejad and Henderson (work in progress) suggests that foreign student advisers (who are likely to pride themselves on their "cultural sensitivity") will often attribute to "cultural differences" maladaptive behavior they would describe as pathological if they saw it manifested by a domestic student. There is a difference, then, between a mindless cultural relativism and a cultural sensitivity that is based on some knowledge of a specific other culture or of the general topic of cultural influences on human behavior, that is, what can be called "cultural competence."

4. Doubts about the appropriateness of conventional Western approaches to counseling. Whether a counselor is an adherent of a particular approach to counseling or therapy (psychoanalysis, rational-emotive therapy, behavior modification, etc.) or has an "eclectic" approach, he or she is likely to harbor doubts about the appropriateness of any approach that clearly arises from Western values and ideas. It has become fairly widely recognized that the nondirective approach advocated by the late Carl Rogers may be less effective with foreign clients whose upbringing leads them to expect clear answers and firm guidance from older people or people perceived as having authority. Freud's ideas are often considered applicable only in the West and perhaps only among certain groups of educated Westerners. How should a counselor approach a Middle Eastern student who is convinced that a cabal of local coeds is conspiring to cause his public humiliation? Typical Western approaches might not readily apply to such a case.

Some Findings from the Literature

The preceding paragraphs have outlined some of the factors that make foreign students unique clients compared to their domestic counterparts. Also, some critical issues in counseling foreign students have been identified. This section focuses on literature that addresses some of these concerns.

In recent years interest has increased in the issues and problems involved when a counselor and client do not share a similar cultural background. This interest has been expressed in the proliferation of books and articles about cross-cultural counseling. It has been spurred by the mandate to integrate schools and workplaces, the new populations of immigrants and refugees, and the increased numbers of foreign students studying outside their home countries. These situations have raised questions about the applicability of Western models of counseling in working with foreign students.

Concern for the appropriate treatment of individuals whose personal and cultural values are not reflected or emphasized in the majority Western society has become salient for several professional associations, and some have addressed the issue of cross-cultural counseling competencies. The most explicit statement of cross-cultural counseling competencies is in an American Psychological Association (APA) (Sue et al. 1982) position paper that suggested that such competencies be considered among the criteria for the accreditation of graduate training programs. The APA competencies include specific beliefs or attitudes, knowledge areas, and skills considered essential for the culturally skilled counseling psychologist. It is useful for counselors at all levels to review these criteria to appreciate the complexity of the field and the task confronting those individuals who work in a counseling capacity with foreign students.

Most cross-cultural counseling studies do not deal with the foreign student population but with domestic minority populations. There are few studies that evaluate counseling outcomes beyond the first counselor-client session. A review of the literature reveals that some of the basic questions concerning the counseling of foreign students still need to be empirically addressed. These basic questions include, Is counseling helpful for foreign students? If so, what counseling strategies are most effective for specific types of clients with what types of problems? If not, what sources and types of help are appropriate for foreign students? Despite these shortcomings, reviewing the literature can be useful for those seeking answers to some critical questions posed by those counseling foreign students.

What Are Some of the Dimensions of Adjustment Stress Seen in Foreign Student Clients?

The most typical problem confronting foreign students has to do with adjusting to the culture they are visiting. The stress of this adjustment affects individuals in different ways and to varying degrees. Counselors working with foreign students would be wise to look for signs of stress caused by efforts to function effectively in the host culture.

Culture shock and adjustment stress are terms that must be viewed in the larger context of cultural adjustment. Cultural adjustment is a psychosocial process. The psychological process focuses on the attitudinal and emotional adjustment of the individual to the new environment. The social process focuses on how the individual integrates into the social interaction of the new culture (Church 1982; Martin 1984).

Cultural adjustment has been described as occurring in a number of different ways. Lysgaard (1955) and Sewell and Davidsen (1961) spoke of a "U" curve of adjustment whereby a curvilinear relationship exists between level of adjustment and amount of time spent in the host country. Lysgaard (1955) studied 200 Norwegian Fulbright scholars in the United States and concluded that individuals go through three phases that he describes as initial adjustment, crisis, and regained adjustment. Although he does not specifically describe these stages, he suggests that after a period of initial satisfaction and well-being, an individual experiences a decline in adjustment shortly after entering the foreign culture. At the time they must interact with the culture to carry out their day-to-day purpose. This is followed by a recovery stage after learning how best to cope with the new environment. Gullahorn and Gullahorn (1963, 1966) extended the "U" curve to the "W" curve to account for a similar readjustment process that occurs when an individual returns to the home country. Church (1982), in his extensive review of the sojourner adjustment literature, reports that support for the U-curve hypothesis is inconclusive and perhaps overgeneralized. Brislin (1981), too, finds research on the U curve inconclusive.

Oberg (1960), Smalley (1963), Garza-Guerrero (1974), Adler (1975), and Torbiorn (1982) have described stages of adjustment that people go through while in the host country for an extended period of time. Even though different labels have been used by the authors, they generally agree on three distinct stages. In the first stage the individual is excited by the experience and generally finds things good and interesting. This is often referred to as the "honeymoon" stage. The second stage is characterized by confusion and disintegration as the individual confronts new values, behaviors, beliefs, and lifestyles. This is the stage at which the negative aspects of culture shock are experienced most profoundly and can be termed the crisis stage. The third stage is one of recovery, and the individual experiences an appreciation and understanding of and sensitivity to the new culture. In other words, the individual accommodates both the positive and negative aspects of the new culture and can function in it with a degree of effectiveness or even comfort. Oberg (1960) added a fourth stage that he called the adjustment stage; the individual can begin to work and play in the new culture and perhaps enjoy it, even though there may be occasional moments of anxiety and frustration.

Two other conceptualizations of the cultural adjustment process are worthy of mention. Some authors (Nash 1970; Sewell and Davidson 1961) developed the notion that different types of personalities respond to new cultures in systematically different ways. Using various terms to designate the adjustment patterns they discerned, they found sojourners who actively sought incorporation into the new society, those who resisted such incorporation, and those who showed some of each response.

Grove and Torbiorn (1985) have proposed a "new conceptualization of intercultural adjustment" that involves three variables: level of mere adequacy, applicability of behavior, and clarity of the mental frame of reference. The level of mere adequacy has to do with the standards to which one holds oneself in daily functioning. Applicability of behavior relates to the appropriateness of one's actions in various situations. Clarity of the mental frame of reference has to do with the accuracy of one's understanding of what is going on in one's social environment. Grove and Torbiorn discuss various means by which orientation programs, and presumably counseling, can modify each of these variables to minimize the difficulties of adjustment to a new culture.

Not all authors prefer to use the term "adjustment" to describe the process of feeling comfortable in a new cultural environment. Furnham and Bochner (1986) prefer the theoretical model of "cultural accommodation," which does not rely on the concept of adjustment. This term eliminates the implication that the failures and problems that sojourners experience are symptoms of some underlying pathology that requires treatment. Also, it eliminates the notion of cultural chauvinism that implies that adjusting to the new culture requires one to abandon one's culture of origin.

Berry, Trimble, and Olmedo (1986) speak of "acculturation," which occurs when two or more different cultures come into contact, resulting in changes in the original cultural patterns of one or both of the individuals or groups. These changes can be both behavioral and attitudinal on the part of both cultures or individuals involved. Acculturative stress is often a consequence of the process of acculturation and is characterized by a qualitative change in the life of the individual or community.

Culture shock is the popular label for the negative aspect of cultural adjustment. However, it is commonly viewed as a normal process of adaptation to cultural stress that generally involves such symptoms as depression, anxiety, helplessness, irritability, and a longing for a more predictable and gratifying environment (Church 1982; Adler 1975; Arensberg and Niehoff 1964; Gullahorn and Gullahorn 1963; Lundstedt 1963; Foster 1962; Oberg 1960). Oberg (1960) is generally credited with introducing the term. He believed that culture shock is precipitated by the anxiety that results from losing all one's familiar signs and symbols of social intercourse. Redden (1975), in developing the Culture Shock Inventory, defined culture shock as a psychological disorientation caused by misunderstanding or not understanding the cues of the new culture. It arises from a lack of knowledge, limited prior experience, personal rigidity, and other factors.

Adler (1975) suggests that there are five stages an individual goes through in the development of culture shock. In the contact stage differences are deemed intriguing, and the individual is still insulated by his or her own culture. The second stage is the disintegration stage, during which cultural differences become very apparent and begin to intrude on the individual's sense of well-being. In the third, or reintegration, stage differences are rejected, and the individual becomes preoccupied with likes and dislikes. The fourth is the autonomy stage, in which differences and similarities are legitimized, and the individual is socially and linguistically capable of negotiating most new situations. Fifth is the stage of independence, in which differences and similarities are valued positively, and significant social, psychological, and cultural differences are accepted and enjoyed.

Furnham and Bochner (1986) suggest that there are four traditional features of culture shock that describe the relationship between geographic movement and mental health and account for differences in individuals. The first focus is on grief and bereavement because of the loss of the familiar. The second concerns fatalism versus instrumentalism, or the individual's sense of personal control over the environment. The third is selective migration, which relates to Darwin's theory of natural selection: those sojourners best suited to the new environment will cope better with it. Finally, the fourth notion is that the more realistic an individual's expectations are of the new experience, the greater the ease of adjustment.

Furnham and Bochner (1986) have also identified three other areas of research that have proved useful in offering explanations for culture shock. The areas are negative life events, social support networks, and value differences. The negative life events literature suggests that major life changes often lead to mental and physical illness. Work on social support networks suggests that there is a close positive relationship between the quality and quantity of emotional support one receives from others and an individual's ability to cope with stress. The value difference research offers descriptions of how cultures vary but says little about how and why they may lead to stress or lack of well-being.

A number of other concepts have been used to describe various phenomena related to, but not exactly identical to, culture shock. Guthrie (1966, 1975) used "culture fatigue" to describe the physiological and psychological symptoms of irritability, impatience, depression, loss of appetite, poor sleep, and vague physical complaints often experienced by someone trying to function in a new culture. Smalley (1963) described "language shock" as a significant aspect of cultural adjustment, caused because many cues to social relations lie in the domain of language and are missed when one does not know the local language well.

"Role shock" is used to describe the feeling of ambiguity and loss of personal status often experienced when one tries to transfer one's present role into a new cultural environment and function within that role in the new culture (Byrnes 1966; Higbee 1969). "Education shock" is the term used by Hoff (1979) to describe what frequently happens to foreign students trying to adjust to academic life in the United States. She defines it as a state in which a substantial portion of the learning situation is both new and distressing. Both role shock and education shock are likely to be particularly pronounced among older foreign students who have taken leaves from jobs in their own countries to undertake studies in the United States.

Bennett (1977) uses the term "transition shock" as another way of viewing culture shock. She defines culture shock as a transition involving a state of loss and disorientation requiring adjustment similar to that experienced during any change in one's familiar environment. Cultural adjustment is just one of many experiences that causes transition shock; others include geographic relocation, marriage, divorce, or a death in one's family.

More recently, the cultural adjustment literature has looked to the psychological literature to describe the phenomenon of adjustment in terms of its psychological and physiological impact on the individual. Adjustment stress is defined as the nonspecific state of tension or alarm of the body, causing it to be in a state of readiness for any demand made upon it in the new cultural environment. This definition is based on Selye's (1974) definition of stress. The term stress was first used in conjunction with culture shock by Smith (1955). Recently, however, Adler (1975); Hammer, Gudykunst, and Wiseman (1978); Dyal and Dyal (1981); and Barna (1983) have emphasized the stress factor in cultural adjustment.

What Are Signs of Cultural Adjustment Stress?

It is important for counselors working with foreign students to be aware of the many ways culture shock and adjustment stress can manifest themselves in students. In reviewing the literature on cultural adjustment, culture shock, and adjustment stress, Cort and King (1979) found that most authors view them as a series of psychological reactions developing over time with continued exposure to the new culture. Physiological manifestations are also suggested, but with less frequency. In assessing a student's situation, it is important to develop as complete a picture of the student as possible. For students adjusting to the newness of life in another country, with all that it implies in the way of adjustment stress and culture shock, the stress experienced can manifest itself both physiologically and psychologically.

The literature on cultural adjustment, culture shock, and adjustment stress suggests a number of ways in which stress is manifested psychologically. Thomas (1985) found 21 adaptation psychological correlates of adjustment. Table 2 gives the 21 correlates in the order of their frequency of occurrence in the literature.

Table 2. Psychological Correlates of Adjustment

Depression	David 1971; DuBois 1956; Gullahorn and Gullahorn 1963; Guthrie 1966, 1975; Hojat 1982; Klineberg and Hull 1979; Lin et al. 1982; Melis 1982; Nguyen 1982; Yeh et al. 1979
Helplessness	Adler 1975; Arensberg and Niehoff 1964; Arredondo-Dowd 1981; Bennett 1977; Foster 1962; Gullahorn and Gullahorn 1963; Lundstedt 1963; Oberg 1960
Hostility to host country	Arredondo-Dowd 1981; Church 1982; Cort and King 1979; David 1971; DuBois 1956; Lin et al. 1979; Nash 1970; Oberg 1960
Feelings of anxiety	Bennett 1977; Hojat 1982; Lin et al. 1982; Melis 1982; Nguyen 1982; Spradley and Phillips 1972
Overidentification with one's home country	Arredondo-Dowd 1981; Cort and King 1979; David 1971; DuBois 1956; Oberg 1960
Feelings of with-drawal	Adler 1975; Arredondo-Dowd 1981; Bennett 1977; Cort and King 1979; Lundstedt 1963
Homesickness	Bennett 1977; Church 1982; Klineberg and Hull 1979
Loneliness	Bennett 1977; Hojat 1982; Klineberg and Hull 1979
Paranoid feelings	Lin et al. 1982; Yeh 1972
Preoccupation with cleanliness	Bennett 1977; Church 1982
Irritability	Bennett 1977; Guthrie 1966, 1975
Confusion	Adler 1975; Bennett 1977
Disorientation	Adler 1975; Bennett 1977
Isolation	Bennett 1977
Tension	Bennett 1977
Need to establish continuity	Marris 1975
Psychoticism	Hojat 1982
Neuroticism	Hojat 1982
Defensiveness	Arredondo-Dowd 1981
Intolerance of ambi-guity	Arredondo-Dowd 1981
Impatience	Guthrie 1966, 1975

Physiological correlates are mentioned less frequently, but those mentioned suggest that they closely parallel a physical portrait of a depressive response to stress. Stress occurs when the body stays in a constant state of readiness, even after the arousing stimulus is no longer present and the initial excitement has been replaced (Barna 1983). Selye (1974) suggests that we have only a finite amount of adaptive energy that is both physiological and psychological in nature and that becomes depleted with continual stress. In discussing his concept of the General Adaptation Syndrome, he identified three stages: the alarm stage, in which the person is ready for fight or flight; the resistance stage; and, if stress continues, the person enters a stage of exhaustion in which depression often occurs, seemingly serving to prevent the person from depleting all bodily resources (Selye 1974).

Physiological reactions to the stress of adjustment include loss of appetite, poor sleep, and vague physical complaints. (Guthrie 1966, 1975); physical illness and insomnia or extensive sleep (Barna 1983); and low stamina and energy levels, aching body, a general sense of malaise, and gastrointestinal problems (Melis 1982). It is not uncommon to see recently arrived foreign students with severe headaches and stomach problems and other maladies for which no organic basis can be found.

What Kinds of Problems Do Foreign Students Bring to Counseling?

It is important to distinguish between problems foreign students have and the problems they are likely to bring to counseling. Leong (1984) identified four areas in which foreign students are likely to have problems. These are health, education, vocation, and personal adjustment. Foreign students have been found to be overrepresented as visitors to health services in comparison to their American counterparts (Maha 1964; Rice 1974). Leong (1984) suggests that foreign students, especially Asians, may have a "somatization tendency" when faced with problems of adjustment, preferring to experience and treat them as physical matters rather than psychological ones. Foreign students' educational and vocational problems are similar to those of other students, with some notable exceptions. Foreign students often have language difficulties that affect their academic performance, and they may have a limited understanding of how the host educational system works.

Johnson (1971) found that foreign students rated English-language proficiency, ability to get along financially, separation from family in the home country, and homesickness as their most notable problems. Church (1982) found in reviewing the literature that the most common problems reported by foreign students were language difficulties, financial problems, adjustment to a new educational system, homesickness, and adjustment to social customs and norms. Singh (1963) found that foreign students in Britain experienced unanticipated difficulties in three areas: emotional (loneliness, homesickness); academic (language, oral expression, and teacher-student relationships); and adjustment (place of residence, social class).

Two studies provide interesting data for counselors. A study of Chinese students in the United States was conducted by Chu et al. (1971). It concluded that most Chinese students place a high priority on academic adjustment and consider personal happiness to be far less important. The second study, conducted by Klein et al. (1971), concluded that 90% of 272 incoming foreign students at the University of Wisconsin rated their professional training as more important than personal involvement with Americans or learning about the host culture. Respondents expected their concerns to be centered around finances, courses, schedules, housing arrangements, and academic performance.

These studies suggest that counseling may be most helpful for foreign students, at least for those to whom academic progress is a main concern if it addresses the impediments to successful completion of their studies. Brief behavioral therapy to correct dysfunctional behaviors preventing academic success may be more appropriate than longer-term therapy dealing with the reorganization of the student's personality.

It is rare for a foreign student to initiate a discussion of personal or emotional problems with a counselor. In most cases students request assistance from a faculty member or a foreign student adviser for problems they believe are socially acceptable to discuss with a helper outside the immediate family. Such problems might have to do with finances, a desire to work, or perhaps a legal or immigration question. More personal issues are rarely presented at the outset; it may take the counselor some time to get past the presenting problem to the real counseling issue.

Does Cultural Background Affect How Psychopathology Is Presented?

The literature on psychopathology across cultures is important for individuals working with clients from the non-Western world. Of particular interest is the cross-cultural research on depression, since depression frequently appears as a by-product of adjustment stress (Thomas 1984; Ebbin and Blankenship 1986). Even though people from different cultural groups may have similar physiological symptoms, the recognition, interpretation, and behavioral representation of the problem may vary considerably across cultures (Marsella 1980; Draguns 1985). Kleinman and Good (1985) make the distinction between depression as emotion and depression as disorder. This literature points out some unique cultural differences in how depression is manifested that are helpful for counselors when working with foreign students who are experiencing depression.

A study conducted by Tanaka-Matsumi and Marsella (1976) explored variations in the subjective experience of depression among normal college populations of Japanese nationals, Japanese Americans, and Caucasian Americans. Using word associations to describe their mood when presented with the word "depression," or the Japanese conceptual equivalent *yuutsu*, the experimenters found differences between the Japanese nationals and the Americans. The Japanese nationals used more external referents such as "rain" and "cloud," and somatic terms, such as "headache" and "fatigue." In contrast, the Japanese Americans and Caucasian Americans associated predominantly internal mood-state terms, such as "sad" and "lonely."

Kleinman (1977) conducted a study of 25 patients diagnosed as depressives at a university psychiatric clinic in Taiwan. Of the 25 patients 22 initially complained only of somatic symptoms as compared to emotional or psychological symptoms. After intensive therapy 10 patients still did not admit to psychological affective complaints but rather steadfastly adhered to describing only somatic symptoms. These two studies suggest that a student suffering from somatic complaints that have no organic basis may, in fact, be experiencing depression. Failure to pick up on these cues may mean a delay in proper treatment.

Another important study, reported by Leff (1973) was the International Pilot Study of Schizophrenia, done under the sponsorship of the World Health Organization. The purpose was to study the differentiation of emotional states in nine different countries. It was hypothesized that there would be significant variation in degree of emotional differentiation between countries. Using a semistructured interview to ensure comparability of data, the study found that natives of Western countries showed a greater differentiation of emotion than did people from developing countries, with Nigerians and Chinese showing the least differentiation. There was a strong link between the availability of words for various emotions and the ease with which people distinguish experiences. Cultures that emphasize the individual rather than the group find it more important to describe people's behavior and feelings very specifically. Therefore, more words exist to express feeling states than exist in cultures where the importance of the group is emphasized over that of the individual.

The cross-cultural studies of psychopathology can tell us much about the different ways in which mental illness and stress are manifested across cultures. Perhaps of even greater importance and relevance to those counseling foreign students is the information about the variations in cultural norms. Whereas this literature is valuable and offers important insights into work with foreign students, the special issues and problems of the sojourner population present major challenges to the counselors from whom they seek assistance.

Draguns (1985) cautions counselors against assimilating behavior patterns that are strange, unfamiliar, and different into the category of psychological disturbance or pathology. He gives specific suggestions to counselors who need help in evaluating such behaviors from the client's frame of reference. First, consult research and reviews pertinent to psychopathology across cultures; second, consult colleagues who are familiar with or from the cultural background of the client; third, consult social scientists who have expertise in the culture; fourth, interview members of the cultural group for pertinent cultural information; and finally, the client and his or her family can be enlisted to fill in gaps in information not otherwise available. Consultation with others must be of a general nature to protect the confidentiality of the client, unless the client has specifically given permission to have the case discussed with others.

Overcoming Cultural Differences between Counselor and Client— Is It Possible?

Counselors who work with foreign students continually confront the issue of the degree to which they can overcome cultural barriers that hinder mutual understanding. Can a foreign student ever receive effective, appropriate counseling from a counselor who does not share a similar cultural orientation?

In a counseling relationship one's cultural background plays an important role in how problems and issues are defined, what helping strategies and interventions are employed, and whether successful therapeutic outcomes occur. When the counselor and the client differ in country of origin, cultural background, race, sex, or social class, it is virtually certain that their attitudes, values, and beliefs will be different. In such circumstances communication will be difficult. Counselors are likely to experience misunderstandings, rejection, mutual distrust, and negative transference (Pedersen 1978a). Such problems may prevent the counselor from helping the client.

An issue of even greater importance when cultural differences exist between counselor and client concerns the transmission of values. Counseling is not a value-free process. Rather, it is unusually grounded in the values implicit in the training and in the culture of the counselor. Because of the power differential between the counselor (the help giver) and the client (the one seeking assistance from the one to whom power and authority is attributed), the counselor's values are likely to be given greater credence by the client than they would in a more equal-status interaction. On the other hand, the values may be so discrepant that the client rejects the help and fails to get the needed assistance.

By far the greatest amount of research related to this question has been in the area of counselor-client racial similarity. Most of these studies look at client preference, level of self-exploration, or satisfaction with the first interview as key variables. The evidence is inconclusive as to whether same-race counselor-client pairings are more effective.

Jones (1978) makes an important contribution to this question, and his study deserves further discussion. Unlike other studies that have looked at counselors and clients matched on the variable of race, this study assessed both client and counselor perceptions of the success of 10 counseling sessions. Jones found no significant differences in the outcome of therapy among the different counselor-client racial combinations (black-black, black-white, white-white, white-black) as reported by either counselors or clients. The study suggests that people of different races may effectively work together in counseling provided that there is time to develop a trusting relationship. Analysis of the counseling process in this study found that the course of therapy was changed in a positive direction when the issue of racial difference was openly discussed. Counselor-client trust was enhanced when an implicit difference was made explicit. There is no doubt that cultural differences have an impact on the counseling relationship. These differences were acknowledged and discussed in this study, and the counseling outcomes were not significantly different across various racial combinations. This suggests that acknowledgment of cultural differences might help build a trusting and productive counseling relationship.

Strategies for Effective Counseling with Foreign Students

By now two general points are probably clear. One is that foreign students, as people in transition, are likely to present problems that are sometimes different from those encountered in other populations—specifically, problems of adjustment to a new culture. The second point is that counseling foreign students requires Western-trained counselors to be able to modify their style and approach in various ways. This chapter closes with ideas about what those modifications might be.

Modifying Communicative Style

Barnlund (1975) points out that people prefer to use their accustomed communicative style and will typically try, unconsciously, to enforce it on others because they are more comfortable using their own style. It stands to reason that counselors who wish to put foreign student clients at ease will seek to modify their own communicative styles to accommodate those of their clients. Modifications are possible with respect to a number of aspects of communicative style:

> *Vocal volume.* Malay and Japanese students, for example, typically talk more softly than Americans, but Nigerians speak more loudly. Counselors can adjust their vocal volume accordingly.
>
> *Form of interaction.* Some Germans, Israelis, and Arab students might prefer a more direct approach to interaction. Asians are more likely to prefer consistent politeness and respectfulness.
>
> *Silence.* The typical American proclivity to have someone talking at every moment discomfits people from many other places. Counselors can learn to tolerate periods of silence.
>
> *Length of conversational turn.* Students from many countries are more comfortable than Americans typically are with longer "speeches" from each party in a conversation.
>
> *Eye contact.* Counselors can realize that the eye-contact patterns to which they are accustomed, and from which they make inferences, are culturally based and are not customarily followed by students from elsewhere.
>
> *Degree of explicitness and openness.* By the standards that prevail in many other places, the "openness" that Americans often display is viewed as rudeness or lack of sensitivity. Counselors can take care, if it seems appropriate to do so, not to insist on direct, explicit statements or questions when it seems possible to glean a client's meanings through nonverbal behavior or indirect statements.

These and other such modifications in style can help counselors interact more constructively with students from abroad, no matter what sort of problem is being confronted.

Modifying Counseling Strategies

People's cultural backgrounds provide a "set of lenses" through which they perceive the world. Counselors trained in the United States have been trained with skills and techniques reflecting traditional Western values that place a great deal of emphasis on the individual. Counselors need to be cognizant of and employ special intervention techniques that are oriented to the specific cultural values of their clients.

Knowing a client's value orientation can be most useful in identifying appropriate treatment strategies. Szapocznik et al. (1978) developed an instrument called the Value Orientation Scale, based on the work of Kluckhohn and Strodtbeck (1961), to assess the value orientations of Cuban refugees. They found that Cuban adolescents preferred hierarchical social relationships, subjugation to nature, and had a present time orientation. In contrast, they found that American adolescents preferred individuality in relationships, mastery over nature, and had a future time orientation. Szapocznik and his colleagues have used this information in designing treatment programs to assist Cuban adolescents with chemical dependency problems. Their data have been used to structure a therapy program that better meets the needs of this cultural group. They found that treatment based on the Cubans' own cultural assumptions is significantly more useful to them than the traditional chemical dependency treatment used with white Americans.

A recent study by Thomas (1985) examined the effects of two counseling strategies that reflect different cultural value orientations—an individualistic perspective and an ecological perspective—on perceptions of the counselor by male and female foreign students from five country groups. The individualistic strategy was designed to reflect predominant American values and emphasized the centrality and autonomy of the individual, that is, what the individual wanted and needed for his or her well-being regardless of others in the environment. The ecological strategy reflected contrasting values, specifically, the salience of relationships with family and friends and the responsibilities those relationships carry for the individual. This study found that counselors using the ecological strategy, in which attention was given to the wants, wishes, and the desires of family and community as they related to the student client, were rated as more skillful, knowledgeable about the client's cultural background, trustworthy, understanding, helpful, and attractive. Counselors working with foreign students should be aware that students from many non-Western cultures do not feel it appropriate to set themselves apart from their families or communities and to focus on their individual wants, needs, and desires. Counselors working with this population need to be aware of this and modify their strategies accordingly if they wish to be helpful to their clients.

Modifying Counseling Styles and Client Expectations

Counselors working with foreign students can enhance their credibility with clients by modifying their counseling styles to be consistent with the expectations of the clients. Many students come for help to an expert because they want advice on what to do.

As a group foreign students seem far less likely to come for help in making their own decisions. Two studies by Atkinson, Maruyama, and Matsui (1978) support the idea that racial groups respond differently to directive and nondirective counseling styles. In these studies subjects listened to tapes of the use of the two different styles of counseling. In the first study Asian-American students were the subjects, and in the second study the subjects were Japanese Americans who were members of a Young Buddhist Association. In both studies the counselor was rated as more credible and approachable when employing a directive counseling style. Being more directive can be a useful approach for counselors working with foreign students.

A study by Yuen and Tinsley (1981) compared American students' expectations of counseling with those of a group of Chinese, African, and Iranian students. They discovered that the Americans expected the counselor to be less directive and protective, and they expected to take more responsibility for their own improvement. The Chinese, Africans, and the Iranians, on the other hand, expected to assume a more passive role in counseling and expected the counselor to be a more directive and nurturing figure.

Counselors are likely to be more effective if they vary their styles with culturally different clients. Also, foreign students may need an orientation to counseling to benefit from the experience. This orientation can take place through the interview by the way the counselor gives the client permission to discuss and explore thoughts, feelings, and problems. It may also be useful for the counselor to explain what counseling is and how the counselor can assist the client. It is important for counselors to explore their clients' expectations of counseling in order to respond appropriately to their clients' needs.

Explaining the Adjustment Process

Many foreign students come for help when they feel overwhelmed by the large number of obstacles they perceive to be preventing them from feeling comfortable and effective in the host culture. Foreign students may find themselves with problems they never encountered at home. They may feel strange and also that something is quite wrong with them. Frequently, talking to these foreign student clients about culture shock, the adjustment process, and the stress that is encountered when they try to adapt to a new environment can help them see their feelings as part of the natural process of adaptation. Often this didactic explanation, coupled with emotional support, provides all that is required therapeutically for students to begin feeling better about themselves and their experiences in the host country.

Dealing with Adjustment-related Depression

One can see in the descriptions of the psychological and physiological correlates of culture shock and adjustment stress a number of symptoms that are closely related to the Western concept of depression. Cognitive and behavioral models of depression provide ways to conceptualize the culture shock and stress generally associated with cultural adjustment in foreign students. Therapeutic techniques based on these models of depression can be useful with foreign students undergoing adjustment stress.

Cognitive therapy involves techniques to help clients face three types of cognition that lead to feelings of depression and lack of control. The first type of cognition assumes that outcomes are beyond one's control. An expression of this would be, "No matter how hard I try, I don't think my teaching assistant will let me pass this class." The second type of cognition attributes negative outcomes to internal, stable, and global factors, such as "I'm not smart enough," or "Everyone is smarter than I am." The third cognition subscribes to unrealistic and unattainable goals but continues viewing them as extremely important (Beach, Abramson, and Levine 1981). An example would be a student who insists on pursuing an engineering program despite the fact that he consistently fails all his science and math courses. Cognitive therapy is aimed at changing negative, self-defeating cognitions to help the individual recognize the association between dysfunctional thinking and his or her own feelings and behaviors (Coleman and Beck 1981).

The counselor has three major responsibilities in cognitive therapy. The first is to collaborate with the foreign student to determine whether the student's thoughts, attitudes, or beliefs are contributing to feelings generally associated with depression (Coleman and Beck 1981). The assumption is that one can change one's negative thoughts when presented with evidence that they are counterproductive. The counselor's role is to work with the student in gathering evidence about the impact of the negative thoughts and to help the student accurately interpret it. Small behavioral tasks can be helpful in demonstrating that there is a difference between beliefs about what one can do and one's actual ability to do it. The second counselor responsibility in cognitive therapy is to help the student identify automatic negative thoughts. This can be done by correcting misperceptions and by providing accurate information and feedback to the student about his or her behavior. The third responsibility is to help the student sense some control over the environment. For example, if a foreign student erroneously believes he or she is a social outcast and attributes this to American prejudice, he or she will have a sense of helplessness about ever being able to have an American friend. Also, in all likelihood, the student will act like an outcast and will feel lonely. The counselor can assist such students by helping them monitor the number of times they talk to Americans and by confronting their overgeneralizations. In another example, a student who expects to do poorly in a course will find it difficult to commit to a goal of studying for the course every day. Such students are often helped by having their sense of futility challenged in a supportive atmosphere. They can learn to limit overgeneralizing, drawing negative conclusions from single incidents, making arbitrary inferences, and selectively abstracting details out of context.

Behavioral therapy is generally aimed at increasing the student's activity level, on the assumption that more activity will increase the likelihood of positive reinforcement from the environment. Foreign students experiencing adjustment stress may withdraw and become relatively inactive. Counselors can help students to increase their activity level by contracting them to do certain things within a given timeframe. For example, they might be asked to keep a list of the times they study, exercise, or read a textbook in a given day. This approach provides data as well as reinforcement for the student. Students with study difficulties can be asked to make a list of small, discreet tasks that they should accomplish during a given time period. As each task is accomplished, the student can cross it off the list. Seeing that things can, in fact, be accomplished often acts as a motivator.

Another goal of behavioral therapy is to control behavioral excesses, such as excessive ruminating or verbalizing about negative aspects of oneself, the past, or other people or about somatic complaints. A student who is having problems studying because of worrying about the amount of money parents are spending for school is engaging in a behavioral excess. Helping the student to stop the destructive ruminating by writing down each time he or she does it will help the student be aware of the large amount of time being spent in a fruitless activity. Evidence compiled in this way usually has a substantial effect on reducing destructive behaviors.

Another major goal of behavioral therapy is to help enhance the student's instrumental skills. For foreign students this could mean teaching social skills for interacting appropriately with faculty advisers or classmates, teaching what Americans consider to be the attributes of a good employee, or teaching how to ask Americans to go out on a date. Such behaviors can be taught by modeling and role-playing and can help the student function more effectively in this culture.

Furnham and Bochner (1986) assert that learning about the host culture and learning appropriate social skills for the new environment are effective antidotes to culture shock. They suggest an alternative theoretical model of cultural accommodation that does not rely on the notion of cultural adjustment.

Addressing Presenting Concerns First

Most foreign students come for help because they are experiencing problems that are making it difficult for them to accomplish their educational objectives. Often counselors may see potential areas of growth that we believe would be useful for the student to explore in therapy. For most students the primary purpose in coming to the United States is to complete an educational program. Apart from this goal all else is seen as less important. Counselors need to be aware of this and to focus their therapy on helping the student to deal with the presenting problem first, especially as it relates to the client's educational goal. Failure to focus first on the presenting problem may seriously hinder the establishment of a good working relationship.

Acknowledging Cultural Differences

A trusting relationship between counselor and client is a prerequisite for a successful helping relationship. When the counselor and client are from different cultures, this fact, if not addressed in the interview, can be an impediment to establishing a solid counseling relationship. The counselor can enhance the relationship by making explicit what is already implicit to both parties, that is, that they represent different cultural backgrounds. It is important and indeed essential that the counselor be open and willing to learn and accept the cultural values of the client as the context for the counseling relationship. By using the foreign student client as a cultural resource, the counselor can empower the client and help establish a constructive working relationship.

Conclusion

Foreign students with problems adjusting to their new cultural environment do not often directly seek assistance from a counselor. However, they frequently seek help or information about such logistical matters as finding jobs, getting financial aid, carrying out some immigration procedure, or other less personal concerns. It is possible to simply respond to their inquiries. These presenting concerns, however, are frequently secondary to feelings of homesickness, loneliness, isolation, frustration, sense of failure, and depression. A skillful counselor will create an atmosphere of acceptance and openness by asking questions that convey a concern for the student as a person and convey a willingness to listen. Often questions such as "How are you finding life in the residence hall?" or "What are you doing for fun when you aren't studying?" can show the student a counselor's willingness to know more about him or her. The student can choose whether to use the opportunity to explore other, more personal, concerns with the counselor. Many students will welcome the opportunity to share a part of their personal concerns with a counselor who seems willing to listen, especially if the counselor acknowledges and respects the various attitudes, beliefs, and values the student represents.

References

Adler, P. S. 1975. The transitional experience: An alternative view of culture shock. *Journal of Humanistic Psychology* 15:13–23.

Alexander, A. A., Klein, M. H., Workneh, F., and Miller, M. 1981. Psychotherapy and the foreign student. In P. B. Pedersen, J. G. Draguns, W. J. Lonner, and J. E. Trimble (eds.), *Counseling across cultures.* Honolulu: University of Hawaii Press.

Althen, G. 1984. *The handbook of foreign student advising.* Yarmouth, ME: Intercultural Press.

Althen, G., and Riahinejad, M. 1982. Political depression among students from Iran. In *National Association for Foreign Student Affairs Newsletter.* Washington, DC: National Association for Foreign Student Affairs.

Althen, G., and Stott, F. W. 1983. Advising and counseling students with unrealistic academic objectives. *Personnel and Guidance Journal* 61 (10): 608–611.

Arensberg, C. M., and Niehoff, A. H. 1964. *Introducing social change: A manual for Americans overseas.* Chicago: Aldine.

Arredondo-Dowd, P. M. 1981. Personal loss and grief as a result of immigration. *Personnel and Guidance Journal* 59 (6): 376–378.

Atkinson, D. R. 1983. Ethnic similarity in counseling psychology: A review of research. *Counseling Psychologist* 11 (3): 79–92.

Atkinson, D. R., Maruyama, M., and Matsui, S. 1978. Effects of counselor race and counseling approach on Asian Americans' perceptions of counselor credibility and utility. *Journal of Counseling Psychology* 25:76–83.

Barna, L. M. 1983. The stress factor in intercultural relations. In D. Landis and R. W. Brislin (eds.), *Handbook of intercultural training.* Vol. 2, *Issues in training methodology.* New York: Pergamon Press.

Barnes, G. A. 1984. *The American university: A world guide.* Philadelphia: ISI Press.

Barnlund, D. 1975. *Public and private self in Japan and the United States.* Tokyo: Simul Press.

Beach, S., Abramson, L. Y., and Levine, F. M. 1981. Attributional reformulation of learned helplessness and depression: Therapeutic implications. In J. F. Clarkin and H. I. Glazer, *Depression: Behavioral and directive intervention strategies.* New York: Garland STPM Press.

Bennett, J. 1977. Transition shock: Putting cultural shock in perspective. In N. Jain (ed.), *International and intercultural communication annual,* Vol. 4. Falls Church, VA: Speech Communications Association.

Berry, J. W., Trimble, J. E., and Olmedo, E. L. 1986. Assessment of acculturation. In W. J. Lonner and J. W. Berry (eds.), *Field methods in cross-cultural research.* Beverly Hills: Sage Publications.

Brislin, R. W. 1981. *Cross-cultural encounters: Face to face interaction.* New York: Pergamon Press.

Brislin, R. W., Cushner, K., Cherrie, C., and Yong, M. 1986. *Intercultural interactions: A practical guide.* Beverly Hills: Sage Publications.

Byrnes, F. C. 1966. Role shock: An occupational hazard of American technical assistants abroad. *Annals* 368:95–108.

Chu, H. M., Yeh, E. K., Klein, M. H., Alexander, A. A., and Miller, M. H.

1971. A study of Chinese students' adjustment in the U.S.A. *Acta Psychologica Taiwanica* 13:206–218.

Church, A. T. 1982. Sojourner adjustment. *Psychological Bulletin* 91:540–572.

Coleman, R. E., and Beck, A. T. 1981. Cognitive therapy for depression. In J. F. Clarkin and H. I. Glazer (eds.), *Depression: Behavioral and directive intervention strategies*. New York: Garland STPM Press.

Condon, J. C., and Yousef, F. Y. 1975. *An introduction to intercultural communication*. Indianapolis: Bobbs-Merrill.

Cort, D. A., and King, M. 1979. Some correlates of culture shock among American tourists in Africa. *International Journal of Intercultural Relations* 3:211–225.

David, K. H. 1971. Culture shock and the development of self-awareness. *Journal of Contemporary Psychotherapy* 4:44–48.

Draguns, J. G. 1985. Psychological disorders across cultures. In P. B. Pedersen (ed.), *Handbook of cross-cultural counseling and therapy,* 55–62. Westport, CT: Greenwood Press.

DuBois, C. A. 1956. *Foreign students and higher education in the United States.* Washington, DC: American Council on Education.

Dyal, J. A., and Dyal, R. Y. 1981. Acculturation, stress and coping: Some implications for research and education. *International Journal of Intercultural Relations* 5:301–328.

Ebbin, A., and Blankenship, E. 1986. A longitudinal health care study: International versus domestic students. *Journal of American College Health* 34:177–182.

Foster, G. M. 1962. *Traditional cultures and the impact of technological change.* New York: Harper and Row.

Furnham, A., and Bochner, S. 1986. *Culture shock: Psychological reactions to unfamiliar environments.* London: Methuen.

Garza-Guerrero, A. C. 1974. Culture shock: Its mourning and vicissitudes of identity. *Journal of the American Psychoanalytic Association* 22:408–429.

Goodwin, C. D., and Nacht, M. 1984. *Fondness and frustration.* New York: Institute of International Education.

Grove, C. N., and Torbiorn, I. 1985. A new conceptualization of intercultural adjustment and the goals of training. *International Journal of Intercultural Relations* 9:205–233.

Gullahorn, J. E., and Gullahorn, J. T. 1966. American students abroad: Professional versus personal development. *Annals* 368:43–59.

Gullahorn, J. T., and Gullahorn, J. E. 1963. An extension of the U-curve hypothesis. *Journal of Social Issues* 19 (3): 33–47.

Guthrie, G. M. 1966. Cultural preparation for the Philippines. In R. B. Textor (ed.), *Cultural frontiers of the Peace Corps.* Cambridge: MIT Press.

———. 1975. A behavioral analysis of culture learning. In R. W. Brislin, S. Bochner, W. J. Lonner (eds.), *Cross-cultural perspectives on learning.* New York: John Wiley and Sons.

Hall, E. H. 1959. *The silent language.* New York: Doubleday.

Hammer, M. R., Gudykunst, W. B., and Wiseman, R. L. 1978. Dimensions in intercultural effectiveness: An exploratory study. *International Journal of Intercultural Relations* 2:382–393.

Henderson, S. 1984. Interpreting the evidence on social support. *Social Psychiatry* 19:1–4.

Higbee, H. 1969. Role shock—A new concept. *International Educational and Cultural Exchange* 4 (4): 71–81.

Hoff, B. L. R. 1979. Classroom-generated barriers to learning: International students in American higher education. Ph.D. diss., United States International University, San Diego.

Hofstede, G. 1984. *Culture's consequences: International differences in work-related values.* (Abridged ed.) Beverly Hills: Sage Publications.

Hojat, M. 1982. Loneliness as a function of selected personality variables. *Journal of Clinical Psychology* 38 (1): 137–141.

Horner, D., and Vandersluis, K., et al. 1981. Cross-cultural counseling. In G. Althen (ed.), *Learning across cultures.* Washington, DC: National Association for Foreign Student Affairs.

Institute of International Education. 1987. *Open doors: 1986/87.* New York: Institute of International Education.

Johnson, D. C. 1971. Problems of foreign students. *International Educational and Cultural Exchange* 7:61–68.

Jones, E. E. 1978. Effects of race on psychotherapy process and outcome: An exploratory investigation. *Psychotherapy: Theory, Research, and Practice* 15 (3): 226–236.

Klein, M. H., Alexander, A. A., Tseng, K., Miller, M. H., Yeh, E., Chu, H., and Workneh, F. 1971. The foreign student adaptation project: Social experiences of Asian students in the U.S. *Exchange* 6:77–90.

Kleinman, A. 1977. Depression, somatization, and the "new cross-cultural psychiatry." *Social Science and Medicine* 11:3–9.

Kleinman, A., and Good, B., eds. 1985. *Culture and depression: Studies in the anthropology and cross-cultural psychiatry of affect and disorder.* Berkeley: University of California Press.

Klineberg, O., and Hull, W. F. 1979. *At a foreign university: An international study of adaptation and coping.* New York: Praeger.

Kluckhohn, F. R., and Strodtbeck, F. L. 1961. *Variations in value orientation.* New York: Harper and Row.

Kohls, L. R. 1984. *The values Americans live by.* Washington, DC: Meridian House International.

Leff, J. 1973. Culture and the differentiation of emotional states. *British Journal of Psychiatry* 123:299–306.

Leong, F. 1984. *Counseling international students.* Ann Arbor: ERIC Counseling and Personnel Services Clearinghouse.

Lin, K. M., Masuda, M., and Tazuma, L. 1982. Adaptational problems of Vietnamese refugees: Pt. 3, Case studies in clinic and field: Adaptive and maladaptive. *Psychiatric Journal of the University of Ottawa* 7 (3): 173–183.

Lin, K. M., Tazuma, L., and Masuda, M. 1979. Adaptational problems of Vietnamese refugees: I. Health and mental status. *Archives of General Psychiatry* 36:955–961.

Lockyear, F. 1979. Factors affecting non-sponsored students from Iran. In G. Althen (ed.), *Students from the Arab world and Iran.* Washington, DC: National Association for Foreign Student Affairs.

Lundstedt, S. 1963. An introduction to some evolving problems in cross-cultural research. *Journal of Social Issues* 19 (3): 1–9.

Lysgaard, S. 1955. Adjustment in foreign society: Norwegian Fulbright grantees visiting the United States. *International Social Science Bulletin* 7:45–51.

Maha, G. 1964. Health survey of new Asian and African students at the University of Illinois: *Journal of the American College Health Association* 12:303–310.

Marris, P. 1975. *Loss and change.* New York: Anchor.

Marsella, A. J. 1980. Depressive experience and disorder across cultures. In H. C. Triandis and J. G. Draguns (eds.), *Handbook of cross-cultural psychology.* Vol. 6, *Psychopathology.* Boston: Allyn and Bacon.

Marsella, A. J., and Pedersen, P. B., eds. 1981. *Cross-cultural counseling and psychotherapy: Foundations, evaluation, and cultural considerations.* Elmsford, NY: Pergamon Press.

Marsella, A. J., Sartorius, N., Jablensky, A., and Fenton, F. 1985. Cross-cultural studies of depressive disorders: An overview. In A. Kleinman and B. Good, *Culture and depression.* Berkeley: University of California Press.

Martin, J. 1984. The intercultural reentry: Conceptualization and direction for future research. *International Journal of Intercultural Relations* 8:115–134.

Melis, A. I. 1982. Arab students in Western universities: Social properties and dilemmas. *Journal of Higher Education* 53 (4): 439–447.

Nash, D. 1970. *A community in limbo.* Bloomington: Indiana University Press.

Nguyen, S. D. 1982. Psychiatric and psychosomatic problems among the Southeast Asian refugees. *Psychiatric Journal of the University of Ottawa* 7:163–172.

Oberg, K. 1960. Cultural shock: Adjustment to new cultural environments. *Practical Anthropology* 7:177–182.

Pedersen, P. B. 1978a. Four dimensions of cross-cultural skill in counselor training. *Personnel and Guidance Journal* 56 (8): 480–483.

———. 1978b. Introduction. *Personnel and Guidance Journal* 56 (8): 457.

———, ed. 1985. *Handbook of cross-cultural counseling and therapy.* Westport, CT: Greenwood Press.

Pedersen, P. B., Draguns, J. G., Lonner, W. J., and Trimble, J. E., eds. 1981. *Counseling across cultures.* Honolulu: University of Hawaii Press.

Rahe, R. H., Meyer, M., Smith, M., Kjaer, G., and Holmes, T. H. 1964. Social stress and illness onset. *Journal of Psychosomatic Research* 8:35–44.

Redden, W. 1975. *Culture shock inventory—Manual.* Frederickton, N. B., Canada: Organizational Tests.

Reid, J., ed. 1988. *Building the professional dimension of educational exchange.* Yarmouth, ME: Intercultural Press.

Riahinejad, M., and Henderson, A. Work in progress.

Rice, R. 1974. Foreign student health center visitation: Where does the anomaly lie? *Journal of the American College Health Association* 23:134–137.

Rokeach, M. 1973. *The nature of human values.* New York: Free Press.

Sartorius, N., Davidian, H., Ernberg, G., Fenton, F., Frijii, I., Gastpar, M., Gulbinat, W., Jablensky, A., Kielholz, P., Lehmann, H., Naraghi, M., Shimizu, M., Shinfuku, N., and Takahashi, R. 1983. *Depressive disorders in different cultures.* Geneva: World Health Organization.

Selye, H. 1974. *Stress without distress.* New York: J. B. Lippincott.

Sewell, W. H., and Davidsen, O. M. 1961. *Scandinavian students on an American campus.* Minneapolis: University of Minnesota Press.

Singh, A. K. 1963. *Indian students in Britain.* Bombay: Asia Publishing House.

Smalley, W. A. 1963. Culture shock, language shock, and the shock of self-discovery. *Practical Anthropology* 10:49–56.

Smith, M. B. 1955. Some features of foreign student adjustment. *Journal of Higher Education* 26:231–241.

Spradley, J. P., and Phillips, M. 1972. Culture and stress: A quantitative analysis. *American Anthropologist* 74:518–529.

Steadman, J. 1986. *Malaysia.* Washington, DC: American Association of Collegiate Registrars and Admissions Officers.

Stewart, E. C. 1972. *American cultural patterns: A cross-cultural perspective.* Yarmouth, ME: Intercultural Press.

Sue, D. W. 1981. *Counseling the culturally different: Theory and practice.* New York: John Wiley and Sons.

Sue, D. W., Bernier, J. E., Durran, A., Feinberg, L., Pedersen, P. B., Smith, E. J., and Vasquez-Nuttall, E. 1982. Position paper: Cross-cultural counseling competencies. *Counseling Psychologist* 10 (2): 45–52.

Szapocznik, J., Scopetta, M. A., Aranalde, M., and Kurtines, W. 1978. Cuban value structure. *Journal of Consulting and Clinical Psychology* 46 (5): 961–970.

Tanaka-Matsumi, J., and Marsella, A. J. 1976. Cross-cultural variations in the phenomenological experience of depression: Pt. 1, Word association studies. *Journal of Cross-Cultural Psychology* 7:379–396.

Thomas, K. A. 1982. A pilot study to assess cross-cultural counselor training outcomes. Master's thesis, University of Minnesota, Minneapolis.

———. 1984. Culture shock and adjustment: A special case of depression. Typescript.

———. 1985. A comparison of counseling strategies reflective of cultural value orientations on perceptions of counselors in cross national dyads. Ph.D. diss., University of Minnesota, Minneapolis.

Torbiorn, I. 1982. *Living abroad: Personal adjustment and personnel policy in the overseas setting.* New York: John Wiley and Sons.

Triandis, Harry C., Brislin, Richard, and Hui, C. Harry. 1988. Cross-cultural training across the individualism-collectivism divide. *International Journal of Cultural Inter-Relations* 12 (3): 269–289.

Yeh, E. K. 1972. Paranoid manifestations among Chinese students studying abroad: Some preliminary findings. In W. Lebra (ed.), *Transcultural research in mental health,* vol. 2 of *Mental health research in Asia and the Pacific,* 326–340. Honolulu: University Press of Hawaii.

Yuen, R. K., and Tinsley, H. E. A. 1981. International and American students' expectancies about counseling. *Journal of Counseling Psychology* 28 (1): 66–69.

10

Counseling Refugees:
The North American Experience

HARRIET P. LEFLEY

In the past few decades several million persons have come to the United States and Canada as refugees, émigrés, exiles, entrants, and undocumented aliens—to name a few of the different status labels that have encompassed a similar experience of translocation but have affected its sequelae in terms of acceptance by the new world. We will use the omnibus term "refugees" to describe the experience of involuntarily uprooted people. In today's world few have willingly abandoned their country of origin and elected to live elsewhere. Refugees are characterized as that subset of immigrants who have come under duress, to escape situations perceived as politically, economically, psychologically, and physically threatening to survival.

Because migration histories, acceptance by the host population, and sociocultural distance between clients and counselors may differ substantively in the refugee populations of other countries, this discussion will necessarily focus on the North American experience. Under any condition of migration, however, counseling refugees involves expertise in at least four domains, each embodying both antecedent events and contemporary context. These include: (a) the generic refugee experience of uprooting, loss, and adaptation to an alien culture; (b) the specific antecedents and ongoing events of the translocation experience of the client's group; (c) the contemporary social and familial context, including distal and proximal variables in the host culture that facilitate or impede adjustment; and (d) the adaptive strengths and weaknesses of the individual counselee. The client's subjective culture is the enveloping capsule within which these variables are processed.

The model of subjective culture developed by Triandis et al. (1972) not only includes modal attitudes, norms, roles, and values transported across experience but presumably permits ongoing modification of the criteria used in processing each new domain. As victims of constant flux refugees may interpret and react to their changing realities by holding rigidly to earlier cultural norms or by adjusting their cognitions and behaviors to meet the empirical demands of survival in a highly variable world. As several investigators have suggested (e.g., Szapocznik and

Kurtines 1980), extremes at either end of the continuum may be maladaptive. For most refugees as well as other displaced groups, however, holding fast to cultural norms is both comforting and self-reinforcing. It tends to ensure predictability of response to consensually validated cues and to perpetuate the comforting enclosure of the in-group as support against the outside world (Cassel 1974). Nevertheless, the refugee experience is filled with changing cues and permeable boundaries, and the protective mechanism that facilitates survival of the culture of origin may also militate against optimal adjustment in the culture of final resettlement (see Berry 1986).

Because this process of cultural adaptation has frequently evolved from external threat, it is essential to begin with an understanding that refugee counseling may differ considerably from other types of cross-cultural counseling. Working with foreign graduate students, U.S. citizens going to live abroad, foreign professional families coming to live in the United States, or diverse ethnic groups in the United States of varying socioeconomic levels is different in substance and kind from dealing with refugees. Counseling refugees requires not only an understanding of cultural background and of status and roles within that culture but knowledge of the historical, political, and existential realities attending a particular migration.

The ensuing discussion on counseling refugees will focus on four major areas: (a) contextual issues involving translocation and resettlement, physical health, acculturation, and modes of defining adaptive behavior; (b) generic concerns of all refugee groups; (c) diagnostic assessment, treatment modalities, and parameters of appropriate service delivery; and (d) needs of special populations.

Experiencing Displacement and Translocation

In considering models of counseling refugees, it is essential to begin with generic issues that transect the experience of translocation. Movement from one life, one place, one cultural ambience to another is inherently destabilizing. Moreover, as Cohen (1987) has pointed out, many refugees have experienced a continuum of movement before reaching a terminal point they can call home. Persons may have been in several camps within one country, in several different countries, or in a number of different geographic areas both outside or within the host country. The initial culture shock may have been incurred in movement from rural to urban settings. Indeed, for some groups there may have been a leap across centuries from traditional to modern lifestyles.

Each change brings added ambiguities, with new requirements for psychological adjustment to a life in transition and uncertain expectations of ever attaining even minimal control over one's own destiny.

The sum of these experiences may have conferred an adaptive edge to individuals with (a) high tolerance for frustration or (b) characteristics typically devalued by mental health professionals in the host country. These may include repressors, nonplanners, and those who blend active coping with fatalism (Lin, Masuda, and Tazuma 1982). Conversely, successful adaptation may also accrue to the self-oriented, those who survive by manipulation and selective abandonment of cultural norms. The counselor's countertransferential conflict in dealing with negatively perceived values, always an underlying problem in cross-cultural training (see Lefley 1985b), is particularly salient in this connection. Many refugees have learned survival skills that may be viewed as aversive or even sociopathic by counselors here (see Stein 1986). The task is to help the client apply traditional values in developing behaviors that are equally or more adaptive, an issue discussed further in the final section on counseling models for refugees.

In the midst of this ambience of uncertainty, there are subpopulations with unique features. Groups marginal to a refugee mainstream, such as Cuban or Iranian Jews (Good, Good, and Moradi 1985), may have unique problems of identity or loss. Fragmented families, unaccompanied minors separated from their parents, and refugee children of U.S. servicemen are examples of groups with special counseling needs. Illegal aliens constitute a special risk group. War survivors and persons who have been subjected to starvation, torture, rape, unremitting brutality, and constant fears of impending death require an exceptionally high level of therapeutic skill and sensitivity.

What does it mean to work with people who have endured these conditions? In addition to requiring discrete types of cultural expertise, the task of counseling refugees raises a host of questions regarding commonalities of experience, the parameters of therapeutic intervention, and the types of clients likely to be seen. There are numerous levels of intervention, beginning with generic issues of loss, grieving, difficulty in adjustment, impaired self-concept, familial and generational conflict, and disparity between inflated expectations and disappointing realities. Is the counselor's major objective the building of adaptive strength to cope with these stressful reactions? If so, is this done through insight, behavior management, cognitive restructuring, or other interpersonal, dyadic interventions? Is family therapy the treatment of choice for persons from cultures that are, for the most part, family oriented and therapeutically interdependent? If this is the case, how helpful are contemporary structural or strategic models when they are applied to dealing with uncontrollable external stress? Does the counselor go beyond the clinical role and become an advocate and culture broker for a person who may lack basic skills in negotiating an alien system? Do counselors concern themselves with the client's community, with learning not only the cultural background but the economic and political realities of the client's everyday survival problems in the ethnic enclaves of contemporary U.S. life?

We have suggested that counseling refugees requires tasks and skills over and above those applied to other groups that are culturally divergent from mainstream U.S. norms. However, this population may be unique not only in experience but in personality as well. For most refugees successful exodus is contingent on fortuitous circumstances. This presumably precludes inferences of selective migration of stronger, more psychologically intact individuals. Yet, it has been suggested that considerable strength is required to have transcended the terror and tortures to which many people have been exposed and the long hegira in seeking asylum. For purposes of our discussion we may postulate a continuum of psychological strength, from the very strong to the very weak. These require different sets of counseling skills. Some strong counselees, consonant with their aptitude for survival, may seek out aid for help in adjustment for themselves and their children. In the main, however, the stigma of seeking mental health care is likely to be avoided, and those who come are likely to have been referred for counseling because of problem behaviors of considerable severity (Folkenberg 1986). Although major mental illnesses are infrequent (Lin 1986), counselors must have sufficient cultural expertise to be able to distinguish between adjustment reactions and psychotic decompensation and to triage clients who require psychiatric evaluation, chemotherapy, and possible hospitalization.

Counselors must also become familiar with specific stressors that are a product of cultural, demographic, and experiential differences in the client populations and that affect the individual's capacity for adaptation. The following sections raise issues suggesting that the counselor's role may differ according to level of acculturation of the presenting client or salience of acculturative problems, or both; rural versus urban background; relationship of the client's ethnic group to the host community and to other ethnic groups of indigenous or refugee status; and political issues that affect the client's acceptance and self-perception. Special populations, such as children and adolescents or those who have experienced unusually traumatic events, will be discussed. Finally, commonalities of the refugee experience suggest a stress, coping, and adaptation model as the most fruitful paradigm for intervention.

Initial Adaptation: Dimensions of Culture Shock

Culture shock has been defined by Furnham and Bochner (1986) as a transitory period of confusion and disorientation in adapting to a new culture. In reviewing the literature on migration, these authors suggest that this is the negative part of a "U-curve of adjustment" with three main phases: "an initial stage of elation and optimism, replaced by a period of frustration, depression, and confusion (presumably the period labeled . . . as culture shock), followed by a gradual improvement leading to optimism and satisfaction with the new society" (1986, 234). Furnham and Bochner feel that the cultural stress inherent in this period of disorientation does not warrant interventions by mental health professionals. They state: "There is very little evidence to suggest that culture stress can be regarded as some form of mental illness, or that counseling or 'therapy' is the most appropriate or effective means of alleviating such stress and promoting 'healthy' personalities and satisfactory social relationships" (1986, 234). Rather, they suggest a culture-learning model in which the key idea is not psychologically adjusting to the new culture but learning its salient characteristics. This model is close to the concept of bicultural effectiveness of Szapocznik et al. (*BET,* 1986) and other approaches that emphasize competency building rather than intrapsychic exploration.

These issues are highly germane to the whole question of whether, when, and under what conditions counseling of refugees is indicated and to the intervention model that is most effective for their needs. Although many authors, like Furnham and Bochner, object to "medicalizing" migration and culture change as pathogens, persons who come to the attention of counselors presumably have suffered undue negative effects, and the refugee experience typically has been more stressful than the type of voluntary migration that may also result in the disorientation of culture shock. To a great extent, however, the type and intensity of problems appear to be contingent on how well these persons have resolved their identity feelings and relationships to their own culture and to that of the host society.

Acculturation and Mental Health

For many years the literature on immigrants and indigenous peoples indicated an inverse relationship between psychological health and level of acculturation to the dominant culture (Lefley 1976). These findings seemed intuitively reasonable. They strongly suggested that people who maintained their cultural moorings and still found meaning and stability in traditional ways were less conflicted than persons who were questioning, and perhaps abandoning, old cognitions and values and adopting those of a new culture. It was inferred that the disturbance of former norms and reference points creates ambiguity, a condition that characterizes much of the torment incurred in emotional and mental disorders.

In most of these studies acculturation was defined in terms of various operational indexes, but as a unitary phenomenon of movement away from the pole of one's own culture and toward the pole of another. Berry (1986), noting that acculturation is indeed generally stressful and that refugees may experience greater mental health–related stressors than do other groups, nevertheless has identified four distinct varieties of acculturation. *Assimilation* involves the option of relinquishing cultural identity and moving into the larger society. *Integration* involves movement to join the dominant society but with retention of cultural identity. *Rejection* refers to withdrawal from the mainstream and maintenance of a segregated cultural identity. *Deculturation* characterizes the experience of groups who lack cultural and psychological contact with both their traditional culture and the larger society. Essentially the same schema is cited by Wong-Rieger and Quintana (1987) in their respective four-mode description of assimilation, bicultural integration, ethnic separation, and marginality.

In terms of face validity, integration appears the most healthy and deculturation the least healthy mode of adaptation (other things, such as intergroup power relationships and political realities, being equal). Relevant to Berry's characterization of the rejection and assimilation modes, respectively, are findings by Szapocznik and Kurtines (1980) that both underacculturated and overacculturated Cuban youths in Miami show lower levels of adjustment than bicultural youths who are at ease in both systems. Wong-Rieger and Quintana (1987) similarly found that among Hispanic immigrants and Southeast Asian refugees biculturalism was the most satisfactory form of acculturation. In contrast to previous findings on operation measures of acculturation (Lefley 1976), data from Seelye and Brewer (1970) indicated that greater rather than lesser exposure to the host culture, in terms of work and residence, was related to more positive psychological adjustment.

There is further confirmation in the literature that acculturation is a complex and multidetermined phenomenon. Much of the contemporary research on acculturation has been done in Israel, where the immigration of Jewish groups from widely disparate ethnic backgrounds and levels of modernization permits extensive cross-cultural comparison of the impact of a new cultural system. A major study comparing representative samples of women from five ethnic groups focused on the relationship between traditionalism-modernity and successful adaptation to problems encountered during menopause (Datan, Antonovsky, and Maoz 1981). The investigators found a curvilinear relationship with respect to the traditionalism-modernity continuum. Urban middle-class Israeli Jewish women of Central European origin were best adapted; traditional Israeli Arab village women were close behind. The most poorly adapted were Israeli Jewish women of Turkish, North African, and Persian origin. Antonovsky (1979, 6) noted: "The crucial variable in successful adaptation was not the content of culture and social structure but its relative stability. The Central European and Arab women were rooted in stable cultural contexts; the other three groups were immigrants in transition, uprooted and not yet rerooted." These findings led to Antonovsky's notion of *sense of coherence* as a crucial variable in explaining an individual's resources for tension management and resistance to disease. "The sense of coherence is a global orientation that expresses the extent to which one has a pervasive, enduring though dynamic feeling of confidence that (1) the stimuli deriving from one's internal and external environments in the course of living are structured, predictable, and explicable; (2) the resources are available to one to meet the demands posed by these stimuli; and (3) these demands are challenges, worthy of investment and engagement" (Antonovsky 1987, 19). Attaining this sense of coherence appears to be fundamental for adaptation to the refugee experience.

Although traditional Arab village women appeared to be well adjusted, living within their own coherent world, immigrants who bring with them or develop skills valued in the new culture stand a better chance of making a successful psychological adjustment. Among Indochinese refugees, for example, Nicassio (1983) found that Laotians and Vietnamese showed more favorable adjustment and less alienation from American culture than Hmong and Cambodians, "a finding that is consistent with the better English proficiency, higher socioeconomic status and more positive self-perceptions noted in these refugee groups" (1983, 349). Berry and Blondel (1982) similarly found education and literacy linked to higher psychological functioning. Rumbaut (1985) reported that characteristics of refugees most at risk for mental health problems were lack of education, poor English proficiency, low income and unemployment, advanced age and widowhood, physical health problems, and traumatic migration history. At the environmental level Salvendy (1983) cited sociocultural distance between original and host countries, changes in socioeconomic status, and lack of a large local ethnic community as risk factors. These variables have also been cited with respect to patterns of adaptation of Cuban and Haitian entrants in Miami (Lefley and Bestman 1984; McClellan 1981). Lin, Masuda and Tazuma (1982) reported that Vietnamese refugees with the greatest vulnerability were those with poor social support systems, status inconsistencies, and limited exposure to American culture.

Although studies of cultures in contact have given us valuable reference information, counselors need to know how to adapt these insights to individual cases. Berry, Trimble, and Olmedo (1986) have noted that (a) there are individual differences in the psychological characteristics that each individual brings to the acculturation process, and (b) not every person will participate to the same extent in the process. More-over, both groups and individuals will vary in the degree of change in various domains of cultural attachment. They point out, for example, that attitudes toward the value of traditional technology may change without a parallel change in beliefs and behaviors associated with the old technology—a variability that similarly may obtain for medical and psychological technologies. The presence or degree of acculturative stress is also both a group and individual phenomenon. Describing the reported consequences of societal disintegration and personal crisis, Berry, Trimble, and Olmedo note that "at the group level, previous patterns of authority, of civility, and of welfare no longer operate, and at the individual level, hostility, uncertainty, and depression may set in" (1986, 315). Although societal disintegration almost always has nega-tive group effects, the degree of negative impact on subgroups may vary as a function of age and sex roles in the traditional culture (Lefley 1976). Above all, the salience of culture change operates on an individ-ual organism that brings to the process a certain level of physiological and psychological strength. This truism underlies the opposition of many investigators to a "pseudo-medical model" approach to culture stress (Furnham and Bochner 1986, 233). For those who lack this strength in adaptation to a series of new, often frightening experiences, and particularly to those who become symptomatic, culturally appro-priate counseling becomes a useful mechanism for survival.

Symptomatology

Because of the great diversity among refugee groups, conditions of migration, and types of migrants, the epidemiological picture is far from clear (see Westermeyer 1986). Although the range and intensity of stressors are apparent, parameters of vulnerability and severity of psy-chopathology are not uniformly patterned. Lin (1986), discussing the linkage of psychopathology with stress and social disruption, does not equate the symptomatic behaviors of refugees with those of major men-tal illnesses. Common psychological reactions to the stresses of familial separation and loss, social isolation, and culture shock include depres-sion and anxiety, somatic complaints, marital and intergenerational conflicts, substance abuse, and sociopathic behavior.

Lin notes, however, that most refugees suffer from adaptation, not from disorders that would warrant a psychiatric diagnosis. Moreover, he states that "although common sense tells us that, with the increased levels of stress, refugees would be more vulnerable and more susceptible to developing psychiatric conditions, no reliable epidemiological data have been available to substantiate such assertions" (1986, 67). Kinzie

(1986) indicates that outpatient services for refugees are likely to first serve those with a psychotic disorder. Thus 36% of their first 50 patients had a psychotic diagnosis, but the percentage later dropped to 19% as their caseload expanded.

Periods of Greatest Risk

Westermeyer (1986), evaluating data from various studies of refugee populations, has stated that the highest rates of psychiatric disorders occur in the first year following migration. Rumbaut (1985) suggests that the second year is of significant importance for onset of psychological problems. Regardless of initial episode, symptoms may persist long after arrival. In a study of Hmong refugees Westermeyer (1986) states that about a third experienced increased symptoms one and one-half to three and one-half years after migration, a finding similar to that of Fong and Peskin (1969) for Chinese immigrant students and Lin, Tazuma, and Masuda (1979) for Vietnamese refugees. Sex differences in onset of schizophrenia among refugees were noted by Westermeyer (1986) and by Krupinski (1967). Krupinski found a higher incidence among men one to two years after migration and among women, seven to 15 years after arrival. According to Westermeyer, this finding was attributed to earlier stress experienced by men in job seeking and later isolation of women as they became increasingly alienated from their more acculturated members.

Diagnostic Assessment

Issues in cross-cultural psychiatric diagnosis have been outlined in a number of contexts (Lefley 1986; Westermeyer 1987; Williams 1986). Appropriate use of psychological tests and screening instruments, behavioral observations, linguistic and psycholinguistic interpretation, and distinguishing the parameters of normalcy and deviance are generalizable problem areas in all cross-cultural interactions. Differentiating manifestations of major psychotic disorders from culture-bound syndromes; determining the salience and meaning of seemingly aberrant behaviors in ritual and nonritual contexts (Weidman 1979; Lefley 1979); and teasing out culturally accurate assessments of depression (Kleinman and Good 1985) are difficult tasks for even knowledgeable diagnosticians.

Some unusual anxiety symptoms have been reported for Indochinese refugees, for example, frigophobia, or fear of the cold. "The patient describes a feeling of constant chill, dresses more warmly than neces-

sary, and self-diagnoses the 'chill' as flu or malaria. Using a popular
home remedy known as 'rubbing out the wind,' the refugees will force-
fully rub the forehead, temples, neck, or chest. The treatment is
deemed successful when bruises appear" (Folkenberg 1986, 11).

If most problems of refugees are adjustment reactions, however, as
Lin (1986) suggests, psychiatric diagnosis is secondary to a careful psychosocial assessment. The multiaxial approach of the American Psychiatric Association's (1980) Diagnostic and Statistical Manual (DSM III)
permits some notation of physical problems, severity of stressors, and
functional level. Any psychosocial interview, however, must take an
extensive personal and family history including the client's status and
role in her or his previous life and the correspondence with status and
role here. This includes gender and marital roles and role expectations,
occupational role with respect to educational level, and occupation as a
source of fulfillment or frustration. A systems perspective on client,
family, refugee community, other refugee or indigenous groups, and
mainstream community is essential.

One other area of assessment relates to medical diagnosis and screening out organicity. There is considerable evidence that the stressors and
exposures of migration may lead to a range of health consequences
(Kasl and Berkman 1983). Refugees, including children, often bring
hidden illnesses because of years of deprivation, exposure to toxins and
viral diseases, and malnutrition. Infectious diseases (Dashefsky and
Teele 1983) or intestinal parasitosis (Skeels, Nims, and Mann 1982)
may create malaise and enforce isolation of refugee groups.

Generic Issues in Counseling

Generic issues in service delivery to refugees encompass at least two
broad domains: utilization patterns and content of problems presented.
Reports of Southeast Asian refugees, for example, indicate "immense
stigma against seeing a therapist" and convictions that talking about
feelings and emotions is equivalent to "parading in the nude in public"
(Folkenberg 1986, 10).

Utilization is expected to occur only through referral from the crimi-
nal justice or school systems or in cases of severe, uncontrollable psychotic decompensation in a family member. By and large, refugees are
not expected to personally seek mental health services although acculturated families may do so.

Lin (1986) lists the common stressors among refugees that are likely
to form the content of counseling sessions. These are separation, loss,
and grieving for family members left behind; social isolation; loss or

reversal of social role and status; culture shock and acculturation strain; residual impact of prior traumatic experiences; coping with accelerated modernization; and experiencing minority status in the new world. Changing gender roles are a source of conflict among married couples (see Charles 1986; Sandoval and De la Roza 1986). Among all of these, however, erosion of the family structure through intergenerational conflict is probably the major source of distress.

Changes in traditional relations among the generations are almost inevitable in adapting to modern culture. Because children learn languages and assimilate new experiences more easily, they quickly become the interpreters and "culture brokers" for their parents. For persons accustomed to hierarchical family relationships and a strong parental role, this can be a humiliating experience in the conduct of ordinary business, particularly when parents observe an authority figure communicating with their children rather than with themselves.

Cultural conflict is almost a given when children begin school. Since most refugees are achievement oriented and look to education as an avenue of upward mobility for the children, parents' relationships with schools are intrinsically double-binding. Children are urged to study and respect their teachers. However, public schools, and to a lesser extent private or even parochial schools, are the most prominent sources of value change and acculturation for their children. Here children learn a greater liberality than that found in traditional cultures: less respectful ways of relating to adults, new ideas about boy-girl relationships and sexuality. The boundaries begin to loosen with respect to limits and autonomy; preferences and values may change in modes of dress, music, religious observance, use of intoxicants; and new idols and role models are acquired. In the course of becoming Americanized, children may repudiate the parental culture. This is even more likely to occur if they are told over and over that things were better in the former life at home, with their own adopted culture compared unfavorably with that of their parents. With their diminishing stature and reduced competence in negotiating with the new world, parents in their efforts to counter allegiance to American values may weaken rather than strengthen their own authority.

These changes in children can cause great pain and inevitably lead to family conflict. Parents who have survived untold horrors to build a new life in the United States may very well feel that their efforts have resulted in gross life failure. They may feel guilty for having deluded themselves or chosen the wrong goal. If the reactions are internalized, depression, psychosomatic symptoms, or other disorders may surface. Their children's repudiation or depreciation of the cultural heritage, however, is a greater pain. This may be interpreted not only as a rejection of the parents but as invalidation of their massive struggle for survival.

From the child's viewpoint, however, a common complaint is excessive parental demands and expectations. There appears to be inordinate investment in children's educational attainment among refugees, a projection of all parental hopes and aspirations on the next generation (see Nidorf 1985). For the achiever this can be an incentive and reinforcer, although in communal cultures children may feel responsible for carrying the fortune of the entire family on their narrow shoulders. For the more fragile child, however, attempts to fulfill such expectations may incur tremendous psychological costs and even precipitate decompensation.

Special Populations

Children and Adolescents

The family problems previously discussed are considered generic in refugees' transition from traditional to modern cultural settings. In resettlement in the United States, however, specific problems arise as a function of a particular migration that creates discontinuity in families. In current years we have seen problems of separated children, particularly unaccompanied minors. Carlin (1986) has discussed some of the survival skills adopted by these children. Szapocznik and Cohen (1986) have described their work in assessment and intervention with Cuban unaccompanied adolescents who came in the 1980 *Mariel* boat lift. In cases in which children have been left behind and are later reunited with parents, there are experiential and often status differentials with younger siblings born in the host country, who are now seen as "American" and therefore superior (Charles 1985). Very different psychological problems are characteristic of Amerasian children of American fathers. These are discussed here in some depth because they involve special psychodynamic issues as well as the more typical adjustment problems.

Refugee children of U.S. servicemen. Vietnamese children of American servicemen came to the United States in 1982 through the United Nations–backed Orderly Departure Program. From the fall of 1982 until May 1986, when the Vietnamese government suspended their exodus, 3,700 of these Amerasian children came, with 5,200 family members, mostly mothers and siblings.

The problems of Amerasian children in their home countries are well known by now through media exposure. Vietnamese children were particularly at risk. Called *bui doi* (children of dust), many were openly despised and discriminated against not only by peers but by teachers, government officials, and other authority figures. Viewed as children of the enemy, many were not allowed to go to school; their mothers were refused employment; and lives of poverty, deprivation, and uncertain futures were the norm.

The move to the United States thus represented fulfillment of family dreams, often bringing disappointment to those who had fantasized dramatic changes in life scenarios. Many of these children had long entertained fantasies about their American fathers, typically in the form of redemption by a hero figure. These notions may have been superimposed on an underlying resentment at abandonment and anger at the implicit contrast of their own extreme deprivation with the assumed luxury of their fathers' lives. In a few cases long-term investments of energy in attempting to find the fathers were successful, but only a few ended happily; most of the children met with open rejection (see Terris 1987).

As ongoing psychodynamic issues the identification problems of mixed-race children in their openly hostile home cultures were thus compounded by the ambiguity of feelings toward the perpetrator of their differentness, the father. Fantasies of being redeemed by unknown royal parentage, common among adoptees, were nonetheless grounded in the realities of vastly different lifestyles in Vietnam and the United States. These fantasies were then dashed by the inability to reunite or attain closure with the absent father. In counseling it may be helpful to recognize dissonant love-hate feelings that may be projected onto all males, interfering with normal sexuality and interpersonal relating in both boys and girls.

Additional difficulties found among these and other refugee children are the obvious changes of culture and language, prejudice, homesickness, and the adjustment of going back to school in a strange country. For the most part Amerasian children are being raised in single-parent homes with continuing poverty, albeit less than before. On the plus side the children learn to be survivors; those with strong personalities and talents go on to attain education and upward mobility. Commitment to their families may also be a plus, an incentive to achieve. The obverse side of the family as support system in traditional cultures is the family member's mandate to be a support system for others. This powerful motivator must be recognized and dealt with in any counseling effort. For the person with overpoweringly negative life experiences and inadequate personality resources, such expectations may lead to decompensation. For the counselee with a basically strong personality structure, they may be a powerful incentive for overcoming temporary adjustment reactions to the problems and ambiguities of the new life.

Illegal Aliens

For many refugees life has been a series of traumatic events: mistreatment in the home country, difficulties in exodus, agony on the high seas, culture shock upon arrival in a strange land. For undocumented aliens, however, the traumas do not end there: life continues to be a Sisyphean experience of sliding back two steps for each step forward. Fear of deportation; unanticipated sequelae, such as lack of documentation, which interferes with eligibility for work, school, and social services; and even unanticipated dangers accompanying the long-awaited amnesty continue to reinforce the perilous quality of their lives.

Under the amnesty provision of the Immigration Reform and Control Act of 1986, illegal aliens who can prove they arrived prior to and have lived in the United States continuously since January 1, 1982, are now allowed to apply for temporary resident status and may eventually apply for permanent resident status and citizenship. The deportation fears of those who arrived after this date are extremely stressful. As in their original emigration, lives of these refugees are typically subject to political events beyond their control; their futures are in limbo as powerful others battle over whether they stay or go. For example, a publicized May 1987 letter to President Reagan from President Duarte of El Salvador estimated that some 400,000 to 600,000 Salvadorans, almost $\frac{1}{10}$ of its population, have entered the United States illegally since January 1982. Duarte requested special amnesty for these émigrés, since their return would cripple El Salvador's economy (Pear 1987). Similar pleas were received from the government of Guatemala. A conflict ensued among the Immigration and Naturalization Service, U.S. State Department, and Congress on whether to honor these requests, raising and then dashing hopes with their subsequent rejection.

Even with the amnesty, separation of married couples and of other family members with disparate eligibility, together with the U.S. government's arbitrary designation of degrees of kinship appropriate for reunification, continues to have traumatic impact. A new stressor has emerged in the form of a demand from the Internal Revenue Service that aliens who legalize their status under the Immigration Reform and Control Act of 1986 are liable for back taxes, including interest and penalties for failing to file tax returns. Since most aliens living illegally in the United States have held underground economy, subsistence-level jobs for which they did not dare file tax returns, this retroactive demand creates an enormous burden on typically penniless refugees now seeking to work openly. Regardless of how this issue is resolved, the added burden of choosing between legal status and a penurious, debt-ridden future can conceivably lead to decompensation in already severely stressed persons whose agonies never seem to end.

Victims of Extreme Trauma

Refugees who have been subjected to concentration camp experiences, torture, rape, murder of loved ones, and other inordinately traumatic events frequently show symptomatology of nightmares, startle reactions, sleep and appetite disturbances, and often recurrent intrusive thoughts. Boehnlein et al. (1985) advocate treatment with tricyclic antidepressant medications and long-term supportive therapy for this group. In a study of Cambodian children who have experienced similar traumas, Kinzie et al. (1986) reported that four years after leaving Cambodia, 50% developed Post–Traumatic Stress Disorder. Psychiatric effects were most severe when the children did not reside with a family member. Grief reactions, including prolonged crying, recurrent nightmares, obsessive rumination, and depression, were reported among Kampuchean refugees; these reactions are similar to those of survivors of Nazi concentration camps (van der Westhuizen 1980).

Fortunately, the majority of refugees have not endured the type of searing events that have generated Post–Traumatic Stress Disorder, and many have been able to adjust to one degree or another, although a significant minority will need long-term psychiatric intervention. It is apparent that refugees have undergone a range of experiences and reactions and that therapeutic interventions must be tailored to the specific needs of each situation.

Therapeutic Modalities

Therapeutic models for refugees may be based on one or more (and frequently a combination) of the following types of interventions: aid with environmental stressors; reinforcement of acculturation skills; individual or family counseling or therapy; or "medical model" culturally sensitive psychiatric treatment, including supportive counseling. Although these appear to be listed in large to small systems order, each is interactional in its effects, and all may be appropriate for a particular case. Some examples of each are given below.

A successful social systems intervention was initiated by the Haitian unit of the University of Miami–Jackson Memorial Community Mental Health Center (now New Horizons CMHC) to ensure access to school for children of illegal aliens. Many Haitian children were involuntarily idle and without formal education because their parents, fearing disclosure, could not provide the documents required for entry into school. Both to ease the distress of Haitian clients and as a preventive mental health measure, the Haitian unit negotiated with the Board of Education to allow them to register the children without documentation and in one year successfully enrolled 750 Haitian children in school. Later they were instrumental in changing rules that were unwittingly depriving many refugee children of the potential for literacy and development of productive skills.

Refugee children frequently suffer from interethnic conflict in the larger community, rivalry and harassment in the schools, and relegation to the lowest rung in the pecking order of minority status. Community organization of multicultural task forces, intercultural communication efforts in the schools, interethnic clubs, and programs in cultural heritage are examples of services offered refugees in the community mental health model depicted above (see Lefley and Bestman 1984).

Orientation and acculturation classes are an ongoing component of this mental health center's services for Cuban and Haitian entrants. At the more clinical level, a therapeutic modality for Cuban refugee families was empirically derived from research on acculturation by Szapocznik et al. (*FET,* 1986) at the University of Miami's Spanish Family Guidance Center. Based on validation of a biculturalism and cultural involvement scale that showed greater health in bicultural youth, the authors developed Bicultural Effectiveness Training (BET), which incorporated values clarification and enhancement of communication and negotiation skills in both Hispanic and mainstream U.S. cultures. Later, Family Effectiveness Training (FET) was developed to resolve problems of intergenerational and intercultural conflict within a strategic structural systems framework (Szapocznik et al., *FET,* 1986).

Most refugees are from traditional, family-oriented cultures, where it would be culturally incongruent *not* to involve the family in information and decisions regarding the patient (Lefley 1985a). Thus, family therapy would seem to be the treatment of choice. Much depends, however, on which formulas and models of family therapy are applied. Landau (1982), describing work with cultures in transition, suggests the need of a comprehensive map of the family's development phase of migration and relationships with the larger system, including degree of harmony between cultures and availability of community support systems. The map "should extend beyond that of the individual's and family's life cycle to include the transitional position of the multigenerational family in society" (1982, 558). Lappin and Scott (1982), restoring competency to a widowed, depressed Vietnamese refugee mother, reversed the child interpreter process by having the mother teach both her children and the counselors Vietnamese. They felt this would not only restore pride in heritage, but "most importantly, the mother would be in charge" (1982, 488). Restoration of competency and confidence not only reestablished maternal authority but reaffirmed for the children ethnic pride and linguistic proficiency in their native language.

At the individual level, staff of the Indochinese Psychiatric Clinic of

Oregon Health Sciences University, directed by cultural psychiatrist D. David Kinzie, purposively use an active, directive, authoritative approach to bridge the cultural gap between Western clinicians and Southeast Asian refugee patients. "The medical model of psychiatry practiced at the clinic emphasizes reducing symptoms, alleviating pain, and curing illness. Psychological interpretations are kept to a minimum" (Gold Award 1986, 1145). In this approach the clinician establishes credibility as an authoritative, caring figure in the initial interview. The second step is a detailed psychosocial history covering five areas: "life in the homeland, including education, socioeconomic status, health, family relationships, and war-related problems; experiences during the escape process; life in the refugee camp; adjustment to the United States; and current problems and worries about the future" (Gold Award 1986, 1145). Using a psychoeducational approach in supportive counseling sessions, clinicians recapitulate the stresses endured by the patient, explaining how the brain and body have reacted to them. Symptoms, side effects of medications, children, financial problems, and other current stresses are discussed, and the clinician models positive social behavior and clear communication. Staff also educate the patient's family members and answer their questions. Indochinese mental health counselors function as bilateral cultural and linguistic interpreters.

A Counseling Model for Refugees

Counseling and psychotherapy models have been predicated by and large on models of maladjustment, dysfunction, or psychopathology— on some deficit in the individual or the family that requires revision and improvement. Even models that strengthen skills for negotiating the new culture, like F.E.T., are rooted in premises of a basically dysfunctional family unit that projects cultural and generational conflict onto the so-called identified patient (Szapocznik et al., *FET,* 1986; Szapocznik et al., *BET,* 1986).

Most refugees, however, have endured experiences that make them closer to disaster victims than to persons embodying personality or systemic deficits. Their experiences, moreover, have typically involved a series of inordinately stressful life events rather than a single catastrophe. If their legal status in the new country is uncertain, they face ambiguities, current dangers, and the threat of future catastrophes that automatically make the world a hostile and threatening place. This is a perception of the world that psychoanalytic thinkers used to consider reflective of psychopathology. For refugees, as for other deprived groups, this reality-rooted perception may instead be quite adaptive and even necessary for survival. It is the task of the sensitive counselor to be able to differentiate between paranoia and a well-grounded alertness to potential threat.

Approaches to counseling refugees should thus eschew notions of psychopathology and focus on a model of stress, coping, and adaptation—a paradigm specifically relevant to coping with uprooting and modernization (Coelho and Ahmed 1980) and applicable even in Kinzie's "medical model" psychiatry (Gold Award 1986). Counselors would do well to root themselves in that literature (e.g., Kessler, Price, and Wortman 1985; Taylor 1983), determining those coping styles that are relevant to their work. Traditional value orientations (Spiegel and Papajohn 1986) may also be applied advantageously for adaptation to a current world of ambiguity and strangeness. Present time orientation, for example, is a valuable cognitive mode for persons with unfortunate pasts and demonstrably uncertain futures. Indeed, Beiser (1987) has indicated that this is a common adaptive strategy among Southeast Asian refugees in British Columbia. Leading a client through day-to-day planning may be a valuable addition to his coping skills. If treatment goals are required by a funding source, the concentration should be on short-term rather than long-range objectives. Relational modes that facilitate development and retention of human support systems are strong aids in coping. This includes utilization of traditional healing systems (Sandoval 1979) and membership in "cult houses" as fictive extended family (Garrison 1978). In Sandoval's (1979) analysis supernatural belief systems have been viewed as conferring mastery on the helpless through enabling them to negotiate with the powerful gods. Lefley (1984b) has discussed levels of application of traditional healing modalities (*espiritismo, obeah,* root work, *santeria, vodun*) in community mental health work, and Hiegel (1983) described collaboration with traditional healers in mental health care of refugees in Thailand. Perceptions of locus of illness control appear to be culturally specific, contingent on prior experience with levels of capability for prevention and treatment (Coreil and Marshall 1982). Since refugees have a relatively higher rate of medical problems, these differential perceptions should be explored in dealing with utilization of the health system in the United States.

In this context the counselor should be required to learn about resource availability and even acquire case management skills for dealing with clients' reality problems. Many refugee communities are rife with rumors and wrong or unsubstantiated information regarding their eligibility for services. Yet the human service network is often filled with disparities and inconsistencies which in some cases may even be beneficial. In some communities persons whose children require documentation for school may nevertheless receive medical services at the county hospital without producing papers. Social security cards have been obtained for undocumented aliens through a service agency, enabling them to work (Lefley and Bestman 1984). If counselors of refugees are to be optimally useful, it is incumbent on them to know these regulations and the availability of adaptive resources in their communities.

Above all, in helping refugee clients cope with the ambiguities and frustrations of their new lives, counselors should learn how to utilize cultural variables that foster adaptive skills. Charles (1986), writing about counseling Haitian refugees, has suggested focusing on certain cultural strengths. As an example he states that Haitians feel pride in a value system exemplified as "I am Haitian—I won't lie; I won't steal." The depressed, unskilled patient who has difficulty finding work can be motivated to attend vocational training through the moral insight that the alternative for survival is to become a thief. In addition, Charles emphasizes a focus on family as support system rather than as pathogen or disturbed system; on creating social networks or even a fictive family among mental health center staff when kin are lacking; on ethnic traditions as a source of identity, stability, and continuity; on using the refugee's more flexible margin for survival as an asset in adaptation; and on achievement orientation and group commitment as powerful incentives to overcome dysphoria and despair. In contrast to most counseling approaches, anthropologist Charles (1986), like psychiatrist Kinzie (1986), emphasizes caring authoritativeness, directive education, and guidance as the culturally appropriate modalities to which most refugees are likely to respond.

Finally, it is important to conceptualize counseling as an integral component of an array of basic services vitally relevant to refugee mental health. Boehnlein (1987) has called for the development of separate services for refugees responsive to their political, social, economic, and cultural needs. He emphasizes close integration of medical and mental health services as a culturally appropriate form of service delivery, since traditional cultures do not dichotomize physical and mental illness, and emotionally based somatic complaints are typically addressed to medical healers. His model reflects the National Institute of Mental Health's position that mental health services for refugees be integrated closely with health, education, English-language training, employment, social service, justice, and other services that may enhance adaptation. Although Boehnlein suggests that refugee-oriented services be developed in existing medical institutions, with access to primary care clinicians, specialty consultants, and translators with mental health training, this is essentially an open-systems community mental health model (Lefley 1984b). Research on utilization patterns is now in order to determine the most culturally acceptable sites of service delivery and the counseling modes and service mix correlated with positive outcomes for refugee groups.

References

American Psychiatric Association. 1980. *Diagnostic and statistical manual of mental disorders.* Washington, DC: American Psychiatric Association.

Antonovsky, A. 1979. *Health, stress, and coping.* San Francisco: Jossey-Bass.

————. 1987. *Unraveling the mystery of health.* San Francisco: Jossey-Bass.

Beiser, M. 1987. Changing time perspective and mental health among Southeast Asian refugees. *Culture, Medicine, and Psychiatry* 11:437–464.

Berry, J. W. 1986. The acculturation process and refugee behavior. In C. L. Williams and J. Westermeyer (eds.), *Refugee mental health in resettlement countries,* 25–37. Washington, DC: Hemisphere.

Berry, J. W., and Blondel, T. 1982. Psychological adaptation of Vietnamese refugees in Canada. *Canadian Journal of Community Mental Health* 1:81–88.

Berry, J. W., Trimble, J. E., and Olmedo, E. L. 1986. Assessment of acculturation. In W. J. Lonner and J. W. Berry (eds.), *Field methods in cross-cultural research,* 291–349. Beverly Hills: Sage Publications.

Boehnlein, J. K. 1987. A review of mental health services for refugees between 1975 and 1985 and a proposal for future services. *Hospital and Community Psychiatry* 38 (7): 764–768.

Boehnlein, J. K., Kinzie, J. D., Ben, R., and Fleck, J. 1985. One-year follow-up study of posttraumatic stress disorder among survivors of Cambodian concentration camps. *American Journal of Psychiatry* 142:956–959.

Carlin, J. E. 1986. Child and adolescent refugees: Psychiatric assessment and treatment. In C. L. Williams and J. Westermeyer (eds.), *Refugee mental health in resettlement countries,* 131–139. Washington, DC: Hemisphere.

Cassel, J. C. 1974. Psychiatric epidemiology. In S. Arieti (ed.), *American handbook of psychiatry.* Vol. 2, G. Caplan (ed.), 401–409. New York: Basic Books.

Charles, C. 1985. New dimensions of physical and sexual child abuse within the Haitian community in diaspora. Paper presented at the 15th Biennial conference of the Caribbean Federation for Mental Health, 21–26 July, Nassau, Bahamas.

————. 1986. Mental health services for Haitians. In H. P. Lefley and P. B. Pedersen (eds.), *Cross-cultural training for mental health professionals,* 183–198. Springfield, IL: Charles C. Thomas.

Coelho, G. V., and Ahmed, P. I., eds. 1980. *Uprooting and development: Dilemmas of coping with modernization.* New York: Plenum Press.

Cohen, R. E. 1987. Stressors: Migration and acculturation to American society. In M. Gaviria and J. D. Arana (eds.), *Health and behavior: Research agenda for Hispanics.* Simon Bolivar Research Monographs Series, no. 1, 59–71. Chicago: University of Illinois.

Coreil, J., and Marshall, P. A. 1982. Locus of illness control: A cross-cultural study. *Human Organization* 41:131–137.

Dashefsky, B., and Teele, D. W. 1983. Infectious disease problems in Indochinese refugees. *Pediatric Annals* 12 (3): 232–244.

Datan, N., Antonovsky, A., and Maoz, B. 1981. *A time to reap: The middle age of women in five Israeli subcultures.* Baltimore: Johns Hopkins University Press.

Folkenberg, J. 1986. Mental health of Southeast Asian refugees. *ADAMHA News* 12 (1): 10–11.

Fong, S. L. M., and Peskin, H. 1969. Sex-role strain and personality adjustment of China-born students in America: A pilot study. *Journal of Abnormal Psychology* 74:563–567.

Furnham, A., and Bochner, S. 1986. *Culture shock: Psychological reactions to unfamiliar environments.* London: Methuen.

Garrison, V. 1978. Support systems of schizophrenic and nonschizophrenic Puerto Rican migrant women in New York City. *Schizophrenia Bulletin* 4 (4): 561–596.

Gold Award. 1986. Mental health treatment that transcends cultural barriers: Indochinese psychiatric clinic, Oregon Health Sciences University, Portland. *Hospital and Community Psychiatry* 37:1144–1147.

Good, B. J., Good, M. D., and Moradi, R. 1985. The interpretation of Iranian depressive illness and dysphoric affect. In A. Kleinman and B. Good (eds.), *Culture and depression: Studies in the anthropology and cross-cultural psychiatry of affect and disorder,* 369–428. Berkeley: University of California Press.

Hiegel, J. P. 1983. Collaboration with traditional healers: Experience in refugees' mental care. *International Journal of Mental Health* 12 (3): 30–43.

Kasl, S. V., and Berkman, L. 1983. Health consequences of the experience of migration. *Annual Review of Public Health* 4:69–90.

Kessler, R. C., Price, R. H., and Wortman, C. B. 1985. Social factors in psychopathology: Stress, social support, and coping processes. *Annual Review of Psychology* 36:531–572.

Kinzie, J. D. 1986. The establishment of outpatient mental health services for Southeast Asian refugees. In C. L. Williams and J. Westermeyer (eds.), *Refugee mental health in resettlement countries,* 217–231. Washington, DC: Hemisphere.

Kinzie, J. D., Sack, W., Angell, R., Manson, S., and Rath, B. 1986. The psychiatric effects of massive trauma on Cambodian children: Pt.1, The children. *Journal of American Academy of Child Psychiatry* 25:370–376.

Kleinman, A., and Good, B., eds. 1985. *Culture and depression: Studies in the anthropology and cross-cultural psychiatry of affect and disorder.* Berkeley: University of California Press.

Krupinski, J. 1967. Sociological aspects of mental ill-health in migrants. *Social Science and Medicine* 1:267–281.

Landau, J. 1982. Therapy with families in cultural transition. In M. McGoldrick, J. K. Pearce, and J. Giordano (eds.), *Ethnicity and family therapy,* 552–572. New York: Guilford Press.

Lappin, J., and Scott, S. 1982. Intervention in a Vietnamese refugee family. In M. McGoldrick, J. K. Pearce, and J. Giordano (eds.), *Ethnicity and family therapy,* 483–491. New York: Guilford Press.

Lefley, H. P. 1976. Acculturation, childrearing, and self-esteem in two North American Indian tribes. *Ethos* 4:385–401.

———. 1979. Prevalence of potential falling-out cases among the black, Latin and non-Latin white populations of the city of Miami. *Social Science and Medicine* 13B (2): 113–114.

————. 1984a. Cross-cultural training for mental health professionals: Effects on the delivery of services. *Hospital and Community Psychiatry* 35:1227–1229.

————. 1984b. Delivering mental health services across cultures. In P. B. Pedersen, N. Sartorius, and A. J. Marsella (eds.), *Mental health services: The cross-cultural context,* 135–171. Beverly Hills: Sage Publications.

————. 1985a. Families of the mentally ill in cross-cultural perspective. *Psychosocial Rehabilitation Journal* 8:57–75.

————. 1985b. Mental health training across cultures. In P. B. Pedersen (ed.), *Handbook of cross-cultural counseling and therapy,* 259–266. Westport, CT: Greenwood Press.

————. 1986. Why cross-cultural training? Applied issues in culture and mental health service delivery. In H. P. Lefley and P. B. Pedersen (eds.), *Cross-cultural training for mental health professionals,* 11–44. Springfield, IL: Charles C. Thomas.

Lefley, H. P., and Bestman, E. W. 1984. Community mental health and minorities: A multi-ethnic approach. In S. Sue and T. Moore (eds.), *The pluralistic society: A community mental health perspective,* 116–148. New York: Human Sciences Press.

Lin, K. M. 1986. Psychopathology and social disruption in refugees. In C. L. Williams and J. Westermeyer (eds.), *Refugee mental health in resettlement countries,* 61–73. Washington, DC: Hemisphere.

Lin, K. M., Masuda, M., and Tazuma, L. 1982. Adaptational problems of Vietnamese refugees: Pt. 3, Case studies in clinic and field: Adaptive and maladaptive. *Psychiatric Journal of the University of Ottawa* 7:173–183.

Lin, K. M., Tazuma, L., and Masuda, M. 1979. Adaptational problems of Vietnamese refugees: Pt. 1, Health and mental health status. *Archives of General Psychiatry* 36:955–961.

McClellan, G. S., ed. 1981. *Immigrants, refugees, and U.S. policy.* New York: H. W. Wilson.

Nicassio, P. M. 1983. Psychosocial correlates of alienation: Study of a sample of Indochinese refugees. *Journal of Cross-Cultural Psychology* 14:337–351.

Nidorf, J. F. 1985. Mental health and refugee youths: A model for diagnostic training. In T. C. Owan (ed.), *Southeast Asian mental health: Treatment, prevention, services, training, and research,* 391–430. Washington, DC: National Institute of Mental Health.

Pear, R. 1987. Duarte appeals to Reagan to let Salvadorans stay. *New York Times* 136 (47, 121): 1, 8.

Rumbaut, R. G. 1985. Mental health and the refugee experience: A comparative study of Southeast Asian refugees. In T. C. Owan (ed.), *Southeast Asian mental health: Treatment, prevention, services, training, and research,* 433–486. Washington, DC: National Institute of Mental Health.

Salvendy, J. T. 1983. The mental health of immigrants: A reassessment of concepts. *Canada's Mental Health* 31:9–12, 16.

Sandoval, M. C. 1979. *Santeria* as a mental health care system: An historical overview. *Social Science and Medicine* 13B (2): 137–151.

Sandoval, M. C., and De la Roza, M. 1986. A cultural perspective for serving the Hispanic client. In H. P. Lefley and P. B. Pedersen (eds.), *Cross-*

cultural training for mental health professionals, 151–181. Springfield, IL: Charles C. Thomas.

Seelye, H. N., and Brewer, M. B. 1970. Ethnocentrism and acculturation of North Americans in Guatemala. *Journal of Social Psychology* 80:147–155.

Skeels, M. R., Nims, L. J., and Mann, J. M. 1982. Intestinal parasitosis in Southeast Asian immigrants in New Mexico. *American Journal of Public Health* 72:57–59.

Spiegel, J. P., and Papajohn, J. 1986. Training program in ethnicity and mental health. In H. P. Lefley and P. B. Pedersen (eds.), *Cross-cultural training for mental health professionals,* 49–71. Springfield, IL: Charles C. Thomas.

Stein, B. N. 1986. The experience of being a refugee: Insights from the research literature. In C. L. Williams and J. Westermeyer (eds.), *Refugee mental health in resettlement countries,* 5–23. Washington, DC: Hemisphere.

Szapocznik, J., and Cohen, R. E. 1986. Mental health care for rapidly changing environments: Emergency relief to unaccompanied youths of the 1980 Cuban refugee wave. In C. L. Williams and J. Westermeyer (eds.), *Refugee mental health in resettlement countries,* 141–156. Washington, DC: Hemisphere.

Szapocznik, J., and Kurtines, W. 1980. Acculturation, biculturalism, and adjustment among Cuban-Americans. In A. M. Padilla (ed.), *Recent advances in acculturation research: Theory, models, and some new findings,* 914–931. Boulder, CO: Westview Press.

Szapocznik, J., Rio, A., Perez-Vidal, A., Kurtines, W., Hervis, O., and Santisteban, D. 1986. Bicultural effectiveness training (BET): An experimental test of an intervention modality for families experiencing intergenerational/intercultural conflict. *Hispanic Journal of Behavioral Sciences* 8:303–330.

Szapocznik, J., Rio, A., Perez-Vidal, A., Kurtines, W., and Santisteban, D. 1986. Family effectiveness training (FET) for Hispanic families. In H. P. Lefley and P. B. Pedersen (eds.), *Cross-cultural training for mental health professionals,* 245–261. Springfield, IL: Charles C. Thomas.

Taylor, S. E. 1983. Adjustment to threatening events: A theory of cognitive adaptation. *American Psychologist* 38:1161–1173.

Terris, D. 1987. What place can there be for me? The Southeast Asian immigrant youth. *Boston Globe Magazine* 14 June: 14–15, 32–44, 50–56.

Triandis, H. C., Vassiliou, V., Vassiliou, G., Tanaka, Y., and Shanmugam, A. V. 1972. *The analysis of subjective culture.* New York: John Wiley and Sons.

van der Westhuizen, M. 1980. Kampuchean refugees: An encounter with grief. *Australian Nurses Journal* 10:53–56.

Weidman, H. H. 1979. Falling-out: A diagnostic and treatment problem viewed from a transcultural perspective. *Social Science and Medicine* 13B (2): 95–112.

Westermeyer, J. 1986. Migration and psychopathology. In C. L. Williams and J. Westermeyer (eds.), *Refugee mental health in resettlement countries,* 39–59. Washington, DC: Hemisphere.

————. 1987. Clinical considerations in cross-cultural diagnosis. *Hospital and Community Psychiatry* 38 (2): 160–165.

Williams, C. L. 1986. Mental health assessment of refugees. In C. L. Williams and J. Westermeyer (eds.), *Refugee mental health in resettlement countries,* 175–188. Washington, DC: Hemisphere.

Wong-Rieger, D., and Quintana, D. 1987. Comparative acculturation of Southeast Asian and Hispanic immigrants and sojourners. *Journal of Cross-Cultural Psychology* 18 (3): 345–362.

PART FOUR

Research and
Practical Considerations

The ten chapters in the first three sections of this book have been concerned with practical applications. Those chapters have, we hope, acquainted the reader with a wide range of problems and issues in cross-cultural counseling. This final section is concerned with the technicalities of behavioral counseling, issues relating to assessment, and future research on multicultural counseling.

It can be persuasively argued that behavioral counseling and therapy are the most "culture-general" or "culture-neutral" of all approaches to behavior change, despite the fact that their theoretical fountainhead of behaviorism is decidedly rooted in Western experimental psychology. Junko Tanaka-Matsumi and H. Nick Higginbotham, in Chapter 11, take such a behavioral perspective. However, they also recognize that even the technicalities and "scientific credibility" of the behavioral perspective cannot be applied blindly across cultures. Their chapter provides a valuable orientation to counseling from the behavioral approach, while at the same time emphasizing that a culturally appropriate mode must be found if such an approach has any hope of yielding desired changes in behavior.

In Chapter 12 Walter J. Lonner and Farah A. Ibrahim provide a general guide to the major problems that are involved whenever tests, scales, and other appraisal devices are used in multicultural settings. If used incorrectly or inappropriately, data and information yielded by standardized tests and inventories can be damaging to both the unsuspecting client and the technically unsophisticated counselor. There are several basic principles and problem areas in assessment with which the cross-cultural counselor should be familiar. These principles and problem areas are discussed, along with a brief overview of specific tests and other assessment tools that highlight many of the potential difficulties as well as the possibilities for valuable information.

There are many more questions than there are answers about the practice, process, and efficacy of cross-cultural counseling. Compared with more traditional modes of counseling, for example, behaviorism or psychoanalysis, the very young area of cross-cultural counseling suffers from an almost complete lack of research that could guide counselors in their interactions with clients from cultures other than their own. It is therefore fitting that the last chapter in the book, creatively and competently written by Norman D. Sundberg and David Sue, is entirely devoted to the importance of conducting research in multicultural counseling. The reader will be impressed by the great variety of intriguing hypotheses to be examined in this growing field. These hypotheses will no doubt stimulate many well-designed research projects and dissertations, all progressively leading to an increased understanding of the hundreds of issues and unanswered questions raised throughout this book.

11

Behavioral Approaches to Counseling across Cultures

Junko Tanaka-Matsumi
H. Nick Higginbotham

The application of behavioral strategies to help people of diverse sociocultural backgrounds has advanced markedly in recent years. This chapter reviews cross-cultural studies of behavior modification and therapy among groups in the United States and other countries that have appear since the 1981 edition of *Counseling across Cultures*.

Behavior modification became a visible social movement in the early 1960s (Kazdin 1978; Krasner 1971; Ullmann 1969). It began largely as an attack against the "disease model" conceptualization of abnormal behavior (Bandura 1969; Eysenck 1959; Ullman and Krasner 1965; Wolpe 1958, 1982). The therapeutic focus is the direct change of overt behavior rather than underlying or "disease" factors that produce symptomatic behaviors. Ullmann and Krasner (1969, 244) define behavior modification as "treatment deducible from the sociopsychological model that aims to alter a person's behavior directly through application of psychological principles."

Central to behavior modification is the assessment of functional relationships between the person's behavior and the environment (Baer, Wolf, and Risley 1968). Thus, cultural factors should be evaluated carefully in context of functional analysis. Skinner (1953, 1971) also states that culture is very much a part of one's social environment. Ideas underlying the functional analysis of behavior are consistent with the development of an interactional model of personality (e.g., Draguns 1979; Mischel 1973; Staats 1980), an ecological view of human behavior (Bernstein 1982; Rogers-Warren and Warren 1977), and the concept

---

In this paper the terms "behavior modification" and "behavior therapy" are used interchangeably. "Behavioral approaches" signify those major concepts and procedures associated with classical and operant conditioning, applied behavioral analysis, the psychosocial influence model, social behaviorism, and social learning theory. The authors recognize the operational and sometimes theoretical diversity of these learning models. Yet for the purpose of this chapter, we have subsumed them under the generic title "behavioral approaches," recognizing their common origin in experimental studies of behavior.

of "environmental design" (Krasner 1980). In short, the functional view, in concert with the situational analyses, examines the adequacy of intervention programs from a broad social and cultural perspective (Krasner 1982). Indeed, Stolz (1986) advocates applying behavior analysis to environmental problems of developing countries, such as high infant mortality rates because of malnutrition and unsafe hygiene practices.

In the past decade an increasing number of reports on the development of programs in behavior modification have appeared by authors from both Western and non-Western regions. These regions include Europe (Agathon 1982; Meazzini and Rovetto 1983), Latin America (Ardila 1982), South America (De Rosemberg and Delgado 1985; Queroz, Guilhardi, and Martin 1976), Japan (Uchiyama 1985; Yamagami et al. 1982), Sri Lanka (De Silva and Samarasinghe 1985), Thailand (Mikulas 1983), the Philippines (Guthrie et al. 1982), Australia (Sheehan and White 1976), Ghana (Danquah 1982), and South Africa (Dowdall 1982). Although the specific content and the extent of the programs adopted in each of these countries and regions vary, they share the common goal of directly changing problem behaviors.

The application of behavior modification across cultures underscores the need for increasing trained personnel and developing effective behavior change agents within the client's social milieu (e.g., Stumphauzer and Davis 1983). To achieve this goal it is important to examine the basic difference between the medical model, which looks "inside" the person for problem causes, and applied behavior analysis, which analyzes the relationship between the person and the environment.

The Medical Model of Abnormal Behavior

Until behavior modification emerged as a competitive theoretical basis for the scientific research of behavior, the medical model dominated the mental health field (Kazdin 1978). Independently, the medical model was also attacked by Szasz (1961), who claimed that mental illness is a myth and not a disease. Further, the works of Goffman (1961) and Scheff (1966) argued that abnormal behaviors are socially deviant behaviors; therefore, such behaviors should be evaluated within the specific social contexts of individuals and their social roles.

Contrary to the behavioral and sociological formulations of abnormal behavior, the medical model views maladaptive behaviors as symptoms of an underlying illness (Kendall 1975; Ullmann and Krasner 1965) and uses psychiatric diagnosis for the purpose of developing a universal classification of mental disorders (Kiev 1972; Kleinman 1977; Yap

1974). The third edition of the Diagnostic and Statistical Manual of Mental Disorders (APA 1980) is currently the most frequently employed system of classification of mental disorders in the United States.

Both the first and second editions of the manual met major criticisms in several important points (Draguns and Phillips 1971; Phillips and Draguns 1971). Reliability of diagnosis using these systems was poor for many of the specific disorder categories because of (1) a lack of clear definitions of the disorders, so that diagnosticians had to depend on their own judgment in making a diagnosis (Beck et al. 1962); (2) symptoms overlapping across different diagnostic categories (Zigler and Phillips 1961); (3) patients with the same diagnosis displaying heterogeneous symptom patterns (Enright and Jaeckle 1963); (4) the training backgrounds of the diagnosticians influencing reliability because clinicians tended to make different interpretations of symptomatic behaviors depending on their theoretical training backgrounds (Langer and Abelson 1974); and (5) the same patients being given different diagnostic labels depending on the context in which they were interviewed (Temerlin 1968). These observations led Rosenhan (1973) to conduct a study using pseudopatients in psychiatric hospitals. He concluded that it is not possible to distinguish normal from abnormal behaviors by using psychiatric diagnosis.

The third edition of the Diagnostic and Statistical Manual was developed with the purpose of remediating the problems of poor reliability and of making the system compatible with the ninth revision of the International Classification of Diseases (World Health Organization 1978). Diagnostic reliability of the manual improved considerably because of several innovative features (Spitzer, Williams, and Skodol 1980). First, explicit diagnostic criteria were established for each of the diagnostic categories. Explicit criteria help make objective, rather than subjective, diagnostic judgments. Second, the development of the multiaxial system provides for the evaluation of an individual's condition in terms of information relating to psychiatric condition, medical condition, psychosocial stressors, and adaptive functioning. As more information is systematically evaluated by trained clinicians, it is expected that the final diagnosis is more reliable. Third, large-scale field trials, involving professionals from psychiatry, psychology, and social work regardless of their theoretical orientations, were conducted to test the reliability of the manual's categories (APA 1980).

The Diagnostic and Statistical Manual has been translated into Chinese, Danish, Dutch, Finnish, French, German, Greek, Italian, Japanese, Norwegian, Portuguese, Spanish, and Swedish (APA 1987). The availability of translations does not necessarily mean that the manual is cross-culturally valid: "It is important that the clinician not employ DSM-III-R in a mechanical fashion, insensitive to differences in language, values, behavioral norms, and idiomatic expressions of distress. When applied in a non-Western-language community, DSM-III-R should be translated to provide equivalent meaning, not necessarily dictionary equivalence" (APA 1987, xxvii).

Conrad and Schneider (1980) state that cultures that have had no contact with Western psychiatry rarely define "madness" as an "illness." In fact, even within the same culture there is no single community criterion for "mental illness" (Draguns 1977b; Marsella 1979; Westermeyer and Wintrob 1979). The classification system itself tends to impose categories and criteria regardless of different social contexts (Kleinman 1977). Cross-cultural differences in the evaluative judgments of mental health professionals pose reliability problems in diagnosing culturally different clients. For example, the same client behavior pattern may be seen as indicative of "depression" in one culture and of "schizophrenia" in another culture because of differences in diagnostic practice of the trained professionals (Cooper et al. 1972). Similarly, affect displayed by the same client may be more subtly discriminated as "anxious" or "depressed" as a function of the sociocultural background of the clinicians (Leff 1973). Such differences in the judgments of clinicians across cultures are not accommodated in the current standardized diagnostic system (Draguns 1982).

The process of diagnosing a person is a complex activity. It involves the interaction of the client's behavior, those who observe him or her, and the specific setting within a given culture (Bandura 1969). Each culture develops norms for expected social role behaviors and judges which behaviors are called "abnormal" (Price and Lynn 1986; Ullmann and Krasner 1975). Cross-cultural therapists must attend to the social meaning and context accompanying presenting problems (Draguns 1982; Kleinman and Good 1985; Tanaka-Matsumi 1979a). Carr (1978) demonstrates this in an analysis of the cognitive-behavioral factors underpinning *amok*, a Malay behavioral disorder of violent aggression, by examining the problem within the unique Malay social context. Cross-cultural therapists need a method of assessment that can identify the functional relationship between the individual's problem behaviors and the social environment (Tanaka-Matsumi 1987).

Behavior therapists in general have acknowledged the improvement made by the third edition of the manual over its predecessors; however, they are highly critical about the overinclusive nature of the many diagnostic categories and the diagnostic criteria that are not always empirically derived (e.g., Schacht and Nathan 1977; Hersen and Turner 1984; Nathan 1987). Most seriously, the medical model underlying psychiatric diagnosis continues to be challenged by behavior therapists in their theoretical formulations of maladaptive behaviors (e.g., Eysenck and Martin 1987).

Functional Analysis of Behavior

Behavior modification emphasizes the direct assessment and empirical monitoring of observable behavior in social situations. Maladaptive behavior is culturally deviant and is acquired in response to social situations.

Selection of target behavior. In behavior modification, functional analysis of behavior (Kanfer and Saslow 1969) is used for the purpose of pinpointing the person's specific presenting problem as it relates to his or her current life circumstances. Changeworthy behaviors and situations are then identified for intervention (Morganstern and Tevlin 1981). The therapist, in collaboration with the client, tries to clarify the nature of the client's concern. Although problems may vary across cultures, the behavior assessment always focuses on specific, observable behaviors in the client's current life. The therapist asks how frequently the presenting problem occurs and what the client has done on his or her own to alleviate the distressful situation. Many clients first tend to describe their problems using subjective, vague, and global terms. For example, Ruiz and Casas (1981, 189) report that the most frequent complaint among Chicano college students in the United States is "subjective discomfort" in the form of "low self-esteem" or "negative self-image." The task is to find out more specifically what the client means by these terms. In what situations does the client have such feelings? What does he or she do to cope with the discomfort? In this way the therapist clarifies the precise nature of "subjective discomfort" in behavioral terms in relation to situational factors.

Each society has its unique "idioms of distress" (Nichter 1981) to publicly communicate subjective discomfort. Among Chinese in Asia and Southeast Asian refugees in the United States, depression is frequently conveyed by means of somatic complaints, such as headaches and chest pains (Kleinman and Kleinman 1985; Nicassio 1985; White 1982). The Japanese associate the concept of depression with environmental or somatic terms, such as "rain" and "headache" (Tanaka-Matsumi and Marsella 1976). How does the cross-cultural behavior therapist make explicit the unique communication styles of a variety of clients?

Higginbotham, West, and Forsyth (1988, chaps. 4, 5) use a "therapy as negotiation" analogy. They suggest four procedures for negotiating both the meaning of client-therapist conversation and the cultural meaning of the client's presenting problem. First, the clinician elicits the client's explanation of the presenting problem. Second, the therapist discloses the explanation, or "explanatory model" (Kleinman 1980), that he or she uses to interpret the problem. Third, the two frameworks are compared for commonalities and discrepancies. Finally, the client and clinician translate each explanatory model in terms of mutually acceptable language, so that they may jointly set the content of therapy, the target behavior, and outcome criteria. Kleinman (1980) also emphasizes the importance of assessing the client's views in developing an effective intervention in different cultures.

The negotiating of problem meaning has direct application to the behavioral assessment of social skills deficits. What constitutes appropriate social skills for different populations depends on the analysis of normative interpersonal behaviors in given situations (McFall 1982). Lack of culture-specific skills is associated with problems of anxiety, depression, a withdrawn lifestyle, and communication problems (Curran et al. 1980). For example, in Goldstein's (1974) case report of a Navajo child, a counselor attempted to develop the child's attending behavior by selecting eye contact as a target behavior. Eye contact among the Navajos, however, is taken as a stare or "evil eye." The target behavior in this instance was culturally not acceptable.

The literature on skills training for American blacks reveals that Caucasians may perceive the same pattern of social behaviors as "assertive" for Caucasians but "aggressive" for blacks (Caldwell-Colbert and Jenkins 1982). That is, "blacks are perceived as aggressive by whites when they express their feelings, raise questions, or are assertive" in interracial situations (Caldwell-Colbert and Jenkins 1982, 192). To develop effective interracial communication, it is necessary to recognize cultural differences in the interpretation of social behaviors.

Identifying controlling stimuli. The second step in functional analysis is to identify those situational and person variables that control the current problematic behaviors. More specifically, the therapist calls attention to the events preceding and following the target behavior (Kanfer and Saslow 1969). This may be achieved by asking what the person was doing immediately prior to the target behavior, whether or not there were people around at that time, and how others responded to the client's problematic behaviors. In cases where the client's perceptions and self-statements are deemed to influence the occurrence of the target behavior, efforts should be made to identify those specific cognitive activities through the use of various techniques (Meichenbaum 1977).

Cross-cultural similarities and differences in social responses to unusual behaviors have been reported (Draguns 1980). Al-Issa's (1977) review of sociocultural factors in "hallucinations" found cultures where such experiences are socially approved in specific situations and under socially prescribed circumstances. Among Balinese and Hawaiians, seeing and speaking with entities from the spirit realm are parts of everyday life for some individuals (Connor 1982; Higginbotham 1987). Abad, Ramos and Boyce (1977) note that some Puerto Ricans freely report experiences akin to auditory and visual hallucinations during heightened religious experiences. Within the Western psychiatric-medical profession, hallucinations are viewed as a sign of mental illness. The public is therefore reluctant to report hallucinatory experiences (Al-Issa 1976). Even if an individual did describe a hallucination, he or she would probably do so with anxiety and terror.

In the West, "self" is viewed as being "individualistic," "analytic," and "deductive" (Johnson 1985). Self is also regarded as an autonomous agent of many of the behaviors. The person's body, feelings, and impulses are assumed to operate on a purely naturalistic basis and cannot be modified by supernatural agents (Fabrega 1982, 56). Hallucinations in this context are considered disturbing and imply abnormality. In contrast, those societies that accept hallucinatory behaviors also provide social influences to regulate the duration and termination of the experience and the places of its occurrence (Al-Issa 1977). Functional analysis enables the therapist to identify specific social conditions under which hallucinations occur and thus suggest an environmental control of hallucinations rather than reducing them by the use of tranquilizing drugs as in medicine (Al-Issa 1976).

Durand and Carr (1987) also demonstrate the importance of evaluating controlling social stimuli in their study of the "self-stimulatory" behavior of developmentally disabled children. They found that the target behaviors of frequent hand flapping and body rocking increased when difficult academic tasks were introduced to the subjects. Further, removing the task demands contingent on stereotyped behavior resulted in increased rates of hand flapping and body rocking. Durand and Carr thus suggest that the social environment of some developmentally disabled persons serves to negatively reinforce stereotyped behavior by removing aversive demands (difficult tasks) contingent on the performance of that behavior. Although "self-stimulatory" behavior has traditionally been viewed as "symptoms" of mental retardation, this research provides data that such behavior may be maintained by social consequences and directly modifiable.

Beyond analyzing the antecedents and consequences of the target behavior, the therapist also asks what the client has done in the past to cope with his or her problem. Appraisal of coping in cross-cultural situations should also include culture-relevant data regarding how the client's social network manages the presenting problem as well as family members' beliefs and attitudes about effective treatment (Danquah 1982; Higginbotham 1984; Sow 1980).

Negotiating treatment strategies. The third purpose of conducting functional analysis is to give client and clinician the basis for negotiating plausible treatment strategies to change the target behavior. The objective nature of behavior therapy permits empirical monitoring of treatment effectiveness because target behaviors and therapeutic conditions are specified. Client and therapist together select appropriate target behaviors and hence the success or failure of therapy is readily apparent. Its effectiveness is manifest in observable behavior change regardless of cultural context.

Many techniques are available for changing behavior (e.g., Bandura 1969; Higginbotham, West and Forsyth 1988; Kanfer and Goldstein 1986). Behavior modification emphasizes changing the consequences of maladaptive behaviors. For example, Guthrie et al. (1982) conducted a field experiment in the rural Philippines to change the feeding practices of mothers. Malnutrition is the most serious health problem of infants in the Philippines. Mothers in the experimental conditions were reinforced by either tickets for a drawing or by a colored photograph of the mother and child for improving the diet of the baby and obtaining a weight gain. Mothers who were assigned to the control group had their babies weighed every three months and received nutrition education. They were not reinforced, however, for compliance with the recommended diet for weight gain of their babies. The results of this community intervention showed that reinforcement of improved feeding practices reduced the number of children who remained seriously underweight after one year of age. Behavior modification literature is replete with positive results of changing the consequences of maladaptive behaviors (e.g., Leitenberg 1976; Kazdin and Wilson 1978).

In the past decade increased attention has been directed to developing self-control skills (Mahoney and Arnkoff 1978; Meichenbaum 1977). Meichenbaum (1977) explains that self-observation and development of new self-statements and behaviors are basic components of cognitive-behavior modification. When cognitive-behavior modification is viewed as a form of self-control (Goldfried and Goldfried 1975), its objective is consistent with the self-regulation techniques associated with such Eastern religious experiences as transcendental meditation, yoga, and trance inducement (Shapiro and Zifferblatt 1976). The increased emphasis placed on controlling one's own behavior by learning to change maladaptive thoughts and attitudes has led some behavior therapists to examine the commonalities of behavior modification and Buddhism.

In Mikulas' (1981) analysis Buddhism and behavior modification both emphasize an objective and practical approach to current problems of living. Individuals are taught to become active agents of behavior change by learning to observe both overt and covert activities through specific techniques. To demonstrate the commonalities of behavior modification and Buddhism, Mikulas presents an analysis of meditation and relaxation. He notes that the initial uses of meditation within behavior modification were primarily to facilitate relaxation. All forms of meditation increase one's ability to exercise either "concentration" or "mindfulness" or both (Mikulas 1981, 33). In the terms of behavior modification, concentration leads to self-control of attention, and mindfulness to objective, nonreactive observation of one's covert and overt behaviors. In other words individuals practicing these techniques develop better self-observation skills, which are essential for self-control. Meditation can be used to counter stress by inducing relaxation and even reducing blood pressure in hypertensive clients (e.g., Benson 1975; Patel 1975).

De Silva (1984) examines the texts of Early Buddhism to demonstrate that the various behavior modification techniques can be found in the practice of Buddhism. These techniques include, for example, setting rules, modeling, positive reinforcement of good behavior, stimulus control of overeating, stopping intrusive thoughts, pain control by meditation, and reducing fear by gradually exposing the person to feared objects. It is reported that the Buddhists in Thailand (Mikulas 1983) and Sri Lanka (De Silva and Samarasinghe 1985) were generally receptive to the ideas of behavior modification. Mikulas (1981) and De Silva (1984) both argue that an explicit recognition of the similarities between Buddhism and behavior modification would facilitate the acceptance and success of behavior modification among Buddhists. It is clear that behavior therapists need to place behavior modification in a culturally compatible context to be accepted.

Cultural Context of Behavior Modification: Issues and Dilemmas

Cultural legitimacy of behavioral intervention. To achieve community legitimacy and acceptance, a therapeutic system should accommodate four principal criteria (Higginbotham 1984, chap. 7). These include culture-specific definitions of deviancy, accepted norms of role behavior, expectations of social influence techniques, and approved behavior change agents. Psychological service systems that fail to encompass these dimensions are discontinuous with the client's social network. Alien service systems are likely to induce dysfunctional culture change and provide reduced or harmful care for those in need (Higginbotham 1979a, 1984; Higginbotham and Marsella 1987). Properly conducted functional analysis of behavior requires attention to cultural accommodation. The training of personnel to demonstrate competency in cultural assessment remains one of the most important goals of behavior modification.

The literature offers excellent examples of behavior therapists' failures and successes regarding cultural accommodation. Bandura (1977a, 116) cautions that societies differ in the extent to which reinforcers are structured on an individual or collective basis. Gallimore and his colleagues (Gallimore 1974; Gallimore, Boggs, and Jordan 1974; Jordan and Tharp 1979) successfully designed a classroom environment consistent with the group affiliation values found in Hawaiian culture. Teachers encouraged group affiliation and delivered reinforcers contingent on group performance rather than individual performance.

Guthrie et al.'s (1982) extensive experience in implementing a large-scale community intervention of maternal feeding practices supports the importance of fully analyzing the culture's belief systems and naturally available reinforcement contingencies so that they do not interfere with a newly introduced system of behavior change. Dowdall (1982) also states that behavior therapy's effectiveness in an indigenous African culture depends on achieving an integration with cultural and religious values and beliefs. Furthermore, just as socialization practices and values differ among groups, the effectiveness and delivery of different reinforcers vary depending upon the person's culture-specific learning history (Gallimore, Weiss, and Finney 1974; Guthrie et al. 1982; Schultz and Sherman 1976; Sidman 1960, 385; Staats 1975). In sum, cross-cultural behavior therapists must evaluate the client's immediate problem behaviors through functional analysis of his or her social network and the associated cultural accommodation criteria of that group.

Cross-cultural behavior therapists and the selection of behavior change agents. It is essential to consider therapist variables when working with people from diverse cultural backgrounds. Who is qualified or competent to serve as the change agent for different ethnic and cultural groups is a major concern (Higginbotham 1984, 236–239). There are different views of cross-cultural competency. Ruiz and Casas (1981) advocate bilingualism and biculturalism as requirements for working with American Chicano clients. Draguns (1981) cautions that in situations where therapeutic verbal communication is essential the use of the second language may lose subtle meanings specific to the primary language. Goldstein (1981), on the other hand, cautions against eliminating potential helpers based on static factors, such as ethnicity and age.

In behavior therapy only those trained in principles of behavior change and in skills to practice those principles should deliver treatment. At the same time, the extent to which the therapist is capable of enhancing the credibility and expectancy of cross-cultural therapy should be evaluated (Higginbotham 1977). Because behavior therapy is primarily a social influence process, behavior therapists should actively attend to culture-relevant role behaviors during client contact to establish an effective helper-client relationship (Wilson and Evans 1976). This means that therapists need to accommodate cultural rules of interaction that help define appropriate role behaviors as therapists (Johnson 1981).

Behavior therapy actively trains those significant others in the client's environment to be part of the intervention. Tharp and Wetzel's (1969) triadic model of behavioral consultation views therapy as a chain of interpersonal influences. This model consists of three parties: consultants, mediators (behavior change agents), and target clients. Qualified behavior therapists act as consultants and train mediators, who maintain direct and continuous contact with the client. Both the consultant and the mediator need recognition as a legitimate source of influence in the client's environment for the problem under consideration (Higginbotham 1976). Training of behavior change agents has proved effective in such areas as behavioral management of children at home by the parents (e.g., Forehand and King 1977; Patterson 1974) and in school by the teachers (e.g., Bavermeister and Jamail 1976; Jones 1982; Tanaka-Matsumi and Tharp 1977). Psychiatric hospital personnel have also been effectively trained as behavior change agents to modify severely maladaptive behaviors of chronic mental patients (e.g., Paul and Lentz 1977).

Bernstein (1982) emphasizes the need for broadening our ecological perspective in selecting and training appropriate behavior change agents to reduce competing variables in the naturalistic environment. The use of behavior change agents selected from the client's own environment should also increase the probability of the target behavior's maintenance and generalization in the naturalistic environment (Higginbotham, West, and Forsyth 1988, chap. 7; Stokes and Baer 1977; Tanaka-Matsumi, in press). In non-Western countries behavior therapy programs tend to develop initially within Western-oriented settings, such as medical schools (e.g., Danquah 1982; De Rosemberg and Delgado 1985). It is important, therefore, to seek an integration with the client's naturalistic environment through the use of culturally resourceful and trained behavior change agents (Higginbotham 1984).

Treatment Efficacy and Research Needs

Single-subject research model in behavior therapy. The strength of behavior therapy as a model for cross-cultural counseling lies in its advanced methods for empirically evaluating environment and person conditions and monitoring the degree of behavior change produced by treatment. Therapy is conceptualized as a single-subject experiment that includes a continuous monitoring of treatment variables and target behaviors (Baer, Wolf, and Risley 1968; Kazdin 1982). Effects of therapy are measured in terms of behavior change relative to the unique baseline of the individual or group. There is no imposed theoretical criterion independent of the client's own progress.

Wolf's (1978) idea of "social validation" is important for cross-cultural intervention. This notion incorporates social criteria for evaluating the treatment focus, procedures, and effects (Kazdin 1982). The therapist must be aware of the expected social behaviors of the client's cultural group in order to evaluate treatment using "social comparison" (Kazdin 1977). For example, when depression was defined as a behavioral communication of the person's dejected state and experiences, it was necessary to employ a group of untrained observer-judges, rather than mental health experts, to socially validate those behaviors communicated by the actor-subjects (Tanaka-Matsumi 1983). By incorporating the components of social validation, behavior therapists may develop a socially accepted intervention plan within the client's cultural context.

More specific explanations for failures in cross-cultural counseling. The field of cross-cultural counseling should stand or fall on its ability to demonstrate the viability of its procedures (Higginbotham 1979b, 65). The literature is replete with competing notions of why cross-cultural counseling is inherently prone to failure. A partial list includes such factors as patient-therapist "barriers" of social values, culture, and language (Sue 1981; Vontress 1981); cognitive or behavioral incongruity (Carkhuff and Pierce 1967; Wohl 1981); resistance (Alexander et al. 1981); negative countertransference and stereotypic therapist response to clients (Atkinson, Morten and Sue 1979; Bloombaum, Yamamoto, and James 1968; Safilios-Rothschild 1969); incongruent therapy expectations (Goldstein 1973; Higginbotham 1977); and distrust (Maultsby 1982).

Careful inspections of the social influence processes involved in work with clients from unique cultures reveal conditions that predictably elicit "countercontrol" (Goldfried and Davison 1976) or "resistance" to behavior change. There are several ways to reduce client resistance to change and enhance expectations for improvement of the presenting problem.

First, enhancement of the therapist's interpersonal attraction contributes significantly to an attenuation of client resistance (Goldstein, Heller, and Sechrest 1966). Under conditions of high interpersonal attraction, client-therapist communication is more persuasive (Wilson and Evans 1976), and the therapist's ability to function as a model for the client increases because of his discriminative and reinforcing behaviors (Krasner 1962; Staats 1975). Goldstein and Myers (1986) systematically increase client attraction to the therapist by creating specific occasions for the client to observe others expressing positive qualities of the therapist. This method enhances the credibility and ascribed status of the therapist and communicates facilitative messages (e.g., empathy and warmth) to the client.

A second method to enhance the therapist's social influence lies in the identification of situation variables that evoke client expectations of positive treatment outcomes. Such an expectation is called situation-outcome expectancy (see Higginbotham, West, and Forsyth 1988, chap. 6, for a typology of client expectancies). Clients actively evaluate the helper's qualities. They also try to find out if specific treatment leads to an improvement of their problem. A high situation-outcome expectancy results when the client believes that treatment contains the conditions sufficient to bring about improvement. Expectancies serve several functions: (1) they influence therapist instructions (Lick and Bootzin 1975); (2) they elicit positive affect, such as hope and delight, that help counteract anxiety, depression, and helplessness (Frank 1973); and (3) they motivate clients to persist in their efforts to achieve improvement of the problem and to learn coping skills. Higginbotham, West, and Forsyth (1988) argue that the therapist's expectancies are more powerful determinants of counseling events and outcomes than those of the client. Even when the client perceives poor chances for behavior change, the therapist's positive expectancies can overcome this lack of hope. Therapists have a host of procedures at their disposal to elevate low situation-outcome expectancies. One way is to elicit and actively discuss the client's discrepant expectations. In addition, cultural assessment knowledge enables the clinician to (1) construct a plausible problem interpretation tied to a potent-sounding intervention; (2) use subtle nonverbal and language cues to promote treatment credibility; and (3) increase therapist-client congruence based on perceived similarities (e.g., Goldstein and Myers 1986; Higginbotham 1977).

In sum, research indicates that prior to implementing intervention techniques, it is imperative to thoroughly assess the cultural determinants of client outcome expectancy. Behavior therapists should adhere to an empirical monitoring of culturally relevant variables that enhance interpersonal attraction, reduce client countercontrol, and elevate situation-outcome expectancies of both client and therapist.

Ethical considerations. Ethical and value considerations in selecting therapy goals and techniques are advocated by virtually all investigators of principles of behavior modification (e.g., Bandura 1969; Krasner and Ullmann 1965; Stolz 1978). In his book *Walden Two*, Skinner (1948) anticipated the issue of behavioral control and value judgments in the design of a culture. Under a "medical" model of "mental illness," the activities of the professional are justified by the goal of the model— removal of symptoms and cure of illness (Ullmann and Krasner 1965). In behavior therapy, however, since no behavior is considered normal or abnormal in itself, social values are inherent considerations in behavior modification. They determine who should treat the person and what should be the goal of therapy (Goldiamond 1974). When therapists operate across cultural and ethnic boundaries, criteria for ethical value judgments become even more problematical and require careful reviews (Draguns 1981; Higginbotham 1979b; Korman 1974).

Broadly speaking, behavior therapy involves cultural learning with distinct moral and epistemological underpinnings (Bandura 1974). Woolfolk and Richardson (1984) argue that it is embedded in the ideology of modernity and the values of modern technological society. Science is enshrined as the ultimate source of knowledge and the model for all forms of intellectual activity (Winner 1977). The rationality of behavior therapy ran counter to two currents of Western thought: (1) the Freudian notion that irrational forces motivate behavior, and (2) the idealized view of self as detached from social context and the distaste for viewing people as pawns of the environment. Consequently, behavior therapists in the early days were met with resistance from parents who interpreted reward contingencies as "bribes," who could not "see the point of" keeping detailed records of behavior when it was the child's "attitude" that was bad. Moreover, these professionals had to persuade middle- and upper-class clients reared on "Romantic humanism" that self-control was not gained through exploration of feelings, confessions of fantasies, and cultivation of passions. Rather, behavioral self-regulation was strengthened by "extinction" of inappropriate emotion, "thought stopping" of undesirable fantasies, and adoption of rational problem-solving techniques in various situations (Woolfolk and Richardson 1984, 780).

Behavior therapists recognize that cultural sentiments underlying behavioral methods are transmitted in a context of intense cultural learning and social influence. Uchiyama (1985) notes that progress of behavior therapy in Japan can be impeded by the unique Japanese cultural sentiment that does not encourage deductive empiricism. In any therapy the therapist directly and indirectly shapes the client into a mode of problem definition consistent with the therapy's underlying principles (Higginbotham et al. 1988, chap. 4; Meichenbaum 1977). For example, the Japanese therapeutic method of introspection and self-observation called Naikan therapy, shapes the client to focus his or her entire attention on specific interpersonal behavioral exchanges through a set of instructions (Tanaka-Matsumi 1979b).

Ethical practice is ensured when the clinician is familiar with the culture within which he or she operates and competently applies the cultural knowledge to case management. The American Psychological Association Vail Conference on Professional Training underscored this point. The conference proclaimed that it is unethical for a professional to offer services to members of a cultural group in which he or she lacks expertise (Korman 1974). If Western-derived treatments are applied to non-Western populations without proved effectiveness, such procedures may lead to unethical practice. Behavior therapy addresses ethical issues by stating that therapy is basically an educational process. Behavior therapists are taught to clearly give the treatment rationale, obtain client-informed consent, and empirically evaluate progress according to social criteria (Higginbotham 1984). This means that the client is expected and encouraged to actively participate in the determination of therapy goals. The questions of "What is good?" and "Who decides?" will continue to challenge behavior therapists.

Counseling American Minorities, Refugees, and Overseas Sojourners: Cross-Cultural Applications of Behavior Modification

To elucidate a behavioral approach to cross-cultural counseling, we present an analysis of problems experienced by minority groups, foreign students, refugees, and overseas sojourners.

Minority Groups

Numerous authors (e.g., Atkinson, Morten, and Sue 1979; Ruiz and Casas 1981; Sue 1977; Sue and Morishima 1982; Vontress 1981; Walz and Benjamin 1978) have aptly described the cultural insensitivity of existing mental health services and their steadfast avoidance by many minority groups. American minorities underutilize formal psychological services for several important reasons. First, ethnic clients have historically received poorer-quality care when they sought help and experienced less satisfactory outcomes (Sue 1977). They were often assigned nonprofessional helpers and received treatment requiring less staff time, that is, medication (Hollingshead and Redlich 1958). Second, Padilla, Ruiz, and Alvarez (1975) identified inflexible intake procedures, long waiting lists, and geographic isolation of the clinic from those it serves. Similarly, mental health centers that do not have culturally and linguistically competent workers are frustrating to help seekers who are unable to comprehend clinic operations or communicate readily their reasons for seeking help.

The traditional, middle-class model of counseling itself has drawn the sharpest criticism for its irrelevance to the requirements and lifestyles of minority and non-Western clients. Atkinson, Morten, and Sue (1979) readily point out that the intrapsychic approach of traditional counseling does not lead to the concrete problem solving that clients desire most. Intrapsychic models see dysfunction as the consequence of intrapersonal disorganization rather than social factors, hence change should be at the individual level conforming to an imposed standard of normality. The counseling style according to such a model tends to be highly verbal and office-bound. It perpetuates the very socialization process that creates barriers between culturally different persons.

Another major factor is the service user's attitudes toward receiving professional care. Maultsby (1982, 39) states that "as a group, American blacks have a deeply rooted, long-standing distrust of American psychiatry." Green (1982) argues that when black clients are seen in clinic settings, many of them have acquired maladaptive behaviors typical of learned helplessness and view external social situations to be uncontrollable. Coupled with the negative attitude toward professional psychiatric services, blacks have been a largely underserved population in the United States. For Asian Americans stigmatizing consequences of receiving psychiatric care have tended to prohibit them from seeking desirable help (Sue and Morishima 1982).

Clinicians working with minority groups have recognized the use of behavioral methods as one of the viable alternatives to traditional counseling (e.g., Schinke et al. 1987). They see it as meeting the special requirements of low-income and culturally different clients (Atkinson, Morten, and Sue 1979; Goldstein 1973; Padilla, Ruiz, and Alvarez 1975; Rappaport 1977). It is reported in the clinical literature that native Americans (Ruiz and Casas 1981), Hispanic Americans (Padilla, Ruiz, and Alvarez 1975), and Asian Americans (Sue and Morishima 1982; Sue and Zane 1987) prefer the therapist to take an active, directive role. They prefer explicit directions on how to solve problems and bring immediate relief from distressing conditions. Vontress (1981) asserts that counselors must immediately make clear what, how, and why they intend to do what is planned in therapy in order to reduce uncertainty experienced by clients and their families. Preventing an early dropout is a prime concern for cross-cultural therapists (Sue and Zane 1987).

Research by Folensbee, Draguns, and Danish (1986), however, question the clinical claims that members of Puerto Rican and black American minority groups respond better to directive interventions than to nondirective ones. They stress the need for documenting actual counseling interactions between the therapist and the client for different ethnic groups.

Behavior therapy is goal directed. It is structured into step-by-step procedures through which therapists teach alternative behaviors that can be practiced in the current social context of the client's activities. Because the focus of therapy is on developing new social behaviors, the client can actually observe and monitor the effects of therapy itself. Further, new behaviors should receive positive feedback and reinforcement from people in the client's everyday environment that then maintain the behaviors acquired.

Foreign Students and Overseas Sojourners

An extensive literature has evolved describing the environmental stressors and adjustment reactions experienced by foreign students, Peace Corps volunteers, and other overseas sojourners (e.g., Brein and David 1971; Jones and Popper 1972; Liem and Kehmeier 1980; Ogino and Hoshino 1983; Taft 1977). For foreign students the primary worry is academic difficulties (Sharma 1973), reflecting collateral problems of language and past educational experience. This is predictable for persons who have made a substantial financial and personal investment toward the successful completion of degree studies. Foreign students are reluctant to allow personal considerations (e.g., getting used to local customs, participating in campus activities) to get in the way of their studies, although there is some indication that extensive social interaction with local citizens facilitates their satisfaction (Brein and David 1971; Ferguson 1979).

Overseas sojourners and foreign students experience a "culture shock" (Oberg 1958; Hoshino 1980; Taft 1977) in their struggle to cope with an unfamiliar culture. The behavioral approach provides a comprehensive appraisal of culture shock. Culture shock is a maladaptive response to a new situation in which previous learning is inadequate for coping with the novel environment. Situational and social cues that used to serve as discriminative stimuli for effective actions are no longer effective. Thus, most of the behavior the person has acquired in the previous environment proves useless in his or her new environment. Skinner (1971, 139) analyzes this type of adjustment problem and emphasizes the importance of actually describing the behavior of the individual rather than focusing on the emotional effects of the ineffective behavior. When the environmental outcome is unpredictable because of the inability to respond appropriately to social cues, the individual may stop responding. His behavior is extinguished because of the lack of reinforcement in a new environment. Consequently, his or her perceived self-efficacy (Bandura 1977b) may be reduced, and severe emotional consequences, such as depression and anxiety, may follow (Seligman 1975). Consistent avoidance behavior prevents the person from learning new behaviors. It serves to maintain negative emotional reactions because avoidance reduces the negative emotions associated with the feared environment. Such negative emotional reactions may generalize to similar but innocuous events and situations. Hence, the person with culture shock may come to see a great deal of "danger" in the new environment and come to avoid a broad array of cultural circumstances that might otherwise be found positive.

Remediation of culture shock involves new social learning. Two complementary approaches have been suggested (Brein and David 1971;

David 1976; Ogino and Hoshino 1983; Taft 1977). First, the sojourner needs to learn new intercultural skills that will enable him or her to attain positive effects and avoid negative effects in the new environment. That is, the person learns a new set of behaviors so that negative contingencies of the previous behavior may be replaced by positive contingencies (Skinner 1971). This learning is similar to conducting a functional analysis of behaviors in the new environment, so that one can learn what behavior leads to desirable consequences in a foreign cultural setting through observation and trial-and-error learning (Taft 1977).

Sojourner preparation programs, in contrast, make use of knowledgeable models (like returning Peace Corps volunteers) and guided practice in simulated host country settings. Landis and Brislin (1983) have published a three-volume handbook on various intercultural training programs aimed at successful adjustments to another culture. Also available for training material is a publication of 100 critical incidents involving difficult intercultural encounters that were socially validated by experienced overseas sojourners (Brislin et al. 1986). In short, receiving instructions and behavioral training through modeling, role-playing, and feedback prepares people for what to expect and how to cope within a new culture. Such programs give prior knowledge to the newcomer and prepare him or her to act in such a way that members of the host culture will respond positively. In short, skills training is essential to successful adjustment.

The second method for remediating culture shock is through attenuation of unpleasant experiences. Behavioral research shows a significant relationship between engagement in pleasant activities and self-report of positive moods (Lewinsohn 1974). Thus, to increase one's positive moods, it is necessary to find new reinforcers and learn skills to acquire them in a new environment. David (1976) provides a comprehensive format for counselors to help sojourner clients attain reinforcers and avoid punishers. Four questions are asked: What are your sources of reinforcement back home? Are there any events that might occur but have not that would act as reinforcers? How many potential reinforcers are available in the host culture? What events in the host culture can be used as reinforcers during predeparture training; that is, how can you anticipate good things happening and rehearse your experience with them?

The counselor-trainer is able to focus on specific anticipated problems from the assessment of reinforcers and potentially unpleasant events (cf. MacPhillamy and Lewinsohn 1982). In sum, the behavioral approach analyzes "culture shock" into specific experiences and behaviors of the individual in a new environment. By identifying situations in which the person faces problems, the therapist guides him or her to learn new skills that help reduce stress and increase opportunities to engage in reinforcing activities. This should be done until the person learns new role behaviors consistent with the host culture that will be positively reinforced and maintained by the members of the host culture. This approach is therefore directed toward training people in appropriate social skills and by disseminating culture-related information in a systematic manner.

Refugees

Refugees, such as the nearly 500,000 Indochinese who have sought security in the United States since 1975 (Nicassio 1985), confront serious adjustment obstacles. The literature points out the intense plight of these "persons without a homeland" and the adverse psychological consequences of their flight from Southeast Asia (Aylesworth, Ossorio, and Osaki 1979; Ferguson 1979; Rahe et al 1978; Williams and Westermeyer 1983).

Central to assessing the condition of the Southeast Asians is an appreciation of the profound sense of loss in their lives (Nicassio 1985). The disruption of the family network and the loss of social support during involuntary emigration have been noted as particularly critical in the adjustment of the refugees in the camps and resettlement environment (Nicassio and Pate 1984; Nguyen 1982; Rahe et al. 1978). Inability to speak English and unemployment are further obstacles to successful resettlement. Further, the loss of the traditional practice of ancestor worship disrupts the refugees' contact with their ancestors (Liem and Kehmeier 1980). Finally, government and public attitudes toward their immigration have not been uniformly positive. There have been reports of hostile and indifferent treatment by members of the host country (Liu 1979). Recent clinical and field research indicates that depression is the most common complaint found in refugees who have sought professional psychiatric help (Nicassio 1985).

Nicassio (1985) advocates that some of the refugees' behavior pattern that is similar to that of "learned helplessness" (Garber and Seligman 1980) may be attenuated by guiding them to actively participate in the host culture so that they will once again learn that their behavior and outcome are related and gradually stop withdrawing. There is a need to empirically evaluate the efficacy of various behavioral interventions for the unique problems of refugees.

Summary and Conclusion

Behavior modification advocates an experimental analysis of behavior in the client's own social environment. Contrary to the psychiatric-medical model, in the theoretical models underlying behavior therapy and behavior modification, behavior is neither normal nor abnormal in itself apart from the client's own sociocultural context. The behavioral approach emphasizes specific conditions: the client's cultural conception of problem behaviors, setting specific goals in therapy, arranging conditions to increase the client's expectation of therapy success, minimizing "countercontrol," and using appropriate social influence agents. Cross-cultural behavior therapists must be particularly sensitive to making value judgments concerning the selection of target behaviors for intervention. The progress of therapy is measured relative to the client's own behavioral baseline and through social validation of the target behavior, methods of change, and treatment outcome.

The experience of "culture shock" reported by foreign students, overseas sojourners, and refugees can be analyzed in terms of ineffective responses to unfamiliar social cues and lack of desirable social behaviors in an unfamiliar cultural environment. The behavioral approach emphasizes actual descriptions of problem behaviors in specific situations and training in alternative skills to achieve desirable consequences. Thus, behavior modification offers a strong research and treatment model for cross-cultural counseling.

References

Abad, V., Ramos, J., and Boyce, E. 1977. Clinical issues in the psychiatric treatment of Puerto Ricans. In E. R. Padilla and A. M. Padilla (eds.), *Transcultural psychiatry: A Hispanic perspective*. Los Angeles: Spanish Speaking Mental Health Center, University of California.

Agathon, M. 1982. Behavior therapy in France, 1976–1981. *Journal of Behavior Therapy and Experimental Psychiatry* 13:271–277.

Alexander, A. A., Klein, M. H., Workneh, F., and Miller, M. H. 1981. Psychotherapy and the foreign student. In P. B. Pedersen, J. G. Draguns, W. J. Lonner, and J. E. Trimble (eds.), *Counseling across cultures*, 227–246. Honolulu: University of Hawaii Press.

Al-Issa, L. 1976. Behavior therapy and hallucinations: A sociocultural approach. *Psychotherapy: Theory, Research and Practice* 13:156–159.

———. 1977. Social and cultural aspects of hallucinations. *Psychological Bulletin* 84:570–587.

American Psychiatric Association (APA). 1980. *Diagnostic and statistical manual of mental disorders*. 3d ed. Washington, DC: American Psychiatric Association.

———. 1987. *Diagnostic and statistical manual of mental disorders*. Rev. 3d ed. Washington, DC: American Psychiatric Association.

Ardila, R. 1982. International developments in behavior therapy in Latin America. *Journal of Behavior Therapy and Experimental Psychiatry* 13:15–20.

Atkinson, D. R., Morten, G., and Sue, D. W. 1979. *Counseling American minorities: A cross-cultural perspective*. Dubuque, IA: William C. Brown.

Aylesworth, L. S., Ossorio, P. G., and Osaki, L. T. 1979. Stress and mental health among Vietnamese in the United States. In R. Endo, S. Sue, and N. Wagner (eds.), *Asian-Americans: Social and psychological perspectives.* Palo Alto, CA: Science and Behavior Books.

Baer, D. M., Wolf, M. M., and Risley, T. R. 1968. Some current dimensions of applied behavior analysis. *Journal of Applied Behavior Analysis* 1:91–97.

Bandura, A. 1969. *Principles of behavior modification.* New York: Holt, Rinehart, and Winston.

————. 1974. Behavior therapy and models of man. *American Psychologist* 29:859–869.

————. 1977a. *Social learning theory.* Englewood Cliffs, NJ: Prentice-Hall.

————. 1977b. Self-efficacy: Toward a unifying theory of behavioral change. *Psychological Review* 84:191–215.

Bavermeister, J. J., and Jamail, J. A. 1976. Teachers as experimenters and behavior engineers: An extension and cross-cultural replication. *Inter-American Journal of Psychology* 10:41–45.

Beck, A. T., Ward, C. H., Mendelson, M., Mock, J. E., and Erbaugh, J. K. 1962. Reliability of psychiatric diagnosis 2: A study of consistency of clinical judgments and ratings. *American Journal of Psychiatry* 119:351–357.

Benson, H. 1975. *The relaxation response.* New York: W. W. Norton.

Bernstein, G. S. 1982. Training behavior change agents: A conceptual review. *Behavior Therapy* 13:1–23.

Bloombaum, M., Yamamoto, J., and James, Q. 1968. Cultural stereotyping among psychotherapists. *Journal of Consulting and Clinical Psychology* 32:99.

Brein, M., and David, K. H. 1971. Intercultural communication and the adjustment of the sojourner. *Psychological Bulletin* 76:215–230.

Brislin, R. W., Cushner, K., Cherrie, C., and Yong, M. 1986. *Intercultural interactions: A practical guide.* Beverly Hills: Sage Publications.

Caldwell-Colbert, A. T., and Jenkins, J. O. 1982. Modification of interpersonal behavior. In S. M. Turner and R. T. Russell (eds.), *Behavior modification in black populations,* 171–207. New York: Plenum Press.

Carkhuff, R. R., and Pierce, R. 1967. Differential effects of therapist race and social class upon patient depth of self-exploration in the initial clinical interview. *Journal of Consulting Psychology* 31:632–634.

Carr, J. 1978. Ethno-behaviorism and the culture-bound syndromes: The case of *amok. Culture, Medicine and Psychiatry* 2:269–293.

Connor, L. H. 1982. The unbounded self: Balinese therapy in theory and practice. In A. J. Marsella and G. M. White (eds.), *Cultural conceptions of mental health and therapy.* Dordrecht, Holland: D. Reidel Publishing.

Conrad, P., and Schneider, J. W. 1980. *Deviance and medicalization: From business to sickness.* St. Louis: Mosby.

Cooper, J. E., Kendell, R. E., Gurland, B. J., Sharpe, L., Copeland, J. R. M., and Simmons, R. 1972. *Psychiatric diagnosis in New York and London.* London: Oxford University Press.

Curran, J. P., Miller, I., Zwick, W., Monti, P. M., and Stout, R. L. 1980. The socially inadequate patient: Incidence rate, demographic and clinical features, hospital and post-hospital functioning. *Journal of Consulting and Clinical Psychology* 48:375–382.

Danquah, S. A. 1982. The practice of behavior therapy in West Africa: The case of Ghana. *Journal of Behavior Therapy and Experimental Psychiatry* 13:5–13.

David, K. H. 1976. The use of social-learning theory in preventing intercultural adjustment problems. In P. B. Pedersen, W. J. Lonner, and J. G. Draguns (eds.), *Counseling across cultures.* Honolulu: University of Hawaii Press.

De Rosemberg, F. K., and Delgado, F., Sr. 1985. The establishment of a behavior therapy unit within a general hospital in Venezuela: The first five years. *Journal of Behavior Therapy and Experimental Psychiatry* 16:5–7.

De Silva, P. 1984. Buddhism and behavior modification. *Behaviour Research and Therapy* 22:661–678.

De Silva, P., and Samarasinghe, D. 1985. Behavior therapy in Sri Lanka. *Journal of Behavior Therapy and Experimental Psychiatry* 16:95–100.

Dowdall, T. 1982. Behavior therapy in South Africa. *Journal of Behavior Therapy and Experimental Psychiatry* 13:279–286.

Draguns, J. G. 1977a. Advances in the methodology of cross-cultural psychiatric assessment. *Transcultural Psychiatric Research Review* 14:125–143.

———. 1977b. Problems of defining and comparing abnormal behavior across cultures. In L. L. Adler (ed.), *Issues in cross-cultural research,* 664–675. Vol. 285, Annals of New York Academy of Science. New York: New York Academy of Science.

———. 1979. Culture and personality. In A. J. Marsella, R. G. Tharp, and T. Ciborowski (eds.), *Perspectives in cross-cultural psychology.* New York: Academic Press.

———. 1980. Psychological disorders of clinical severity. In H. C. Triandis and J. G. Draguns (eds.), *Handbook of cross-cultural psychology.* Vol. 6, *Psychopathology,* 99–174. Boston: Allyn and Bacon.

———. 1981. Cross-cultural counseling and psychotherapy: History, issues, current status. In A. J. Marsella and P. B. Pedersen (eds.), *Cross-cultural counseling and psychotherapy: Foundations, evaluation, and cultural considerations,* 3–27. Elmsford, NY: Pergamon Press.

———. 1982. Methodology in cross-cultural psychopathology. In L. Al-Issa (ed.), *Culture and psychopathology,* 33–70. Baltimore: University Park Press.

Draguns, J. G., and Phillips, L. 1971. *Psychiatric classification and diagnosis: An overview and critique.* Morristown, NJ: General Learning Press.

Durand, V. M., and Carr, E. 1987. Social influences on "self-stimulatory" behavior: Analysis and treatment application. *Journal of Applied Behavior Analysis* 20:119–132.

Enright, J. B., and Jaeckle, W. R. 1963. Psychiatric symptoms and diagnosis in two subcultures. *International Journal of Social Psychiatry* 9:12–17.

Eysenck, H. J. 1959. Learning theory and behavior therapy. *Journal of Medical Science* 105:61–75.

Eysenck, H. J., and Martin, I., eds. 1987. *Theoretical foundations of behavior therapy.* New York: Plenum Press.

Fabrega, H. 1982. Culture and psychiatric illness: Biomedical and ethnomedical aspects. In A. J. Marsella and G. M. White (eds.), *Cultural conceptions of mental health and therapy.* Dordrecht, Holland: D. Reidel Publishing.

Ferguson, B. 1979. Vietnamese refugee adjustment in Honolulu. Master's thesis, University of Hawaii, Honolulu.

Folensbee, R. W., Draguns, J. G., and Danish, S. J. 1986. Impact of two types of counselor intervention on black American, Puerto Rican, and Anglo-American clients. *Journal of Counseling Psychology* 331:446–453.

Forehand, R., and King, H. E. 1977. Noncompliant children: Effects of parent training on behavior and attitude change. *Behavior Modification* 1:93–108.

Frank, J. D. 1973. *Persuasion and healing.* Baltimore: Johns Hopkins University Press.

Gallimore, R. 1974. Affiliation motivation and Hawaiian-American achievement. *Journal of Cross-Cultural Psychology* 5:481–492.

Gallimore, R., Boggs, J. W., and Jordan, C. 1974. *Culture, behavior and education: A study of Hawaiian Americans.* Beverly Hills: Sage Publications.

Gallimore, R., Weiss, L. B., and Finney, R. 1974. Cultural differences in delay of gratification: A problem of behavior classification. *Journal of Personality and Social Psychology* 30:72–80.

Garber, J., and Seligman, M. E. P. 1980. *Human helplessness.* New York: Academic Press.

Goffman, E. 1961. *Asylums.* Garden City, NY: Doubleday Anchor.

Goldfried, M. R., and Davison, G. C. 1976. *Clinical behavior therapy.* New York: Holt, Rinehart, and Winston.

Goldfried, M. R., and Goldfried, A. P. 1975. Cognitive change methods. In F. H. Kanfer and A. P. Goldstein (eds.), *Helping people change,* 1st ed., 89–116. New York: Pergamon Press.

Goldiamond, I. 1974. Toward a constructional approach to social problems: Ethical and constitutional issues raised by applied behavior analysis. *Behaviorism* 2:1–84.

Goldstein, A. P. 1973. *Structured learning therapy.* New York: Academic Press.

———. 1981. Expectancy effects in cross-cultural counseling. In A. J. Marsella and P. B. Pedersen (eds.), *Cross-cultural counseling and psychotherapy: Foundations, evaluation, and cultural considerations.* Elmsford, NY: Pergamon Press.

Goldstein, A. P., Heller, K., and Sechrest, L. B. 1966. *Psychotherapy and the psychology of behavior change.* New York: John Wiley and Sons.

Goldstein, A. P., and Myers, C. R. 1986. Relationship-enhancement methods. In F. H. Kanfer and A. P. Goldstein (eds.), *Helping people change,* 3d ed., 19–65. New York: Plenum Press.

Goldstein, G. S. 1974. Behavior modification: Some cultural factors. *Psychological Record* 24:89–91.

Green, L. 1982. A learned helplessness analysis of problems confronting the black community. In S. M. Turner and R. T. Jones (eds.), *Behavior modification in black populations,* 73–93. New York: Plenum Press.

Guthrie, G. M., Guthrie, H. A., Fernandez, T. L., and Estrera, N. O. 1982.

Cultural influences and reinforcement strategies. *Behavior Therapy* 13:624–637.

Hersen, M., and Turner, S. M. 1984. DSM-III and behavior therapy. In S. M. Turner and M. Hersen (eds.), *Adult psychopathology and diagnosis*, 485–502. New York: John Wiley and Sons.

Higginbotham, H. N. 1976. A conceptual model for the delivery of psychological services in non-Western settings. In R. W. Brislin and M. P. Hamnett (eds.), *Topics in culture learning* 4:44–52. Honolulu: East-West Center Press.

————. 1977. Culture and the role of client expectancy in psychotherapy. In R. W. Brislin and M. P. Hamnett (eds.), *Topics in culture learning* 5:107–124. Honolulu: East-West Center Press.

————. 1979a. Culture and mental health services. In A. J. Marsella, R. G. Tharp, and T. Ciborowski (eds.), *Perspectives on cross-cultural psychology*. New York: Academic Press.

————. 1979b. Cultural issues in providing psychological services for foreign students in the United States. *International Journal of Intercultural Relations* 31:49–85.

————. 1984. *Toward world challenge to psychiatry: Culture accommodation and mental health care*. Honolulu: University of Hawaii Press.

————. 1987. The culture accommodation of mental health services of Native Hawaiians. In A. Robillard (ed.), *Contemporary issues in mental health research in the Pacific Islands*. Honolulu: University of Hawaii Press.

Higginbotham, H. N., and Marsella, A. J. 1987. International consultation and the homogenization of psychiatry in Southeast Asia. *Social Science and Medicine* 22.

Higginbotham, H. N., West, S., and Forsyth, D. 1988. *Psychotherapy and behavior change: Social, cultural and methodological perspectives*. New York: Pergamon Press.

Hollingshead, A. B., and Redlich, F. C. 1958. *Social class and mental illness: A community study*. New York: John Wiley and Sons.

Hoshino, A. 1980. Culture shock. In A. Hoshino (ed.), *Culture shock*, 5–30. L'Esprit d'Aujourd'hui No. 161. Tokyo: Shibundo.

Jones, R. J., and Popper, R. 1972. Characteristics of Peace Corps host countries and the behavior of volunteers. *Journal of Cross-Cultural Psychology* 3:233–245.

Jones, R. T. 1982. Academic improvement through behavioral intervention. In S. M. Turner and R. T. Jones (eds.), *Behavior modification in black populations*, 121–147. New York: Plenum Press.

Johnson, F. A. 1981. Ethnicity and interaction rules in counseling and psychotherapy: Some basic considerations. In A. J. Marsella and P. B. Pedersen (eds.), *Cross-cultural counseling and psychotherapy: Foundations, evaluation, and cultural considerations*, 63–84. Elmsford, NY: Pergamon Press.

————. 1985. The Western concept of self. In A. J. Marsella, G. DeVos, and F. L. K. Hsu (eds.), *Culture and self: Asian and Western perspectives*, 91–138. New York: Tavistock Publications.

Jordan, C., and Tharp, R. G. 1979. Culture and education. In A. J. Marsella, R. G. Tharp, and T. Ciborowski (eds.). *Perspectives in cross-cultural psychology.* New York: Academic Press.

Kanfer, F. H., and Goldstein, A. P., eds. 1986. *Helping people change: A textbook of methods.* 3d ed. New York: Pergamon Press.

Kanfer, F. H., and Saslow, G. 1969. Behavioral diagnosis. In C. M. Franks (ed.), *Behavior therapy: Appraisal and status.* New York: McGraw-Hill.

Kazdin, A. E. 1977. Assessing the clinical or applied importance of behavior change through social validation. *Behavior Modification* 1:427–452.

———. 1978. *History of behavior modification.* Baltimore: University Park Press.

———. 1982. *Single-case research designs: Methods for clinical and applied settings.* New York: Oxford University Press.

Kazdin, A. E., and Wilson, G. T. 1978. *Evaluation of behavior therapy.* Cambridge, MA: Ballinger.

Kendell, R. E. 1975. The concept of disease and its implications for psychiatry. *British Journal of Psychiatry* 127:305–315.

Kiev, A. 1972. *Transcultural psychiatry.* New York: Free Press.

Kleinman, A. 1977. Depression, somatization, and the "new-cross-cultural psychiatry." *Social Science and Medicine* 11:3–9.

———. 1980. *Patients and healers in the context of culture.* Berkeley: University of California Press.

Kleinman, A., and Good, B., eds. 1985. *Culture and depression: Studies in the anthropology and cross-cultural psychiatry of affect and disorder.* Berkeley: University of California Press.

Kleinman, A., and Kleinman, J. 1985. Somatization: The interconnections in Chinese society among culture, depressive experiences, and the meanings of pain. In A. Kleinman and B. Good (eds.), *Culture and depression: Studies in the anthropology and cross-cultural psychiatry of affect and disorder,* 429–490. Berkeley: University of California Press.

Korman, M. 1974. National conference on levels and patterns of professional training in psychology: Major themes. *American psychologist* 29:441–449.

Krasner, L. 1962. The therapist as a social reinforcement machine. In H. H. Strupp and L. Luborsky (eds.), *Research in psychotherapy,* Vol. 2. Washington, DC: American Psychological Association.

———. 1971. Behavior therapy. In P. H. Mussen and M. R. Rozenzweig (eds.), *Annual Review of Psychology.* Palo Alto, CA: Annual Reviews.

———. 1982. Behavior therapy: On roots, contexts, and growth. In G. T. Wilson and C. M. Franks (eds.), *Contemporary behavior therapy: Conceptual and empirical foundations,* 11–62. New York: Guilford Press.

———, ed. 1980. *Environmental design and human behavior: A psychology of the individual in society.* Elmsford, NY: Pergamon Press.

Krasner, L., and Ullmann, L. P. 1965. *Research in behavior modification: New developments and implications.* New York: Holt, Rinehart and Winston.

———. 1973. *Behavior influence and personality.* New York: Holt, Rinehart and Winston.

Landis, D., and Brislin, R., eds. 1983. *Handbook of intercultural training,* Vols. 1–3. Elmsford, NY: Pergamon Press.

Langer, E. J., and Abelson, R. P. 1974. A patient by any other name . . . !

Clinical group differences in labeling bias. *Journal of Consulting and Clinical Psychology* 42:4-9.

Leff, J. 1973. Culture and the differentiation of emotional states. *British Journal of Psychiatry* 123:299-306.

Leitenberg, H. 1976. *The handbook of behavior modification and behavior therapy.* Englewood Cliffs, NJ: Prentice-Hall.

Lewinsohn, P. M. 1974. A behavioral approach to depression. In R. J. Friedman and M. M. Katz (eds.), *The psychology of depression: Contemporary theory and research,* 157-178. Washington, DC: V. H. Winston.

Lick, J., and Bootzin, R. 1975. Expectancy factors in the treatment of fear: Methodological and theoretical issues. *Psychological Bulletin* 82:917-931.

Liem, N. D., and Kehmeier, D. F. 1980. The Vietnamese. In J. F. McDermott, W. S. Tseng, and T. W. Maretzki (eds.), *People and cultures in Hawaii.* 2d ed. Honolulu: University of Hawaii Press.

Liu, W. 1979. *Transition to nowhere.* Nashville: Charter House.

McFall, R. M. 1982. A review and reformulation of the concept of social skills. *Behavioral Assessment* 4:1-33.

MacPhillamy, D., and Lewinsohn, P. M. 1982. The Pleasant Events Schedule: Studies on reliability and validity and scale intercorrelations. *Journal of Consulting and Clinical Psychology* 50:363-380.

Mahoney, M. J., and Arnkoff, D. B. 1978. Cognitive and self-control therapies. In S. L. Garfield and A. E. Bergin (eds.), *Handbook of psychotherapy and behavior change: An empirical analysis.* New York: John Wiley and Sons.

Marsella, A. J. 1979. Cross-cultural studies of mental disorders. In A. J. Marsella, R. Tharp, and T. Ciborowski (eds.), *Perspectives on cross-cultural psychology.* New York: Academic Press.

Maultsby, M. C., Jr. 1982. A historical view of blacks' distrust of psychiatry. In S. M. Turner and R. T. Jones (eds.), *Behavior modification in black populations,* 39-56. New York: Plenum Press.

Meazzini, P., and Rovetto, F. 1983. Behavior therapy: The Italian way. *Journal of Behavior Therapy and Experimental Psychiatry* 14:5-9.

Meichenbaum, D. H. 1977. *Cognitive behavior modification: An integral approach.* New York: Plenum Press.

Mikulas, W. 1981. Buddhism and behavior modification. *Psychological Record* 31:331-342.

————. 1983. Thailand and behavior modification. *Journal of Behavior Therapy and Experimental Psychiatry* 14:93-97.

Mischel, W. 1973. Toward a cognitive social learning reconceptualization of personality. *Psychological Review* 80:252-283.

Morganstern, K. P., and Tevlin, H. E. 1981. Behavioral interviewing. In M. Hersen and A. S. Bellack (eds.), *Behavioral assessment,* 71-100. New York: Pergamon Press.

Nathan, P. E. 1987. DSM-III-R and the behavior therapist. *Behavior Therapist* 10:203-205.

Nicassio, P. M. 1985. The psychological adjustment of the Southeast Asian refugee: An overview of empirical findings and theoretical models. *Journal of Cross-Cultural Psychology* 16:153-173.

Nicassio, P. M., and Pate, J. K. 1984. An analysis of problems of resettlement of the Indochinese refugees in the United States. *Social Psychiatry* 19:135–141.

Nichter, M. 1981. Idioms of distress. *Culture, Medicine, and Psychiatry* 5:379–408.

Nguyen, S. D. 1982. Psychiatric and psychosomatic problems among the Southeast Asian refugees. *Psychiatric Journal of the University of Ottawa* 7:163–172.

Oberg, K. 1958. Culture shock and the problem of adjustment to new cultural environments. Washington, DC: U.S. Department of State, Foreign Service Institute.

Ogino, K., and Hoshino, A. 1983. *Culture shock to Nipponjin.* Tokyo: Yuhikaku.

Padilla, A. M., Ruiz, R. A., and Alvarez, R. 1975. Community mental health services for the Spanish-speaking surnamed population. *American Psychologist* 30:892–905.

Patel, C. H. 1975. Yoga and biofeedback in the management of "stress" in hypertensive patients. *Clinical Science and Molecular Medicine* 48:171–174.

Patterson, G. F. 1974. Interventions for boys with conduct problems: Multiple settings, treatments, and criteria. *Journal of Consulting and Clinical Psychology* 42:471–481.

Paul, G., and Lenz, J. 1977. *Psychosocial treatment of chronic mental patients.* Cambridge: Harvard University Press.

Phillips, L., and Draguns, J. G. 1971. Classification of the behavior disorders. *Annual Review of Psychology* 221:447–482.

Price, R. H., and Lynn, S. J. 1986. *Abnormal psychology.* 2d ed. Chicago: Dorsey Press.

Queroz, L. O. S., Guilhardi, H. J., and Martin, G. L. 1976. A university program in Brazil to develop psychologists with specialization in behavior modification. *Psychological Record* 26:181–188.

Rahe, R. H., Looney, J. G., Ward, H. W., Tung, T. M., and Liu, W. T. 1978. Psychiatric consultation in a Vietnamese refugee camp. *American Journal of Psychiatry* 135:185–190.

Rappaport, J. 1977. *Community psychology: Values, research, action.* New York: Holt, Rinehart and Winston.

Rogers-Warren, A., and Warren, S. F., eds. 1977. *Ecological perspectives in behavior analysis.* Baltimore: University Park Press.

Rosenhan, D. L. 1973. On being sane in insane places. *Science* 179:250–258.

Ruiz, R. A., and Casas, J. M. 1981. Culturally relevant behavioristic counseling for Chicano college students. In P. B. Pedersen, J. G. Draguns, W. J. Lonner, and J. E. Trimble (eds.), *Counseling across cultures,* 181–202. Honolulu: University of Hawaii Press.

Safilios-Rothschild, C. 1969. Psychotherapy and patient's characteristics: A cross-cultural examination. *International Journal of Social Psychiatry* 15:120–128.

Schacht, T., and Nathan, P. E. 1977. But is it good for the psychologists?: Appraisal and status of DSM-III. *American Psychologist* 32:1017–1025.

Scheff, T. J. 1966. *Being mentally ill.* Chicago: Aldine.

Schinke, S. P., Schilling, R. F., Palleja, J., and Zayas, L. H. 1987. Prevention research among ethnic-racial minority group adolescents. *Behavior Therapist* 7:151–155.

Schultz, C. B., and Sherman, R. H. 1976. Social class, development and differences in reinforcer effectiveness. *Review of Educational Research* 46:25–59.

Seligman, M. E. P. 1975. *Helplessness: On depression, development and death.* San Francisco: Freeman.

Shapiro, D. H., and Zifferblatt, S. M. 1976. Zen meditation and behavioral self-control: Similarities, differences and clinical applications. *American Psychologist* 31:519–523.

Sharma, S. 1973. A study to identify and analyze adjustment problems experienced by foreign non-European graduate students enrolled in selected universities in the state of North Carolina. *California Journal of Educational Research* 24:135–146.

Sheehan, P. W., and White, K. D., eds. 1976. *Behavior modification in Australia.* Parkville, Victoria: Australian Psychological Society.

Sidman, M. 1960. *Tactics of scientific research.* New York: Basic Books.

Skinner, B. F. 1948. *Walden two.* New York: Macmillan.

———. 1953. *Science and human behavior.* New York: Macmillan.

———. 1971. *Beyond freedom and dignity.* New York: Bantam-Vintage.

Sow, I. 1980. *Anthropological structures of madness in black Africa.* New York: International Universities Press.

Spitzer, R. L., Williams, J. B. W., and Skodol, A. E. 1980. DSM-III: The major achievements and an overview. *American Journal of Psychiatry* 137:151–164.

Staats, A. W. 1975. *Social behaviorism.* Homewood, IL: Dorsey Press.

———. 1980. "Behavioral interaction and interactional psychology." Theories of personality: Similarities, differences, and the need for unification. *British Journal of Psychology* 71:205–220.

Stokes, T. F., and Baer, D. 1977. An implicit technology of generalization. *Journal of Applied Behavior Analysis* 10:349–367.

Stolz, S. B. 1978. *Ethical issues in behavior modification.* San Francisco: Jossey-Bass.

———. 1986. A future role for behavior analysis: A view from afar. Presidential address, Division 25, the annual meeting of the American Psychological Association, Washington, DC.

Stumphauzer, J. S., and Davis, L. C. 1983. Training Mexican American mental health personnel in behavior therapy. *Journal of Behavior Therapy and Experimental Psychiatry* 14:215–217.

Sue, D. W. 1981. *Counseling the culturally different: Theory and practice.* New York: John Wiley and Sons.

Sue, S. 1977. Community mental health services to minority groups: Some optimism, some pessimism. *American Psychologist* 32:616–624.

Sue, S., and Morishima, J. K. 1982. *The mental health of Asian Americans.* San Francisco: Jossey-Bass.

Sue, S., and Zane, N. 1987. The role of culture and cultural techniques in psychotherapy: A critique and reformulation. *American Psychologist* 42:37–45.

Szasz, T. S. 1961. *The myth of mental illness: Foundations of a theory of personal conduct.* New York: Hoeber-Harper.

Taft, R. 1977. Coping with unfamiliar environments. In N. Warren (ed.), *Studies of cross-cultural psychology*. Vol. 1. London: Academic Press.

Tanaka-Matsumi, J. 1979a. Taijin Kyofusho: Diagnostic and cultural issues in Japanese psychiatry. *Culture, Medicine and Psychiatry* 3:231–245.

———. 1979b. Cultural factors and social influence techniques in Naikan therapy: A Japanese self-observation method. *Psychotherapy: Theory, Research and Practice* 16:385–390.

———. 1983. Using behavioral validation strategy in cross-cultural research. Paper presented at the annual meeting of the American Psychological Association, Anaheim, CA.

———. 1987. Values and theories in cross-cultural research: Is depression universal? Paper presented at the annual meeting of the American Psychological Association, New York.

———. In press. The cultural difference model and applied behavior analysis in the design of early childhood intervention. In L. L. Adler (ed.), *Cross-cultural research in human development: Focus on life span*. Westport, CT: Praeger-Greenwood Press.

Tanaka-Matsumi, J., and Marsella, A. J. 1976. Cross-cultural variations in the phenomenological experience of depression: Pt. 1, Word association studies. *Journal of Cross-Cultural Psychology* 7:379–396.

Tanaka-Matsumi, J., and Tharp, R. G. 1977. Teaching teachers of Hawaiian children: Consultation and research strategies. In R. W. Brislin and M. H. Pamnett (eds.), *Topics in culture learning* 5:92–106.

Temerlin, M. K. 1968. Suggestion effects in psychiatric diagnosis. *Journal of Nervous and Mental Disease* 147:349–359.

Tharp, R. G., and Wetzel, R. 1969. *Behavior modification in the natural environment*. New York: Academic Press.

Turner, S. M., and Jones, R. T., eds. 1982. *Behavior modification in black populations*. New York: Plenum Press.

Uchiyama, K. 1985. Bottlenecks in the development of behavior therapy in Japan. *Seishin Ryoho* 11:17–23.

Ullmann, L. P. 1969. Behavior therapy as a social movement. In C. M. Franks (ed.), *Behavior therapy: Appraisal and status*. New York: McGraw-Hill.

Ullmann, L. P., and Krasner, L. 1965. *Case studies in behavior modification*. New York: Holt, Rinehart and Winston.

———. 1969. *A psychological approach to abnormal behavior*. 1st ed. Englewood Cliffs, NJ: Prentice-Hall.

———. 1975. *A psychological approach to abnormal behavior*. 2d ed. Englewood Cliffs, NJ: Prentice-Hall.

Vontress, C. E. 1981. Racial and ethnic barriers in counseling. In P. B. Pedersen, J. G. Draguns, W. L. Lonner, and J. E. Trimble (eds.), *Counseling across cultures*, 87–107. Honolulu: University of Hawaii Press.

Walz, G. R., and Benjamin, L. 1978. *Transcultural counseling*. New York: Human Sciences Press.

Westermeyer, J., and Wintrob, R. 1979. "Folk" criteria for the diagnosis of mental illness in rural Laos: On being insane in sane places. *American Journal of Psychiatry* 136:755–761.

White, G. M. 1982. The role of cultural explanation in "somatization" and "psychologization." *Social Science and Medicine* 5:1519–1530.

Williams, C. L., and Westermeyer, J. 1983. Psychiatric problems among adolescent Southeast Asian refugees. *Journal of Nervous and Mental Disease* 171:79–84.

Wilson, G. T., and Evans, I. M. 1976. Adult behavior therapy and the therapist-client relationship. In C. M. Franks and G. T. Wilson (eds.), *Annual review of behavior therapy.* New York: Brunner/Mazel Publishers.

Winner, M. 1977. *Autonomous technology: Technics-out-of-control as a theme in political thought.* Cambridge: MIT Press.

Wohl, J. 1981. Intercultural psychotherapy: Issues, questions, and reflections. In P. B. Pedersen, J. G. Draguns, W. J. Lonner, and J. E. Trimble (eds.), *Counseling across cultures,* 133–159. Honolulu: University of Hawaii Press.

Wolf, M. M. 1978. Social validity: The case for subjective measurement, or how applied behavior analysis is finding its heart. *Journal of Applied Behavior Analysis* 11:203–214.

Wolpe, J. 1958. *Psychotherapy by reciprocal inhibition.* Palo Alto, CA: Stanford University Press.

———. 1982. *The practice of behavior therapy.* 3d ed. New York: Pergamon Press.

Woolfolk, R., and Richardson, F. C. 1984. Behavior therapy and the ideology of modernity. *American Psychologist* 39:777–786.

World Health Organization (WHO). 1978. *Mental disorders: Glossary and guide to their classification in accordance with the ninth revision of the International Classification of Diseases.* Geneva: World Health Organization.

Yamagami, T., Okuma, H., Morinaga, Y., and Nakao, H. 1982. Practice of behavior therapy in Japan. *Journal of Behavior Therapy and Experimental Psychiatry* 13:21–26.

Yap, P. M. 1974. *Comparative psychiatry: A theoretical framework.* Toronto: University of Toronto Press.

Zigler, E., and Phillips, L. 1961. Psychiatric diagnosis and symptomatology. *Journal of Abnormal and Social Psychology* 63:69–75

12

Assessment in
Cross-Cultural Counseling

WALTER J. LONNER
FARAH A. IBRAHIM

This chapter covers assessment in cross-cultural counseling, including clinical judgments, as well as standardized and nonstandardized assessment to arrive at a diagnosis of client status, progress, change, and growth. A review of the literature reveals that assessment in the domain of cross-cultural counseling is still fairly uncharted territory. There are several reasons for this lag in the field, the most significant being the multiplicity of variables that merit investigation before a conclusive statement can be made about any aspect of cross-cultural counseling and psychotherapy (Lorian 1978; Sundberg 1981). Without appropriate assessment strategies, professionals are unable to diagnose, or name, the problem, which leads to difficulties in the development of appropriate goals or process and ultimately in assessing outcome of the intervention.

Lorian (1978) recommends that the multivariate nature of socioeconomic, racial, and ethnic differences demands that they be studied simultaneously. Further, he recommends that to understand the lifestyles of disadvantaged (or culturally different) clients, it is critical that mental health professionals enter into collaborative research efforts with other social scientists. As is true in "mainstream" counseling and psychotherapy, the critical issues in cross-cultural assessment (as in counseling and psychotherapy) are still the ones incorporated in Paul's (1967, 111) comment: "*What* treatment, by *whom,* is most effective for *this* individual with *that* specific problem, and under *which* set of circumstances?" We may rephrase this statement into "*what* assessment, by *whom,* is most effective for *this* individual with *that* specific problem, under *which* set of circumstances, in *which* specific cultural environment?"

Delivery of effective mental health services to cross-cultural clients has been an area of concern for practitioners, researchers, and educators (Bales 1985; Bernal and Padilla 1982; Ibrahim and Arredondo 1986; Pedersen 1986; Marsella and Pedersen 1981; Sue 1983). Current research indicates that educational programs designed to prepare counseling, school, and clinical psychologists generally overlook providing information to students that would make them culturally effective (Bernal and Padilla 1982; Ibrahim et al. 1986). Programs fail to emphasize knowledge of different cultures and groups, their philosophical and psychological assumptions, beliefs, and values, and an understanding of individual variation within groups. This evidences a lack of desire or initiative to incorporate these concerns in mental health professional preparation programs. As noted in the current literature, this leads to numerous problems in the delivery of adequate and appropriate mental health services (Bales 1985; Sue 1981; Sue 1983).

It is our contention that to provide ethical and appropriate counseling and psychotherapy to clients from different sociocultural backgrounds, the helping professional needs to understand the client's worldview and philosophical and psychological assumptions and as well have adequate knowledge of both the primary and secondary cultural environments (Ibrahim 1984a, 1985; Ibrahim and Arredondo 1986). This implies that each individual client be viewed as a unique "cultural reality" (Ibrahim 1984a), with an emphasis on the individual's "subjective culture" (Triandis et al. 1972) or worldview (Ibrahim 1984b; Sue 1978).

The individual's worldview and behaviors need to be appraised from Lewin's (1935) perspective of behavior as a function of the person in the environment. This orientation suggests that both the individual and the environment need to be evaluated. Generally, the environment is conceptualized as unidimensional. In reality, the client's environment is often multidimensional and multicultural (depending on the nature of the society under consideration). Ibrahim (1985) has proposed a tridimensional model of the environment and its influences on the client. The model proposes three dimensions: Dimension 1 is the client's worldview or personal cultural reality; Dimension 2 is the client's primary group and its cultural influence (including the family); and Dimension 3 reflects the larger environment, which in the case of the United States is the majority group and other cultural groups and their influences on the client. Additionally, the sociopolitical history of the client's cultural group (Sue 1981) needs to be considered to understand his or her beliefs, biases, and perspectives. This requires that the counselor engage in some form of initial client assessment that addresses these different facets of the client.

Initial Client Assessment

The first step in any counseling and psychotherapy encounter is to understand the client and the issues, problems, symptoms, and pain that led the client to seek help and relief. Culturally appropriate initial client assessment should lead to meaningful goals (for the client) and a useful therapeutic intervention. In cross-cultural counseling, because of the paucity of research and assessment methodologies, it is necessary to assess the client as a cultural entity before any intervention can be implemented (Ibrahim 1984a; Ibrahim and Arredondo 1986).

There are two specific approaches to the assessment of client world-views, beliefs, values, and perspectives. These include Sue's (1978) internal/external locus of responsibility and control model (see later in a section on locus of control) and Ibrahim and Kahn's (1984) scale to assess worldviews. Other approaches that facilitate initial client assessment in cross-cultural encounters include Atkinson, Morten, and Sue's (1983) Identity Development model, and Szapocznik et al.'s (1983) Bicultural Effectiveness Training model.

Ibrahim and Kahn (1984, 1987) developed the Scale to Assess World Views (SAWV) based on Ibrahim's (1984a, 1984b, 1985) theoretical approach to cross-cultural counseling and psychotherapy. The scale can be used to assess individual and group worldviews on Kluckhohn's (1951, 1956) five existential categories as outlined in table 1. Kluckhohn believed that these existential categories were universal because every culture has to find a solution to these problems of existence at some time or another (Zavalloni 1980).

The use of the scale assists the counselor in three ways. First, it makes the client's values and assumptions explicit. These values and assumptions have a direct relationship to the client's cognitive, emotional, and social perceptions and interactions with the world. Second, it provides an understanding of the expression and experiences of the issues and problems that the client brings to counseling. Third, when the counselor is knowledgeable about different cultural groups, use of the SAWV provides insight into the client's specific worldview (Ibrahim 1984b, 1985). Based on knowledge of the client's worldview, the client's cultural group and its assumptions, and the client's sociopolitical history, the counselor will be better able to formulate the nature of the therapeutic relationship to be pursued, approaches and techniques to be used in assessment and counseling, and identification of goals and process that would be meaningful and appropriate for the specific client (Ibrahim 1985). One study that used the SAWV to train counselors to assess and access client worldviews confirmed that clients perceived these counselors as more effective and sensitive (Sadlak and Ibrahim 1986).

Clinicians have recommended that in general it is useful to use value instruments to assess client values, beliefs, and dispositions. Kavanaugh (1980) reviewed various values scales that may be useful for the counselor. Although the paper-and-pencil measures mentioned by Kavanaugh were not designed explicitly for cross-cultural assessment, we would underscore his recommendation regarding their use as

Table 1. Five Existential Categories and Range of Variations

1. *Human Nature   What is the character of human nature?*
   Bad: human nature is evil.
   Good and Bad: human nature is a combination of good and evil.
   Good: human nature is good.

2. *Relationships   What is the modality of people's relationships?*
   Lineal-hierarchical: ordered positional succession within the group, continuity through time and primacy of group goals.
   Collateral-Mutual: primacy given to goals and welfare of lateral extended groups.
   Individualistic: primacy given to individual goals.

3. *Nature   What is the relationship of people to nature?*
   Harmony: people and nature coexist in harmony.
   Subjugation and control: people can subjugate and control nature.
   Power of Nature: nature is powerful and controls people.

4. *Time Orientation   What is the temporal focus of human life?*
   Past: a focus on the past.
   Present: a focus on the present.
   Future: a focus on the future.

5. *Activity Orientation   What is the modality of human activity (i.e., self-expression)?*
   Being: preference for activities that provide spontaneous expression of the self.
   Being-in-becoming: emphasis on activity that has as its goal development of all aspects of the self as an integrated being.
   Doing: preference for activities that result in measurable accomplishments by external standards.

Note: Adapted from Kluckhohn and Strodtbeck (1961) and Green and Haymes (1973).

springboards for discussion for a better understanding of client values and assumptions and by inference their modes of problem solving and decision making.

In this chapter, within the context of diagnosis as well as evaluation of outcome, three specific areas will be discussed. These include (1) clinical judgments, (2) standardized assessment, including problems in using measures of intellectual or personality in cross-cultural settings, and (3) nonstandardized assessment.

Problems of Diagnosis and Evaluating Outcome in Counseling and Psychotherapy

In traditional counseling and psychotherapy research and practice, the major issues have been diagnosis, what specific techniques or process to use with which diagnostic category, and evaluating outcome in psychotherapy (Strupp 1978). The most critical issue appears to be diagnosis, or formulation of the therapeutic problem. In this context clinical judgments and both standardized and nonstandardized tests have been used. Torrey (1986) contends that once the problem has been "named" in counseling and psychotherapy, the development of goals and the process of helping become relatively straightforward. The identification of the problem that has brought the client to counseling is difficult in within-group counseling situations and gets understandably more complex in cross-cultural situations. Marsella (1982), in a review of the literature on culture and mental health, presents compelling data to support the hypothesis that culture plays a major role in the etiology, expression, course, and outcome of mental disorders. Further, he stresses that all aspects of mental disorders are inextricably linked to the sociocultural milieu in which they are generated.

Clinical Judgments

Clinical judgments have included "armchair" diagnosis grounded in a theory of personality or psychotherapy and diagnosis based on classification systems such as the American Psychiatric Association's Diagnostic and Statistical Manual and the International Classification of Diseases Number Nine. These approaches have received mixed evaluations by practitioners and theorists alike. Specifically, cross-cultural research has raised a number of questions about the ethnocentricity of these methods (Marsella 1982). It becomes increasingly complex in cross-cultural counseling encounters to determine if the set of symptoms presented really add up to the helper's notion of a specific diagnosis. For instance, Marsella, Kinzie, and Gordon (1973) note that the expression of mental disorders in different cultures varies according to the concept of the self in each individual culture. Additionally, Katz, Gudeman, and Sanborn (1969, 1978) have shown that cultural variations exist in both normal and abnormal group profiles of various ethnic groups.

Studies of interaction of culture and psychosis indicate that ethnic groups differ markedly in the behavioral and effective expression of what appears to be the same underlying psychopathology (Enright and Jaeckle 1963). Draguns (1980) concluded from a review of the literature on psychological disorders of clinical severity that although the extent of shaping by culture is unclear, culture does have an influence on psychopathological expression. Complicating the issue further, clinical judgments are also subject to individual bias (Abramowitz and Dokecki 1977). Torrey (1986) points out that since helpers are immersed in their own cultural contexts, they are unable to see or comprehend the bias and stereotypes they impose upon the client. It is apparent from a review of the current literature and research that an understanding of the specific culture in which the mental or psychological disorder manifests itself is critical in arriving at a meaningful diagnosis. Additionally, it would be a worthwhile strategy to involve clients in the process of arriving at a clinical judgment by having them discuss the meaning of their symptoms and behavior in their own cultural contexts. Higginbotham (1979) presented a four-point culture-specific assessment program, which proposed (a) analysis of the problem from a cultural perspective, specifically the local rules for assigning deviant labels and causation; (b) finding the cultural norms for personal adjustment to assist in the establishment of therapy goals; (c) studying the means of social influence in healing and resocialization; and (d) analyzing the relationship of the community with the agency providing the service, including preferred personnel, location, access, and costs. Use of such a comprehensive culture-specific assessment program would greatly enhance the validity and reliability of clinical judgments.

Standardized Assessment

One of our central concerns in this chapter is to examine the extent to which tests developed in one culture (usually in the United States or some other Western country) can effectively step across cultural boundaries to be useful adjuncts in counseling across cultures.

Cultural bias is inherent in the cross-cultural use of all tests (Frijda and Jahoda 1966). One of the major reasons for this bias is that all tests are isomorphic with the culture or society in which they originated; as such, they are not easily transported to other cultures without at least some modification. Nevertheless, many tests can be properly used across cultures if certain issues are taken into account.

On the following pages are several topics that are important when considering the use of psychological tests among ethnically diverse clients or when looking at test results from such clients.

The distinction between constructs and criteria. Psychological tests have often been described as being either construct related (i.e., they relate to some psychological theory concerning, for example, anxiety or dependency, and are therefore called theoretical) or criterion referenced (that is, they depend upon empirically established relationships and are not necessarily associated with any particular psychological theory). This distinction has been used by Anastasi (1988) and to some extent by Cronbach (1984), the two most widely used textbooks on psychological testing in the United States. Since it may be invalid to assume that psychological constructs constitute a universal template (owing to indigenous thought or value systems, for example, or because most constructs have been developed and inferred by Western scientists), the use of construct-related tests could result in an inappropriate attribution of a construct to a person whose culture of origin may not foster the development of or value the Western-based construct. In the jargon of cross-cultural methodologists this is "imposing an etic"—assuming a construct to be valid everywhere, or at least in the new cultural setting. The counterpart of "etic" is "emic," a term used to describe the nature of the construct from *within* that culture only (for a discussion of the emic-etic distinction, see Berry 1969 and Lonner 1979). Using a similar rationale, the same researchers may maintain that criteria are not transferable from one culture to another.

Consider an example using the popular construct of intelligence, which is undoubtedly a human universal. Probably all cultures have a word for it, and even the most radical cultural relativist could not deny its veridicality as a powerful source of human variation, both within and across cultures or ethnic groups. However, the actual behavioral connotations or ramifications of "intelligence" vary significantly across cultures. In the West, for example, intelligence is usually associated with being smart (knowledge of many things) and fast (ability to relate these known things rapidly to others). Among the Baganda people of Uganda, however, the concept of intelligence, *obugezi,* is associated with wisdom, slow thoughtfulness, and social propriety; it is not important to be fast, but it is important to be right (Wober 1974).

Thus, the conservative solution would be to develop tests based on locally conceived (within-culture) constructs, with locally valid criteria to "prove" the existence of the construct. Berry (1972) has called this approach "radical cultural relativism," as opposed to a position that may presume the universality of the construct. Obviously, the radical extreme would lead to the dilemma of rendering comparisons across cultures impossible; every group of people would have its own noninterchangeable set of constructs and attendant criteria. Carried to an existential extreme, this line of thought would mean that every person would have his or her own set of constructs and criteria.

One way to view the problem would be to assume a high extensional agreement among behavioral scientists (as well as in a client-counselor dyad) as to what a construct is; how criteria document the construct's *particular* cultural manifestation may vary. For example, a counselor and his or her client may agree that "shyness" (extensionally validated by both as at least a personality adjective) is one of the client's characteristics. The counselor, knowing the overt manifestations and social or personal ramifications of shyness in his or her own culture, may falsely attribute these characteristics to his or her client. For the client (and unknown to or overlooked by the counselor), however, shyness may be based on criteria that are more appropriate in an Alpine valley or a Navajo village. The word shyness would be agreed upon, but its culturally determined referents would not (see Zimbardo 1977 concerning cultural variations of shyness). Such differentials are probably used extensively in many intercultural counseling encounters as a ploy, or as an "ice breaker," leading to more effective learning of feeling or affect on the part of both the client and the counselor. Discussing the nature of shyness and its behavioral characteristics in both the client's and the counselor's cultural experiences may lead to better understanding of the cultural parameters of this particular emotion.

Because of such problems associated wtih criteria and their cultural variations, it can be argued that criterion-based tests (such as the Minnesota Multiphasic Personality Inventory [MMPI]) are inappropriate for intercultural use. On the other hand, tests developed on the basis of some culturally invariant construct or construct system are more defensible for use, since they would bridge the gap that exists between the culture of the client and the culture of the counselor. Later in this chapter this problem will arise again in a discussion of the MMPI and several other personality assessment techniques.

The establishment of equivalence. If equivalence of tests is established across cultures, then these stable bases would permit substantial confidence in making intercultural comparisons. However, tests seldom completely satisfy certain standards for equivalence that have been adopted by cross-cultural methodologists (Malpass and Poortinga 1986).

Four types of equivalence are frequently mentioned. The first of these is *functional equivalence.* Cultural artifacts, institutions, rituals, roles, and so forth are variable throughout the world. However, since every society or cultural group must exercise basic functions in order to survive (Aberle et al. 1950), comparativists are obliged to find the common ground among these cultural prerequisites before using tests to measure the presence of traits in one culture as opposed to others. One cultural group's sign of status, for example, may be a small herd of cattle; another group's functional counterpart may be a pickup truck and a chain saw; a third group's equivalent may be a vacation to the Virgin Islands. Or, as Przeworski and Teune (1970, 92) have so colorfully put it: "For specific observation a belch is a belch and nepotism is nepotism. But within an inferential framework a belch is an 'insult' or a 'compliment' and nepotism is 'corruption' or 'responsibility.' " Researchers need to clarify that tests used across cultures are tapping into the same functional characteristics. If they are not, then conclusions drawn from making comparisons of test scores could be flawed.

Conceptual equivalence operates at the individual level, and functional equivalence operates at the level of the group. Conceptual equivalence is concerned with the *meaning* that persons attach to specific stimuli such as test items. This form of equivalence is at the root of the common opinion that it is impossible to develop a truly culture-fair test. Such a test would have to contain items that are either equally familiar or equally unfamiliar to everyone. In the first situation the stimulus object, word, or sentence would have to be so ubiquitous that virtual uniformity of exposure would be guaranteed (the concept of mother comes close to the ideal). In the second situation a visit to another planet would be necessary to find test material that would be totally unfamiliar to all. Without test items that are conceptually equivalent and, at the same time, have relevance to functionally equivalent cultural indicators, accurate interpretations of responses may be impossible.

A variant of conceptual equivalence is linguistic, or translation, equivalence. As implied, this form of equivalence must ensure that words and sentences on tests, questionnaires, interviews, and so forth convey the same *meaning* (Brislin 1986). Back-translation is a term used for a method with which the serious user of tests across cultures should have some familiarity. In back-translation one takes a sentence in the first (or originating) language, translates it into the "target" language, and then has a native speaker of the target language return the translation through a bilingual interpreter. For example, if the phrase "A stitch in time saves nine" were translated, back-translated, and further refined so as to come back unscathed in meaning (i.e., a little preventive maintenance now will save considerable work in the future), then a successful back-translation would have been accomplished.

The fourth type of equivalence has been called *metric* or *scalar equivalence* (see Poortinga 1975a, 1975b, for details). The points to be emphasized here are that tests and scales should be functionally equivalent; that is, they should measure the same behavioral property in different groups of people. Sets of data from different cultures should show the same coherence of structure if they are to be compared legitimately. A test should be measuring the same things, and at the same levels, when employed in other cultural contexts.

Finally, Sechrest, Fay, and Zaidi (1972) discussed the issues of equivalence in terms of the idiomatic, grammatical-syntactical, experiential, and conceptual. They also refer to what they call the paradox of equivalence. The paradox, as Sharma (1977) correctly points out, is as follows: If a test is to yield comparable results across cultures to demonstrate equivalence, then as it becomes *more* equivalent the *less* likely will cultural differences be found. If, in contrast, one looks primarily for cultural differences and ignores the problem of equivalence, then the greater the likelihood of finding cultural differences. In the latter case, however, the differences that are found may reflect inadequacies in the establishment of equivalence rather than real cultural differences. The problem can be stated another way, compatible with a classical anthropological problem associated with making comparisons across cultures: As a test item or stimulus diffuses into (is carried to) another culture, its form, function, and meaning may vary in unknown and perhaps unpredictable ways.

The nature of test content: Verbal versus nonverbal. For many years it was assumed that tests employing nonverbal stimuli were "fairer" than tests relying primarily on verbal material; hence, they were more appropriate for intercultural use. Many tests, for example, used figural analogies, mazes, and other formats that assume that abilities, intelligence, and even personality can be assessed more fairly across cultural groups if only the widely variable linguistic dimension is nullified or transcended.

Research on cultural and ecological influences on perceptual and cognitive style has shown that these factors can influence the way in which simple stimuli such as visual illusions are interpreted (see Deregowski 1980). More relevant for cross-cultural counseling is an earlier study by Bagby (1957). Bagby was concerned with the extent to which the cultural characteristics of conflicting visual presentations are perceived differently by members of different societies. He presented 10 pairs of slides to samples of American and Mexican adults. In each pair one photograph was of a typical Mexican scene and the other was a photograph of a typical American scene. Under these conditions of experimentally induced binocular rivalry, Bagby found that the scenes from the subjects' own culture tended to be perceptually dominant, thus supporting transactional perceptual theory, which holds that perception is fundamentally determined by previous experience.

As mentioned earlier under the establishment of equivalence, it should not be assumed that verbal material—words, phrases, and sentences found in personality and intelligence tests—have the same meanings to all persons everywhere, even if they can read English well. Western-based tests and inventories, particularly those developed in the United States, are liberally endowed with subtle idioms. Before technical advances in translation procedures became available (Brislin 1986), many tests were sometimes translated literally, word for word, without paying much attention to how they were understood in the target culture.

Response sets. In the psychological testing literature there are many response sets (sometimes referred to as response styles) that could affect test scores. The response set of *acquiescence,* for instance, generally refers to the tendency of a subject to agree (or its reverse, to disagree) with extremes, usually on attitude statements. Some clients, the stereotypic Asian for example, may tend to say yes out of politeness, reflecting the norms of his or her culture. The response set of *social desirability* refers to the tendency of subjects to answer in the direction they consider to be the more socially favorable alternative. Other response sets include *evasiveness* (unwillingness to commit oneself) and *carelessness* (the making of inconsistent judgments). Another problem, called *extreme response style,* was the focus of a cross-cultural study by Chun, Campbell, and Yoo (1974). See Fiske (1970) for a summary of various response sets and the types of instruments in which each will most likely be found.

Unless a psychological test or other data-gathering device has a built-in sensor to detect the presence of response sets, any one of these response sets may affect the final score. Any client from another culture will likely possess an assortment of cultural values and general culture-originating personality factors that predispose him or her to respond in ways that appear unique to a United States psychologist or counselor. For example, people who have been conditioned not to take a middle-of-the-road position will likely respond infrequently to the "?" in the "Yes-?-No" response format frequently found in personality tests. Such dispositions could lead to distorted or inflated responses, especially if the test has not been normed on the culture of which the student is a member. Thus, a critical step to be taken before unusual or bizarre profiles or scores are interpreted would be to ascertain how response sets may have influenced the results. If they are even slightly suspect, the safest alternative would be to ignore altogether the results rather than to try to bend interpretations around them.

Response sets tend to invalidate test scores in terms of unicultural norms. There may be times, however, when the response sets themselves could be helpful in assessing particular aspects of a client's personality or attitudinal dispositions. For example, it may be of significant interest to discuss with the client his or her reasons for responding in unexpected ways, and these stated reasons may give clues to ways in which the client approaches life situations.

The above possibilities necessitate a brief summary of a methodological controversy that for many years has surrounded response sets and response styles. As Anastasi (1988) has pointed out, research on these response tendencies has gone through two principal stages. They were first considered irrelevant, a merely unwanted source of error variance. Attempts were therefore made to adjust test formats or scoring procedures to minimize these effects. Later they were regarded as indicators of personality dispositions, worthy of study in their own right. For instance, Crowne and Marlowe (1964) developed an argument that the response set of *social desirability* (or responding to inventories and tests in a manner so as to put up a good front) is related to a person's need for social approval and avoidance of criticism.

The tendency to infer deficits from test score differences. Counselors should be wary of the tendency to overinterpret test score differences, a situation in which the test interpreter is generally motivated to account for lower scores (which may, for example, suggest pathology, lowered intelligence, or some other "deficiency"). Typically, personality tests are constructed to scale both the highs and lows of personality functioning (see below). Hence, any tendency to overinterpret these tests may be to make high scores higher than they really are; similar tendencies may exist for lower scores. Overinterpretation by clinicians is difficult to avoid, for they naturally want to construct a coherent and complete picture of a client's personality. Nature abhors a vacuum; counselors abhor incomplete information about their clients.

When a member of a culture different from one's own does not do well on standardized tests developed by psychologists, then reasons for the differences advanced by test interpreters may fall into an artificially imposed deficit column. Cole and Bruner (1971), for instance, noted that standard intelligence tests tell us what people *cannot* do but fall short in telling us what they *can* do.

A general rule in assessing intelligence across cultures is that unless compelling corroborative evidence from varied external sources suggests that test scores are valid, no inferences suggestive of deficits in ability or in personality should be drawn. Scores on psychological tests are, of course, incomplete representations of a person. But test scores are certainly better than nothing at all. One may argue that reasonably good tests given under optimal conditions to people from different cultural backgrounds are in fact more reliable initial representations of behavioral predispositions than is an initial interview or other information of a highly subjective nature.

Attempts to resolve one or more of the issues. There have been numerous attempts to minimize the Euroamerican bias in many psychological assessment instruments. By devising tests that contain stimuli that cut across cultural lines or by adequately norming existing tests on subjects from many cultures, testers may be able to make tests more useful in counseling and research. But realistically, the problems may never be fully resolved.

To provide culturally appropriate and differentiated interpretation for a culture-bound or -biased test, we thought we would share the following. Recently, one of us (Ibrahim) was called upon by an elementary school to conduct an intellectual assessment of an immigrant child from Pakistan. The school needed to determine if the child was hampered by a language barrier, or perhaps a learning disability, as opposed to the possibility of his not being challenged intellectually. Since none of the available intellectual assessment devices that were available in the school had been developed or normed in Pakistan, any assessment strategy would be biased and inappropriate. Recognizing this fact, the decision was made to select an instrument that would determine if the child's cognitive development was age-appropriate. The purpose of the assessment was made clear to the school: we would not be able to arrive at a clear-cut answer regarding his intellectual development (because a number of the test items were culture-bound and inappropriate for the child), but we would try to assess his cognitive development and provide information on how he compared to his peers in the United States. To achieve these ends, the K-ABC (Kaufman and Kaufman 1983) was selected, a test that is based on Piaget's theory of cognitive development. Although it is a culture-bound test, its use in this context was appropriate, and the interpretation was differentiated to meet the needs of the child and the school. The results were presented to facilitate the teachers' task in teaching the boy from his cognitive-processing perspective and to identify areas that needed work (e.g., he used a simultaneous-processing strategy exclusively and had difficulty in all tasks that demanded a sequential-processing strategy). There was also definitely a language barrier.

The above example underscores two important points we would like to emphasize. First, a test or scale should never be used to limit the client's potential but only to identify potential for growth. Second, if at all possible it would be best to use a test that is somehow linked to a theoretical framework that has been used with some success in cross-cultural research.

We now consider some examples of tests that have enjoyed at least moderate success among persons from various cultural backgrounds. A brief review of some tests that have been designed to measure intelligence or specialized abilities will be followed by an overview of a handful of personality-type tests.

Intellectual assessment. The Cattell Culture-Fair Intelligence Test is one of several attempts to develop a measure of general intelligence through the use of nonverbal material. It consists of various forms, but the format is consistent: items require the subject to complete a series, to classify objects that belong together, and to complete patterns that amount to figural analogies. The Cattell Culture-Fair may exceed some tests in its alleged comprehensiveness in tapping various intellectual dimensions, but it certainly does not exceed the Kohs Blocks or the Raven Matrices for sheer usage. Both of these popular tests capitalize on spatial-perceptual relations; both are assumed to be good measures of the so-called general ("g") factor in intelligence.

The Kohs Blocks, Raven Matrices, Porteus Mazes, and other spatial-perceptual tests and tasks have been used extensively across cultures in attempts to measure and understand cultural and ethnic variations in cognitive style, a useful construct in cross-cultural counseling. Certain cultural and ecological factors foster the development of a field-independent cognitve style (in which characteristics of autonomy, a sense of separate identity, and nonconformity are more apt to be found). Some cultures, however, foster the development of relatively undifferentiated individuals, who are termed field dependent. The cognitive style of field dependence characteristically is associated with such traits or tendencies as group orientation, conformity, and a relatively low sense of separate identity. People who score high on tests measuring spatial skills are usually more field independent. This cognitive style dimension, which cuts across intellectual, social, and personality domains, has received a great deal of cross-cultural attention. It is a useful way to think about skills, abilities, and competencies without reference to standard and generally culturally insensitive intelligence tests. This popular construct and its concomitant cultural and subcultural variations are explained in some detail elsewhere (see Berry 1976; Witkin and Berry 1975; Witkin and Goodenough 1981).

Standard intelligence tests like the Wechsler Adult Intelligence Scale and the Stanford Binet have been used extensively across cultures and ethnic groups, with varying degrees of success. Largely as a reaction against the alleged and implicit cultural unfairness of the Wechsler and similar tests, several years ago there were a number of attempts to develop intelligence tests that are as fair to specific minority groups in the United States as the Wechsler is "fair" to the affluent white. Such tests had the same rationale: by tapping into the ethos of any cultural group, items can be developed that measure "intelligence" in a particular cultural milieu. These "tests" made their point: because every ethnic group has its own slang, idioms, heroes, and cultural legacies, members of the "in-group" will always do better on them than will members of the "out-group." This point can be proven ad infinitum but would hardly be useful for comparative purposes, if comparisons of cognitive variables across ethnic or cultural groups is one's goal.

An interesting alternative to standard intelligence testing is Mercer's (1979) System of Multicultural Pluralistic Assessment, or SOMPA. SOMPA is an assessment program used with young children. It includes the Wechsler scales designed for children but also employs other scales specifically designed to give data about the child's physical condition and social competence within his or her own cultural milieu. The entire SOMPA battery yields an Estimated Learning Potential (ELP). Expressed as a standard score, ELP takes into consideration standardized test results and many other nontest factors that may have a bearing on the child's performance in school.

The assessment of personality and pathology. Assessing personality and pathology across cultures presents even more difficulties than ability testing. A brief look at a few measures of personality and pathology, including their extensions into various cultural and ethnic groups, should alert the reader to some major difficulties associated with the cross-cultural assessment of variables that are often used in clinical assessment. The measures to be considered are the Minnesota Multiphasic Personality Inventory, the California Psychological Inventory, the Locus of Control Scale, the State-Trait Anxiety Inventory, and a few measures of depression.

A vast literature and colorful history surrounds the Minnesota Multiphasic Personality Inventory (MMPI), which is the most widely used paper and pencil personality test ever devised. Paralleling the medical model of disease etiology, its original intent was to measure the extent to which an individual's responses to the 566 items (e.g., "I love to go to dances" or "I have had some very unusual religious experiences") were like the responses of individuals who fell into discrete psychiatric groupings such as schizophrenia and paranoia. Nowadays the names of the scales are not nearly so important as the configuration of responses to the items when the profile is interpreted, often by very sophisticated computer programs. However, the logic now used is similar to the logic of the medical model: people who show similar patterns in personality dysfunction or in poor adjustment to crises tend to respond in highly similar ways to the items. Butcher (1984), Butcher and Keller (1984), Duckworth (1979), and Graham (1977) give excellent overviews of recent developments in the MMPI and how it is typically used in counseling.

As is true of *any* psychological test, in some ways the MMPI is not entirely appropriate for use across different cultures or ethnic groups. It started with a Western system of psychiatric classification; its original normative groups came primarily from small, mostly rural, groups of University of Minnesota hospital patients (and, for contrast, visitors to the hospital); and it is essentially atheoretical or criterion oriented. In other ways, however, there are several reasons why the MMPI can be considered an excellent cross-cultural assessment device, at least on a continuing exploratory basis. First, there is universality in at least some types of mental disorder, especially schizophrenia and depression (Draguns 1980). Second, the voluminous MMPI literature gives clinicians and researchers one of the richest storehouses of psychometric data ever amassed (about 125 translations of the MMPI are reportedly in use). Third, as patterns of complaints and disorders as well as systems of diagnosis diffuse across and within cultures, there may be an increasing tendency to view both symptom and diagnosis in universalistic dimensions (Draguns 1980).

Contemporary cross-cultural and cross-ethnic use of the MMPI generally follows two paths. One path concerns its international use (Butcher and Pancheri 1976; Butcher 1984). The other path monitors its use among ethnic groups in the United States. The best, yet somewhat technical, source of information about this latter strain of MMPI research and applications is Dahlstrom, Lachar, and Dahlstrom (1986). They focus extensively on black-white differences on the MMPI but not to the complete exclusion of other U.S. ethnic groups. For instance, in the 1970s Gynther (1972, 1979) concluded that small but consistent differences in black versus white responses to various items reflect differences between blacks and whites in values, social expectations and perceptions, and roles rather than absolute differences in adjustment. Gynther's reviews suggest that a principal value held by many blacks is "distrust of society and social cynicism." For instance, more whites than blacks endorse the statement, "the police are usually honest," an endorsement that may say something more about "class" differences than "race" differences. Dahlstrom, Lachar, and Dahlstrom maintain that there is no "serious bias or distortion in the use of the MMPI in mental health settings for the assessment of the emotional status of black clients" (1986, 205), but at the same time they lament the rather low level of accuracy for both blacks and whites.

Finally, the MMPI is currently experiencing a major restandardization (Butcher and Keller 1984), an overview of which can be found in the September 1986 issue of *Science* magazine.

The California Psychological Inventory (CPI) is a 480-item self-report measure of 18 personality dimensions (such as dominance, sociability, responsibility, self-control, and femininity). While many of its items come directly from the MMPI, Harrison Gough, the developer of the CPI, claims that the items tap important dimensions of social interaction that occur every day. These "folk concepts," as Gough calls them, are to be found in all cultures and societies. Thus, unlike the development of the MMPI and many other personality inventories, one factor considered during the development of the CPI was its potential usefulness in a variety of cultural settings, both in the United States and abroad. A comprehensive CPI handbook has been compiled by Megargee (1972).

Several CPI scales have received considerable attention across cultures; this attention usually focuses on whether or not selected scales are invariant across cultures. The Femininity (Fe) scale, for instance, was studied in Japan by using 600 students in a Japanese university (Nishiyama 1975). Since 30 of the 38 scale items that make up the Fe scale yielded differences in the same direction as in the original normative group, the author concluded that the scale is sufficiently robust for use in Japan. Similar conclusions have been reached by individuals studying the Socialization (So) scale and other scales in many different countries.

The Locus of Control Scale, otherwise known as the I-E (internal-external) Scale, is a popular, quick method to measure the "locus of control" of reinforcement. When he developed the concept, Rotter (1966) suggested that some persons, by virtue of the nature of the social environment that fosters achievement and autonomy, can be characterized as "internals"—that is, they perceive reinforcement accruing from the result of their own efforts since they control the environment. Where reinforcement is random or capricious and in general not under one's control, an "external" person may believe that fate, luck, or chance is the rule of thumb in life. This construct led to the development and widespread use of both the generic I-E Scale and many variations of it that have been developed for use with different populations (Lefcourt 1981).

Phares (1984) maintains that beliefs of internality or externality have three sources: (1) *family antecedents,* wherein families that have warm and protective child-rearing practices tend to develop individuals who are "internal"; (2) *consistency of experience,* which implies that inconsistent discipline may teach children that the world is capricious and unpredictable, thereby fostering an "external" orientation; and (3) *social,* an antecedent whereby individuals who have little access to power or opportunities for financial or personal growth would likely develop an "external" belief system. These sources are generally based on Western research; whether they would hold up in non-Western cultures is an open question.

Numerous studies have examined the nature of the I-E Scale in a variety of sociocultural settings, subjecting the responses to factor and other statistical analyses. The results of these studies suggest that when subjects from widely differing cultures are given the scale, their responses might form their own unique clusters. The reasons underlying such different clustering can be traced to differing perceptions of the social, political, and interpersonal environment. Dozens if not hundreds of "cross-cultural" locus of control studies can be found in recent literature. For instance, Nagelschmidt and Jakob (1977) gave the I-E Scale to a sample of Brazilian women. Two factors, "externality" and "fatalism," emerged, casting doubt (as have many other studies) over the unidimensionality of the construct as originally conceived. Munro (1979) made similar conclusions from his South African study, and Jones and Zoppel (1979) concur and add that the I-E Scale lacks equivalent meaning between blacks in Jamaica and blacks in the United States. Many studies uncover numerous factors underlying locus of control. For instance, Trimble and Richardson (1982) found five factors when they analyzed responses from a large sample of American Indians. These were trust, personal control, race ideology, ideological control, and a residual fate ideology. Hui and Triandis (1983), in a contrast study of Hispanic subjects and U.S. mainstream male navy recruits, found that the Predictable-Unpredictable World factor was equivalent for the two groups and that at least one other aspect of control, which has been called the Difficult-Easy World factor, is conceptually and functionally equivalent for both groups.

A particularly valuable review of the locus of control concept across cultures and ethnic groups is Dyal (1984), which appeared in a major book of readings dealing with this popular concept.

Using locus of control along with the concept of locus of responsibility (Jones et al. 1972), Sue (1978, 1981) proposed a conceptual model that is useful in discussing cultural identity during initial client assessment. Sue placed locus of control and locus of responsibility on a continuum in such a manner that they intersect to form four quadrants or worldviews: internal locus of control–internal locus of responsibility (IC-IR); external locus of control–internal locus of responsibility (EC-IR); internal locus of control–external locus of responsibility (IC-ER); and external locus of control–external locus of responsibility (EC-ER). The assumption here is that once the counselor is able to determine the loci of control and responsibility of the client, along with an understanding of the client's sociopolitical history and racial and cultural background, appropriate goals and process for counseling can be developed. However, while there are many different measures of locus of control, there are as yet no measures of locus of responsibility. Therefore, this framework will currently have to be viewed as a heuristic perspective for cross-cultural counselors.

The State-Trait Anxiety Inventory (STAI) is one of nearly a hundred measures that have been developed to assess anxiety, probably the most common "condition" that the counselor will see in his clients. Charles Spielberger and his colleagues developed the STAI to measure both situation- or state-induced anxiety (a temporary state that anyone can experience) and anxiety as a general and enduring characteristic of a person (trait anxiety). The A-State scale consists of 20 statements that describe current feelings, such as "I am worried" or "I am jittery." The 20 items on the A-Trait scale are more general, such as "I lack self-confidence."

A three-volume set of books edited by Spielberger and Diaz-Guerrero (1976, 1983, 1986) contains research reports concerning the use of the inventory among a wide assortment of cultural and ethnic groups. A comprehensive bibliography has been published (Spielberger 1984). The cross-cultural research program followed by STAI devotees parallels the efforts of those who work with the MMPI across languages and cultures: Translate the scale into another language, administer it to a sample of individuals from another culture, and then determine its factor structure, or its correlation with variables such as academic performance and self-concept. Often missing in these "static group comparisons" is a discussion of "emic" or culture-relative conceptions of anxiety (or whatever local term is functionally equivalent to the Western construct of anxiety). Different situations, such as actual physical danger, ambiguous circumstances, and daily routines, will evoke different levels of anxiety for different people, and these factors can vary widely across cultures as well. That problem aside, the STAI is never-theless the most widely used device to measure "anxiety" across cul-tures; therefore, the data that it stimulates can be of considerable help to the cross-cultural counselor.

A serious psychometric problem arises whenever a scale such as the STAI or any other paper-and-pencil scale of anxiety (or virtually any other psychological construct) is translated, administered to people in or from other cultures, and its absolute scale values used for direct com-parison with scale values from the culture of origin or from other cul-tures. The problem is that a way to calibrate anxiety scale values with absolute levels of anxiety has not yet been found. If comparisons of scale scores are restricted to groups within a new culture or ethnic commu-nity, there would be no problem. But if comparisons are to be made across cultures, the absence of an absolute (common) reference scale presents difficulties. For tests or scales to be directly interpretable on mean scale values across culture-linguistic groups, several things must be achieved: (1) each item's validity as an indicator of the underlying trait should remain unchanged; (2) the scale values and probability of endorsement at the item level should be the same; and (3) all the items taken together should have the same average validity, the same average absolute scale value, and the same operating characteristics in all cul-tures to which the inventory is extended. It is most unlikely that all of these conditions can be met in an absolute sense. This is another way of saying that norms developed in one culture should never be used in interpreting test scores from another culture unless all of the psychome-tric properties warrant such direct comparisons.

Depression and its measurement. Disorders of affect and mood, in particu-lar depression (the "common cold" of psychological disorders), are among the more controversial phenomena that the cross-cultural coun-selor will observe in his or her clients. In one of the more recent books dealing with the topic, Kleinman and Good (1985) consider culture and depression from historical, anthropological, psychiatric, and psycholog-ical perspectives. In that text Carr and Vitaliano (1985) present theoret-ical implications of converging research on depression and the culture-bound syndromes. They challenge the view that depression is a universal psychobiological disorder, arguing that culture conditions behavioral repertoires. Further, they challenge the disease model and propose a distress approach and an extended cognitive-behavioral inter-pretation of depression. Beiser (1985) presents a study of depression among Africans, North Americans, and Southeast Asians and con-cludes that the experience of depression is more similar than different across cultures. He proposes that future research needs to consider both cultural and genetic explanations as alternative hypotheses. However, Beiser notes that depression as illness is not the same across cultures.

Marsella et al. (1985), in an overview of cross-cultural studies of depressive disorders, underscore that depression involves the totality of human functioning—biological, psychological, and sociocultural. Further, they conclude that different cultures conceptualize the problem of depressive disorders in different ways. A recent contribution in the understanding of depression is the development of a culturally informed and interactionist model (Weiss and Kleinman 1988).

Many different techniques and scales have been developed to measure depression. These include the Beck Depression Inventory (see Beck 1978; Beck et al. 1979), which is probably the most widely used depression scale in the United States. Others are the Zung Self-Rating Scale (Zung 1969), the Depression Adjective Checklist (Levitt and Lubin 1975), the MMPI (Butcher and Pancheri 1976), the Hamilton Depression Scale (Binitie 1975; Teja and Narang 1970), the World Health Organization's Schedule for Standardized Assessment of Depressive Disorders (World Health Organization 1983), and various versions of the Hopkins Symptom Checklist (Derogatis et al. 1974). Also, because the diagnoses of the *Diagnostic and Statistical Manual* of the American Psychiatric Association give specific criteria for depression, several other self-report scales have recently appeared. For instance, see Zimmerman et al. (1986) for details on a scale to diagnose major depressive disorders, and Klein, Depue, and Slater (1986) for a new inventory designed to identify cyclothymia.

There are also several nonsymptom measures of psychological characteristics associated with depression. One is the Attributional Style Questionnaire designed to measure the constructs associated with depression as predicted by the reformulated learned helplessness model (see Seligman et al. 1979, as well as Peterson et al. 1982, which describes a questionnaire designed to measure "helplessness"). Beck also developed a questionnaire tapping attitudes, which measures "hopelessness," and is appropriately called the Hopelessness Scale. It is a 20-item true-false measure of an individual's negative expectancies about himself or herself and his or her future (see Beck et al. 1974).

However, the symptoms of depression and its related behavioral and cognitive dimensions may vary widely across cultures. For instance, Kleinman (1982) found that in China depressed patients did not in the majority of cases show the loss of ability to experience pleasure or the helplessness, hopelessness, guilt, and suicidal thoughts so characteristic of depressives in North America. Thus, a counselor could make a big mistake by translating a scale for depression and giving it to clients from another cultural or ethnic group unless, of course, the scale's psychometric properties are shown to be identical across the different groups. Since this will not likely be the case, the counselor should "determine indigenous definitions of depression, take cognizance of different syndromes of depressive behavior, be aware of biased samples due to case-finding procedures, and examine the meanings of various symptoms within the shared belief systems of the population under study" (Guthrie and Lonner 1986, 263).

A note on projective techniques. The previous version of this chapter (Lonner 1981) devoted several pages to projective methodology as a special technique in cross-cultural assessment. There is no doubt that projective methodology is potentially very fruitful and that adherents of such procedures across cultures (e.g., some ethnopsychiatrists and clinical psychologists) make good use of such tests as the Rorschach, the Thematic Apperception Test, and especially the Holtzman Inkblot Technique when assessing clients from other cultural perspectives. If we had the space to do so in this chapter, it would have been interesting to explore the use of projective techniques across cultures. However, we believe that projective techniques are used very infrequently if at all by the type of counselor who may be using this particular book as a guide in counseling and assessment across cultures. One must keep in mind that (1) it takes special training, to say nothing of a more or less doctrinaire viewpoint (usually psychodynamic), to use such methods ethically, and (2) people who engage in what might be called "generic" cross-cultural counseling have relatively little need to employ projective methodology. On the other hand, those who may want to consider using these rather unstructured and potentially fruitful devices should not be deterred from exploring their potential. But their use should be preceded by a careful reading of the important literature in this area. Somewhat dated but still valuable sources of information about the cross-cultural use of projectives include the classic book in this area (Lindzey 1961) and a review of their use in psychological anthropology (Spain 1974). Additionally, Holtzman's (1980) review of projective techniques and their place in cross-cultural research and application should be considered a key reference.

We have completed an overview of several issues and problems surrounding the use of psychological tests in assessing clients from other cultures or ethnic groups. More information on these topics can be found in Irvine and Berry (1983; in press), Lonner (1985), Guthrie and Lonner (1986), and Sundberg and Gonzales (1981).

Nonstandardized Assessment

The problems posed by standardized assessment methods have led to the extended use of nonstandardized assessment methodologies. These methodologies emerged from the application of principles derived from behavioral approaches and were proposed as an alternative to "traditional" approaches for understanding human behavior (Mash 1979;

Nay and Nay 1984). Shertzer and Linden (1979) state that a large variety of nonstandardized techniques are available for collecting information about an individual. When these techniques are used judiciously and appropriately they can enhance a counselor's understanding of the client. Further, they state that "a major difference between standardized and nonstandardized measures is that the latter group of assessment tools and techniques is usually not developed or normed by means of data obtained from well-defined populations" (1979, 364). It is clear that even when information is gathered from both standardized and nonstandardized sources, the result, although it may seem comprehensive, is only providing a small portion of the descriptive information about the complex of temperament and "personality" reflected in each unique client.

Jones (1977) recommends against the utilization of fixed-response formats, preselected vocabularies, and other measurement deterrents to a client's full expression. Instead he recommends the use of free-response approaches, open-ended interviews, and participant-observer techniques. In response to these recommendations, Goldstein (1981, 94–95) proposes specific cross-cultural client assessment using a "multi-method, multisource measurement strategy, in which behavioral, self-report, other report, and projective information is gathered not only from the participants themselves, but also from such relevant figures as the client's family, the counselor's supervisor, independent interview-rating judges, and appropriate others." Since nonstandardized approaches are also vulnerable to bias and stereotype by the helper, it is critical that the counselor be well versed in understanding the culture of the client. Nonstandardized approaches include structured interviews for specific disorders, observation, rating scales, assessment of social and environmental behavior, and self-report measures.

Interviews fall in the category of structured observations, according to Shertzer and Linden (1979). They define an interview as "an undisguised controlled observation of an individual's behavior, obtained usually in a one-to-one conversation" (1979, 375). Diagnostic interviewing necessitates that interviewers have a formal theoretical position from which they investigate the client's presenting problem. Structured interview schedules are available that can assist a practitioner in arriving at a diagnosis (Houck and Hansen's Diagnostic Interviewing Schedule 1972; Woody's Clinical Assessment Interview Format 1972). Specific to anxiety disorders is the Anxiety Disorders Interview Schedule by Dinardo et al. (1983). These structured interviews may be used with caution with cross-cultural clients to arrive at some tentative hypothesis regarding the problem the client is facing.

Self-report and self-observation have been used to the widest extent in counseling and psychotherapy. This method involves a paper and pencil or other self-endorsement made by the client to reflect on past behavior or to carry out ongoing self-evaluations (Nay and Nay 1984). Self-report measures include free-response measures, checklists, and rating approaches. A major limitation is that self-report measures are subject to bias and response sets (see pp. 308–309). Well-known self-report measures used in counseling and psychotherapy include fear and avoidance hierarchies, most commonly used for anxiety and phobia treatment based on Wolpe's (1973) subjective degree of discomfort scale; behavioral checklists; and simple methods for recording observations. An example of a cross-culturally fruitful structured checklist is the Adjective Checklist (Gough and Heilbrun 1980). Williams and Best (1982) and their colleagues in many countries have used it extensively to assess cultural variations in sex-role stereotypes, ego states, self concept, and other psychological phenomena.

Self-observation measures include daily and weekly logs, autobiography, and biographical inventory, which can be used to gain self-report information when it is not possible to conduct an interview. Additionally, value scales, studies of goal orientation, and long-range planning have been used as self-regulation measures. Further, self-monitoring devices such as mechanical counters, self-monitoring cards, and videotaping are also useful (Bergin and Lambert 1978). Well-known questionnaires that have been used in counseling and psychotherapy research and practice include the Fear Questionnaire (Marks and Mathews 1979), a brief one-page form that yields three major scales (scores for agoraphobia, social phobia, and blood and injury phobia), enabling one to examine the relative severity of phobic response as compared to standardized norms; the Beck Depression Inventory (Beck 1978); the Hamilton Depression Scale (Hamilton 1960); the State-Trait Anxiety Inventory (Speilberger, Gorsuch, and Lushene 1970); the Taylor Manifest Anxiety Scale (Taylor 1953); the Fear of Negative Evaluation Scale (Watson and Friend 1969); the Social Avoidance and Distress Scale (Watson and Friend 1969); and the Client Posttherapy Questionnaire (Cartwright, Kirtner, and Fiske 1963).

Evaluation of the intervention involves using the assessment tools that originally assisted in the diagnosis phase. Generally, instruments from the nonstandardized domain are utilized by clinicians to evaluate how effective the counseling intervention is during the process of counseling and at termination.

Counseling Evaluation Issues

Counseling and psychotherapy have multiple effects on the client, as emphasized by Strupp and Hadley (1977). They propose a tripartite model to evaluate the diverse changes that result from counseling and psychotherapy: (1) the outcome, viewed from the vantage point of society (behavior); (2) the individual (sense of well-being), and (3) the mental health professional (theories of healthy functioning). Further, they emphasize that these three perspectives be assessed simultaneously.

Bergin and Lambert (1978), after reviewing the literature on psychotherapy outcome, make the following recommendations. First, since change is multidimensional, research and practice should continue to study the divergent processes of change, that is, the kinds of change, implying a more rigorous specification of the variables underlying clients', therapists', and others' ratings of outcome. Further, careful comparison is indicated of outcome factors, such as thinking habits, overt behavior, physiological changes, and the feeling states.

Second, outcome evaluation must include assessment of changes in both behavior and internal states. Additionally, they recommend that "situational" measures be employed and be given preference over the "less promising personality assessment" (1978, 174). Further, the therapist should individualize change criteria rather than use global improvement indices. Procedures that would prove useful in implementing an individualized strategy include Goal Attainment Scaling (Kiresuk and Sherman 1968), and the Problem-Oriented System (Weed 1968; Klonoff and Cox 1975).

Third, suggestions should be followed regarding useful techniques for outcome evaluation. This information comes from a number of sources and includes:

The client (self-report, both standardized and nonstandardized assessment, and situational tests);

Therapist evaluation, such as the Therapist Change Report (Lorr et al. 1962), the Psychiatric Evaluation Form (Spitzer, Endicott, and Cohen, 1967), the Use of Target Complaints as the criterion for improvement (Battle et al. 1966), and the Interpersonal Behavioral Inventory (Lorr and McNair 1965);

Expert "trained observers," using devices such as the Timed Behavior Checklist for Performance Anxiety (Paul 1966), the Behavior Rating Category System (Becker et al. 1967), the Behavior Checklist of Interpersonal Anxiety (Diloreto 1971), and Analogue Procedures (Williams and Brown 1974);

Evaluation by relevant others using such scales as the Katz Adjustment Scale (Katz and Lyerly 1963).

Assessment of Process

Success in counseling is highly dependent on the process that the client experiences. This process needs to be consistent with the cultural assumptions and beliefs of the client. If this occurs, the client will believe that the counselor understands him or her and will therefore be effective in providing relief (Torrey 1986). Torrey supports the view that the client has to experience the counselor as someone who understands and who will be effective in helping to provide relief for the client's presenting problem. We believe that basic to this process of interpersonal influence is a shared worldview (Ibrahim 1984b, 1985; Torrey 1986). The counselor can use the SAWV (Scale to Access World Views) to develop a shared worldview with the client (Ibrahim 1985; Sadlak and Ibrahim 1986; Schroeder and Ibrahim 1982). In "generic" counseling and psychotherapy the closest correlate of what the client experiences as a shared worldview is Rogers' (1957) proposition regarding the necessary and sufficient conditions for effective therapy, that is, nonpossessive warmth, genuineness, and accurate empathy.

The most commonly used instruments to assess process in counseling have involved those that assess the facilitative conditions experienced by the client. These have traditionally included the Truax and Carkhuff Scale (1967) or the Carkhuff modified scale (1969) rating empathy, warmth, and genuineness. The most commonly used scales to get client input have been the Barrett-Lennard Relationship Inventory (Barrett-Lennard 1962) and the Truax Relationship Inventory (Truax and Carkhuff 1967). We emphasize that in using these instruments in a cross-cultural context the counselor and the judges providing ratings need to be knowledgeable regarding the client's worldview and primary and secondary cultures to understand the data and information yielded by these assessment techniques.

Summary and Conclusions

In summary, arriving at an accurate judgment regarding the nature of the concerns that have brought the client to counseling involves a three-step process. The first step is understanding the client's worldview, beliefs, values, assumptions, and unique way of approaching the world, including problem-solving and decision-making strategies. The second step involves an understanding of the client's specific "norm" group, that is, with which specific cultural or ethnic group does the client identify, and understanding the advantages and disadvantages that the client faces from that perspective. The third step involves the use of a combination of approaches to understand further the nature of the problem, that is, clinical judgment, standardized assessment tools (where applicable), and nonstandardized assessment techniques that may be appropriate. It is our belief that the better the counselor's understanding regarding the client's worldview and primary identification group, the better the diagnostic process, which in turn increases the probability of culturally appropriate interventions.

In using standardized assessment instruments, counselors need to be aware of the following problems or issues before assessment is begun: the distinction between constructs and criteria, establishment of equivalence, the nature of verbal and nonverbal stimuli in assessment, the role of response sets, and the tendency to infer deficits from test score differences. Although there have been many attempts to reduce or minimize the bias inherent in Western psychological instruments, the issue of bias in testing and assessment may never be fully resolved.

The history of psychological assessment is long and colorful. Many thousands of procedures and techniques have been developed in both standardized and nonstandardized modes to assess the various ways in which people differ. Generally, the "successes" in this controversial area far outweigh the "failures." Critics of testing, however, often contend that tests, scales, inventories, and questionnaires fail to capture the essence of a person, and often will force a client into convenient (for the assessor) categories in which the client may not really belong. The critics of cross-cultural assessment might add that attempts to cross cultural and ethnic lines only contribute to the problem.

We agree that tests, scales, questionnaires, and other tools of assessment are incomplete representations of the client and in the wrong hands can be deadly. We also agree that the cultural or ethnic variable is difficult to transcend. However, in any kind of counseling it is impossible to avoid assessment; even a rather casual and unstructured conversation between counselor and client is a form of assessment. Because it is impossible to avoid appraisal, the position we have explicitly and implicitly taken throughout this chapter can be stated simply: Assess, if you must, but do so with the utmost of caution, and *always* give the benefit of any doubt to the client. Assessment can provide the counselor with interesting and informative material, and with insights that are difficult to develop by other means. On the other hand, faulty, hasty, or incomplete assessment can cut deeply the other way and lead to unfortunate, perhaps even tragic, consequences.

In this chapter we have not actually *advocated* assessment; rather, we have outlined some useful frameworks and have pointed out some areas of controversy and difficulty that should be taken into account in cross-cultural assessment. Tests and related devices are only tools. Ultimately, it is the cross-cultural counselor who will have to decide what to assess, when and by which method to assess it, and how to weigh the risks involved against the possible benefits. Nothing will ever replace the counselor's careful consideration of what is best for the client.

References

Aberle, D. F., Cohen, A. K., Davis, A. K., Levy, M. J., and Sutton, F. X. 1950. The functional prerequisites of society. *Ethics* 60:100–111.

Abramowitz, C. V., and Dokecki, P. R. 1977. The politics of clinical judgment: Early empirical returns. *Psychological Bulletin* 84:460–476.

Anastasi, A. 1988. *Psychological testing.* 6th ed. New York: Macmillan.

Atkinson, D. R., Morten, G., and Sue, D. W. 1983. *Counseling American minorities.* 2d ed. Dubuque, IA: William C. Brown.

Bagby, J. W. 1957. A cross-cultural study of perceptual predominance in binocular rivalry. *Journal of Abnormal and Social Psychology* 54:331–334.

Bales, J. 1985. Minority training falls short. *APA Monitor* 16:7.

Barrett-Lennard, G. T. 1962. Dimensions of therapist response as causal factors in therapeutic change. *Psychological Monographs* 76 (562, entire issue).

Battle, C. C., Imber, S. D., Hoehn-Saric, R., Stone, A. R., Nash, C., and Frank, J. D. 1966. Target complaints as criteria for improvement. *American Journal of Psychotherapy* 20:184–192.

Beck, A. T. 1978. *Depression inventory.* Philadelphia: Center for Cognitive Therapy.

Beck, A. T., Rush, A. J., Shaw, B. F., and Emery, G. 1979. *Cognitive theory of depression.* New York: Guilford Press.

Beck, A. T., Weissman, A., Lester, D., and Trexler, L. 1974. The measurement of pessimism: The hopelessness scale. *Journal of Consulting and Clinical Psychology* 42:861–865.

Becker, W. C., Madsen, C. H., Arnold, C. R., and Thomas, D. R. 1967. The contingent use of teacher praise and attention in reducing classroom behavior problems. *Journal of Special Education* 1:287–307.

Beiser, M. 1985. A study of depression among traditional Africans, Urban North Americans, and Southeast Asian refugees. In A. Kleinman and B. Good (eds.), *Culture and depression: Studies in the anthropology and cross-cultural psychiatry of affect and disorder.* Berkeley: University of California Press.

Bergin, A. E., and Lambert, M. J. 1978. The evaluation of therapeutic outcomes. In S. L. Garfield and A. E. Bergin (eds.), *Handbook of psychotherapy and behavior change.* New York: John Wiley and Sons.

Bernal, M. E., and Padilla, A. M. 1982. Status of minority curricula and training in clinical psychology. *American Psychologist* 37:780–787.

Berry, J. W. 1969. On cross-cultural comparability. *International Journal of Psychology* 4:119–128.

———. 1972. Radical cultural relativism and the concept of intelligence. In L. J. Cronbach and P. J. D. Drenth (eds.), *Mental tests and cultural adaptation.* The Hague: Mouton.

———. 1976. *Human ecology and cognitive style: Comparative studies in cultural and psychological adaptation.* Beverly Hills: Sage-Halsted.

Binitie, A. 1975. A factor-analytical study of depression across cultures (African and European). *British Journal of Psychiatry* 127:559–563.

Brislin, R. W. 1986. The wording and translation of research instruments. In W. J. Lonner and J. W. Berry (eds.), *Field methods in cross-cultural research.* Newbury Park, CA: Sage Publications.

Butcher, J. N. 1984. Current developments in MMPI use: An international perspective. In J. N. Butcher and C. D. Spielberger (eds.), *Advances in personality development.* Vol. 4. Hillsdale, NJ: Erlbaum.

————, ed. 1979. *New developments in the use of the MMPI.* Minneapolis: University of Minnesota Press.

Butcher, J. N., Hama, H., and Matsuyama, Y. 1979. Proceedings of the Sixth International Conference on Personality Assessment, Doshisha University, Kyoto, Japan.

Butcher, J. N. and Keller, L. 1984. Objective personality assessment: Present status and future directions. In G. Goldstein and M. Hersen (eds.), *Handbook of psychological assessment.* New York: Pergamon Press.

Butcher, J. N., and Pancheri, P. 1976. *A handbook of cross-national MMPI research.* Minneapolis: University of Minnesota Press.

Carkhuff, R. 1969. *Helping and human relations.* New York: Holt, Rinehart and Winston.

Carr, J. E., and Vitaliano, P. P. 1985. The theoretical implications of converging research on depression and the culture-bound syndromes. In A. Kleinman and B. Good (eds.), *Culture and depression: Studies in the anthropology and cross-cultural psychiatry of affect and disorder.* Berkeley: University of California Press.

Cartwright, D., Kirtner, W. L., and Fiske, D. W. 1963. Method factors in changes associated with psychotherapy. *Journal of Abnormal and Social Psychology* 66:164–175.

Chun, K., Campbell, J., and Yoo, J. 1974. Extreme response style in cross-cultural research: A reminder. *Journal of Cross-Cultural Psychology* 5:465–480.

Cole, M., and Bruner, J. S. 1971. Cultural differences in and inferences about psychological processes. *American Psychologist* 26:867–876.

Cronbach, L. J. 1984. *Essentials of psychological testing.* 4th ed. New York: Harper and Row.

Cronbach, L. J., and Drenth, P. J. D., eds. 1972. *Mental tests and cultural adaptation.* The Hague: Mouton.

Crowne, D. P., and Marlowe, D. 1964. *The approval motive: Studies in evaluative dependence.* New York: John Wiley and Sons.

Dahlstrom, W. G., Lachar, D., and Dahlstrom, L. E. 1986. *MMPI patterns of American minorities.* Minneapolis: University of Minnesota Press.

Deregowski, J. B. 1980. Perception. In H. C. Triandis and W. J. Lonner (eds.), *Handbook of cross-cultural psychology.* Vol. 3, *Basic processes.* Boston: Allyn and Bacon.

Derogatis, L. R., Lipman, R. S., Rickels, K., Uhlenhuth, E. H., and Covi, L. 1974. The Hopkins Symptoms Checklist (HSCL): A measure of primary symptom dimensions. In P. Pichot (ed.), *Psychological measurement in psychopharmacology: Modern problems in psychopharmacopsychiatry* 7:79–110. Basel, Switzerland: S. Karger.

Diloreto, A. O. 1971. *Comparative psychotherapy: An experimental analysis.* Chicago: Aldine-Atherton.

DiNardo, P. A., O'Brien, G. T., Barlow, D. H., Waddell, M. T., and Blanchard, E. B. 1983. Reliability of DSM-III anxiety disorder categories using a structured interview. *Archives of General Psychiatry* 40:1070–1075.

Draguns, J. G. 1980. Psychological disorders of clinical severity. In H. C. Triandis and J. G. Draguns (eds.), *Handbook of cross-cultural psychology.* Vol. 6, *Psychopathology.* Boston: Allyn and Bacon.

Duckworth, J. 1979. *MMPI interpretation manual for counselors and clinicians.* 2d ed. Muncie, IN: Accelerated Development.

Dyal, J. A. 1984. Cross-cultural research with the locus of control construct. In H. Lefcourt (ed.), *Research with the locus of control construct.* Vol. 3, *Extensions and limitations.* New York: Academic Press.

Enright, J., and Jaeckle, W. 1963. Psychiatric symptoms and diagnoses in two subcultures. *International Journal of Social Psychiatry* 9:12–17.

Fiske, D. W. 1970. *Measuring the concepts of personality.* Chicago: Aldine-Atherton.

Frijda, N., and Jahoda, G. 1966. On the scope and methods of cross-cultural research. *International Journal of Psychology* 1:109–127.

Goldstein, A. P. 1981. Evaluating expectancy effects. In A. J. Marsella and P. B. Pedersen (eds.), *Cross-cultural counseling and psychotherapy: Foundations, evaluation, and cultural considerations.* Elmsford, NY: Pergamon Press.

Gordon, L. V. 1963. *The survey of interpersonal values.* Chicago: Science Research Associates.

Gough, H. G., and Heilbrun, A. B. 1980. *The Adjective Checklist bibliography (1980 edition).* Palo Alto, CA: Consulting Psychologists Press.

Graham, J. R. 1977. *The MMPI: A practical guide.* New York: Oxford University Press.

Green, L. S., and Haymes, M. 1973. Value orientation and psychosocial adjustment and norms levels of marijuana use. *Journal of Youth and Adolescence* 2:213–231.

Guthrie, G. M., and Lonner, W. J. 1986. Assessment of personality and psychopathology. In W. J. Lonner and J. W. Berry (eds.), *Field methods in cross-cultural research.* Newbury Park, CA: Sage Publications.

Gynther, M. D. 1972. White norms and black MMPIs: A prescription for discrimination? *Psychological Bulletin* 78:386–402.

———. 1979. Ethnicity and personality: An update. In J. N. Butcher (ed.), *New developments in the use of the MMPI.* Minneapolis: University of Minnesota Press.

Hamilton, M. 1960. Development of a rating scale for primary depressive illness. *British Journal of Social and Clinical Psychology* 6:278–296.

Higginbotham, H. N. 1979. Culture and the delivery of psychological services in developing nations. *Transcultural Psychiatric Research Review* 16:7–27.

Holtzman, W. H. 1980. Projective techniques. In H. C. Triandis and J. W. Berry (eds.), *Handbook of cross-cultural psychology.* Vol. 2, *Methodology.* Boston: Allyn and Bacon.

Houck, J. E., and Hansen, J. C. 1972. Diagnostic interviewing. In R. H. Woody and J. D. Woody (eds.), *Clinical assessment in counseling and psychotherapy,* 119–186. Englewood Cliffs, NJ: Prentice-Hall.

Hui, C. H., and Triandis, H. C. 1983. Multistrategy approach to cross-cultural research: The case of locus of control. *Journal of Cross-Cultural Psychology* 14:65–83.

Ibrahim, F. A. 1984a. *Cross-cultural counseling and psychotherapy: Initial client assess-*

ment. Paper presented at the annual meeting of the Association of Counseling and Development, Houston.

―――. 1984b. Cross-cultural counseling and psychotherapy: An existential-psychological perspective. *International Journal for the Advancement of Counseling* 7:559–569.

―――. 1985. Effective cross-cultural counseling and psychotherapy: A framework. *Counseling Psychologist* 13:625–638.

Ibrahim, F. A., and Arredondo, P. M. 1986. Ethical standards for cross-cultural counseling: Counselor preparation, practice, assessment, and research. *Journal of Counseling and Development* 64:349–351.

Ibrahim, F. A., and Kahn, H. 1984. *Scale to assess world views* (SAWV). Typescript. University of Connecticut.

―――. 1987. Assessment of world views. *Psychological Reports* 60:163–176.

Ibrahim, F. A., Stadler, H. A., Arredondo, P. M., and McFadden, J. 1986. Status of human rights issues in counselor preparation: A national survey. Paper presented at the annual meeting of the American Association of Counseling and Development, Los Angeles.

Irvine, S. H., and Berry, J. W., eds. 1983. *Human assessment and cultural factors*. New York: Plenum Press.

―――. In press. *Cultural context of human abilities*. New York: Cambridge University Press.

Jones, E. E., Kanouse, D. E., Kelley, H. H., Nisbett, R. E., Valins, S., and Weiner, B. 1972. *Attribution: Perceiving the causes of behavior*. Morristown, NJ: General Learning Press.

Jones, E. E., and Zoppel, C. 1979. Personality differences among blacks in Jamaica and the United States. *Journal of Cross-Cultural Psychology* 10:435–456.

Jones, R. A. 1977. *Self-fulfilling prophecies*. Hillsdale, NJ: Erlbaum.

Katz, M. M., Gudeman, H., and Sanborn, K. 1969. Characterizing differences in psychopathology among ethnic groups in Hawaii. In F. Redlich (ed.), *Social psychiatry*. Baltimore: Williams and Wilkins.

―――. 1978. Ethnic studies in Hawaii: On psychopathology and social deviance. In L. Wynne, S. Matthyse, and R. Cromwell (eds.), *The nature of schizophrenia*. New York: John Wiley and Sons.

Katz, M. M., and Lyerly, S. B. 1963. Methods for measuring adjustment and social behavior in the community: Pt. 1, Rationale, description, discriminative validity, and scale development. *Psychological Reports* 4:1503–1555.

Kaufman, A. S., and Kaufman, N. L. 1983. *K-ABC: Kaufman Assessment Battery for Children*. Circle Pines, MN: American Guidance Services.

Kavanaugh, H. B. 1980. Some appraised instruments of values for counselors. *Personnel and Guidance Journal* 58:613–616.

Kiresuk, T. J., and Sherman, R. E. 1968. Goal attainment scaling: A general method for evaluating comprehensive community mental health programs. *Community Mental Health Journal* 4:443–453.

Klein, D. N., Depue, R. A., and Slater, J. F. 1986. Inventory identification of cyclothymia. *Archives of General Psychiatry* 43:441–445.

Kleinman, A. 1982. Neurasthenia and depression: A study of socialization and culture in China. *Culture, Medicine, and Psychiatry* 6:117–190.

Kleinman, A., and Good, B., eds. 1985. *Culture and depression: Studies in the anthropology and cross-cultural psychiatry of affect and disorder.* Berkeley: University of California Press.

Klonoff, H., and Cox, B. A. 1975. A problem-oriented approach to analysis of treatment outcome. *American Journal of Psychiatry* 132:186–191.

Kluckhohn, C. 1951. Values and value orientations in a theory of action. In T. Parsons and E. A. Shields (eds.), *Toward a general theory of action,* 388–433. Cambridge: Harvard University Press.

———. 1956. Toward a comparison of value-emphases in different cultures. In L. D. White (ed.), *The state of social sciences,* 116–132. Chicago: University of Chicago Press.

Kluckhohn, F. R., and Strodtbeck, F. L. 1961. *Variations in value orientations.* Evanston, IL: Row, Patterson.

Lefcourt, H. M., ed. 1981. *Research with the locus of control construct.* Vol. 1, *Assessment methods.* New York: Academic Press.

Levitt, E., and Lubin, B. 1975. *Depression: Concepts, controversies and some new facts.* New York: Springer.

Lewin, K. 1935. *A dynamic theory of personality.* New York: McGraw-Hill.

Lindzey, G. 1961. *Projective techniques and cross-cultural research.* New York: Appleton-Century-Crofts.

Lonner, W. J. 1979. Issues in cross-cultural psychology. In A. J. Marsella, R. Tharp, and T. Ciborowski (eds.), *Perspectives on cross-cultural psychology.* New York: Academic Press.

———. 1981. Psychological tests and intercultural counseling. In P. B. Pedersen, J. G. Draguns, W. J. Lonner, and J. E. Trimble (eds.), *Counseling across cultures,* 203–226. Honolulu: University of Hawaii Press.

———. 1985. Issues in testing and assessment in cross-cultural counseling. *Counseling Psychologist* 13:599–614.

Lorion, R. P. 1978. Research on psychotherapy and behavior change in the disadvantaged. In S. L. Garfield and A. E. Bergin (eds.), *Handbook of psychotherapy and behavior change: An empirical analysis,* 2d ed., 903–938. New York: John Wiley and Sons.

Lorr, M., and McNair, D. M. 1965. Expansion of the interpersonal behavioral circle. *Journal of Personality and Social Psychology* 2:823–830.

Lorr, M., McNair, D. M., Michaux, W. M., and Raskin, A. 1962. Frequency of treatment and change in psychotherapy. *Journal of Abnormal and Social Psychology* 64:281–292.

Malpass, R. S., and Poortinga, Y. H. 1986. Strategies for design and analysis. In W. J. Lonner and J. W. Berry (eds.), *Field methods in cross-cultural research.* Newbury Park, CA: Sage Publications.

Marks, I. M., and Mathews, A. M. 1979. Brief standard self-rating for phobics. *Behavior Therapy and Research* 17:263–267.

Marsella, A. J. 1982. Culture and mental health. In A. J. Marsella and G. M. White (eds.), *Cultural conceptions of mental health and therapy,* 359–388. Hingham, MA: Reidel.

Marsella, A. J., Kinzie, D., and Gordon, P. 1973. Ethnic variations in the expression of depression. *Journal of Cross-Cultural Psychology* 4:435–458.

Marsella, A. J., and Pedersen, P. B., eds. 1981. *Cross-cultural counseling and psychotherapy: Foundations, evaluation, and cultural considerations.* Elmsford, NY: Pergamon Press.

Marsella, A. J., Sartorius, N., Jablensky, A., and Fenton, F. R. 1985. Cross-cultural studies of depressive disorders: An overview. In A. Kleinman and B. Good (eds.), *Culture and depression: Studies in the anthropology and cross-cultural psychiatry of affect and disorder.* Berkeley: University of California Press.

Mash, E. J. 1979. What is behavioral assessment? *Behavioral Assessment* 1:23–29.

Megargee, E. I. 1972. *The California Psychological Inventory handbook.* San Francisco: Jossey-Bass.

Mercer, J. R. 1979. *SOMPA: Technical and conceptual manual.* New York: Psychological Corporation.

Merluzzi, T. V., Merluzzi, B. H., and Kaul, T. J. 1977. Counselor race and power base: Effects on attitudes and behavior. *Journal of Counseling Psychology* 24:430–436.

Munro, D. 1979. Locus of control attribution: Factors among blacks and whites in Africa. *Journal of Cross-Cultural Psychology* 10:157–172.

Nagelschmidt, A., and Jakob, R. 1977. Dimensionality of Rotter's I-E scale in a society in the process of modernization. *Journal of Cross-Cultural Psychology* 8:101–111.

Nay, W. R., and Nay, R. E. 1984. Issues for behavioral assessment in psychotherapy research. In M. Hersen, L. Michelson, and A. S. Bellack (eds.), *Issues in psychotherapy research.* New York: Plenum Press.

Nishiyama, T. 1975. Validation of the CPI Femininity Scale in Japan. *Journal of Cross-Cultural Psychology* 6:482–489.

Osgood, C. E., May, W., and Miron, W. 1975. *Cross-cultural universals of affective meaning.* Champaign: University of Illinois Press.

Paul, G. L. 1966. *Effects of insight, desensitization, and attention placebo treatment of anxiety.* Stanford: Stanford University Press.

———. 1967. Strategy of outcome research in psychotherapy. *Journal of Consulting Psychology* 31:109–118.

Pedersen, P. B. 1986. Are the APA ethical principles culturally encapsulated? Typescript. Syracuse, NY.

Petersen, C., Semmel, A., von Bayer, C. L., Abramson, L. Y., Metalsky, G. I., and Seligman, M. E. P. 1982. The attribution style questionnaire. *Cognitive Theory and Research* 6:287–300.

Phares, E. J. 1976. *Locus of control in personality.* Morristown, NJ: General Learning Press.

———. 1984. *Introduction to personality.* Columbus, OH: Merrill.

Poortinga, Y. H. 1975a. Limitations on intercultural comparisons of psychological data. *Nederlands Tijdschrift voor de Psychologie* 30:23–39.

———. 1975b. Some implications of three different approaches to intercultural comparison. In J. W. Berry and W. J. Lonner (eds.), *Applied cross-cultural psychology.* Amsterdam: Swets and Zeitlinger.

Przeworski, A., and Teune, H. 1970. *The logic of comparative social inquiry.* New York: John Wiley and Sons.

Rogers, C. R. 1957. The necessary and sufficient conditions of therapeutic personality change. *Journal of Consulting Psychology* 21:95–103.

Rotter, J. 1966. Generalized expectancies for internal versus external control of reinforcement. *Psychological Monographs* 80 (1, Whole no. 609).

Sadlak, M. J., and Ibrahim, F. A. 1986. *Cross-cultural counselor training: Impact on counselor effectiveness and sensitivity.* Paper presented at the annual meeting of the American Psychological Association, Washington, DC.

Samuda, R. J. 1975. *Psychological testing of American minorities.* New York: Dodd, Mead.

Schroeder, D. G., and Ibrahim, F. A. 1982. *Cross-cultural couple counseling.* Paper presented at the national meeting of the American Association for Marriage and Family Therapy, Dallas.

Sechrest, L., Fay, T. L., and Zaidi, S. M. H. 1972. Problems of translation in cross-cultural research. *Journal of Cross-Cultural Psychology* 3:41–56.

Seligman, M. E. P., Abramson, L. Y., Semmel, A., and von Bayer, C. L. 1979. Depressive attributional style. *Journal of Abnormal Psychology* 88:242–247.

Sharma, S. 1977. Cross-cultural comparisons of anxiety: Methodological problems. *Topics in Culture Learning* 5:166–173.

Shertzer, C. D., and Linden, J. D. 1979. *Fundamentals of individual appraisal.* Boston: Houghton Mifflin.

Shostrom, E. L. 1963. *The personal orientation inventory.* San Diego: Educational and Industrial Testing Service.

Spain, D. H. 1972. On the use of projective techniques for psychological anthropology. In F. L. K. Hsu (ed.), *Psychological anthropology.* New ed. Cambridge, MA: Schenkman.

Spielberger, C. D. 1972. Anxiety as an emotional state. In C. D. Spielberger (ed.), *Anxiety: Current trends in theory and research.* Vol. 1. New York: Academic Press.

———. 1975. The measurement of state and trait anxiety: Conceptual and methodological issues. In L. Levi (ed.), *Emotions—Their parameters and measurement.* New York: Raven Press.

———. 1984. *A comprehensive bibliography for the State-Trait Anxiety Inventory.* Palo Alto, CA: Consulting Psychologists Press.

Spielberger, C. D., and Diaz-Guerrero, R., eds. 1976. *Cross-cultural anxiety.* Vol. 1. Washington, DC: Hemisphere.

———. 1983. *Cross-cultural anxiety.* Vol. 2. Washington, DC: Hemisphere.

———. 1986. *Cross-cultural anxiety.* Vol. 3. Washington, DC: Hemisphere.

Spielberger, C. D., Gorsuch, R. L., and Lushene, R. G. 1970. *The State-Trait Anxiety Inventory.* Palo Alto, CA: Consulting Psychologists Press.

Spitzer, R. L., Endicott, J., and Cohen, G. 1967. *The psychiatric status schedule: Techniques for evaluating social and role functioning and mental status.* New York: New York State Psychiatric Institute and Biometrics Research.

Strong, S. R. 1968. Counseling: An interpersonal influence process. *Journal of Counseling Psychology* 15:215–224.

Strupp, H. H. 1978. Psychotherapy research and practice: An overview. In

S. L. Garfield and A. E. Bergin (eds.), *Handbook of psychotherapy and behavior change: An empirical analysis.* New York: John Wiley and Sons.

Strupp, H. H., and Hadley, S. W. 1977. A tripartite model of mental health and therapeutic outcomes: With special reference to negative effects in psychotherapy. *American Psychologist* 32:187–196.

Sue, D. W. 1978. World views and counseling. *Personnel and Guidance Journal* 56:458–462.

————. 1981. *Counseling the culturally different: Theory and practice.* New York: John Wiley and Sons.

Sue, S. 1983. Ethnic minority issues in psychology: A reexamination. *American Psychologist* 38:583–592.

Sundberg, N. D. 1981. Cross-cultural counseling and psychotherapy: A research overview. In A. J. Marsella and P. B. Pedersen (eds.), *Cross-cultural counseling and psychotherapy: Foundations, evaluation, and cultural considerations*, 28–62. Elmsford, NY: Pergamon Press.

Sundberg, N. D., and Gonzalez, L. R. 1981. Cross-cultural and cross-ethnic assessment: Overview and issues. In P. McReynolds (ed.), *Advances in psychological assessment.* Vol. 5. San Francisco: Jossey-Bass.

Szapocznik, J., Santisteban, D., Kurtines, W., Perez-Vidal, A., and Hervis, D. 1983. Bicultural effectiveness training: A treatment intervention for enhancing intercultural adjustment in Cuban-American families. Paper presented at the Ethnicity, Acculturation, and Mental Health among Hispanics Conference. Albuquerque, New Mexico.

Taylor, J. A. 1953. A personality scale of manifest anxiety. *Journal of Abnormal and Social Psychology* 48:285–290.

Teja, J., and Narang, R. 1970. Pattern of incidence of depression in India. *Indian Journal of Psychology* 12:33–39.

Torrey, E. F. 1986. *Witchdoctors and psychiatrists: The common roots of psychotherapy and its future.* New York: Harper and Row.

Triandis, H. C. 1975. Culture training, cognitive complexity and interpersonal attitudes. In R. W. Brislin, S. Bochner, and W. J. Lonner (eds.), *Cross-cultural perspectives on learning.* New York: John Wiley and Sons, Halsted.

————, ed. 1976. *Variations in black and white perceptions of the social environment.* Champaign: University of Illinois Press.

Triandis, H. C., Vassiliou, V., Vassiliou, G., Tanaka, Y., and Shanmugam, A. V. 1972. *The analysis of subjective culture.* New York: John Wiley and Sons.

Trimble, J. E., and Richardson, S. 1982. Locus of control measures among American Indians: Cluster structure analytic characteristics. *Journal of Cross-Cultural Psychology* 13:228–238.

Truax, C., and Carkhuff, R. 1967. *Toward effective counseling and psychotherapy: Training and practice.* Chicago: Aldine.

Watson, D., and Friend, R. 1969. Measurement of social evaluation anxiety. *Journal of Consulting and Clinical Psychology* 43:382–395.

Weed, L. I. 1968. Medical records that guide and teach. *New England Journal of Medicine* 278:593–657.

Weiss, M. G., and Kleinman, A. 1988. Depression in cross-cultural perspective: Developing a culturally informed model. In P. R. Dasen, J. W. Berry, and N. Sartorius (eds.), *Health and cross-cultural psychology: Toward applications.* Newbury Park, CA: Sage Publications.

Williams, J. E., and Best, D. L. 1982. *Measuring sex stereotypes.* Beverly Hills: Sage Publications.

Williams, R. J., and Brown, R. A. 1974. Differences in baseline drinking behavior between New Zealand alcoholics and normal drinkers. *Behavior Research and Therapy* 12:287–294.

Witkin, H. A., and Berry, J. W. 1975. Psychological differentiation in cross-cultural perspective. *Journal of Cross-Cultural Psychology* 6:4–87.

Witkin, H. A., Dyk, R. B., Faterson, H. F., Goodenough, D. R., and Karp, S. A. 1974. *Psychological differentiation.* Potomac, MD: Erlbaum.

Witkin, H. A., and Goodenough, D. R. 1981. *Cognitive styles: Essence and origins.* New York: International Universities Press.

Wober, M. 1974. Towards an understanding of the Kiganda concept of intelligence. In J. W. Berry and P. R. Dasen (eds.), *Culture and cognition.* London: Methuen.

Wolpe, J. 1973. *The practice of behavior therapy.* New York: Pergamon Press.

Woody, R. H. 1972. The counselor-therapist and clinical assessment. In R. H. Woody and J. D. Woody (eds.), *Clinical assessment in counseling and psychotherapy,* 1–29. Englewood Cliffs, NJ: Prentice-Hall.

World Health Organization. 1983. *Depressive disorders in different cultures.* Geneva: World Health Organization.

Zavalloni, M. 1980. Values. In H. C. Triandis and R. W. Brislin (eds.), *Handbook of cross-cultural psychology.* Vol. 5, *Social Psychology.* Boston: Allyn and Bacon.

Zimbardo, P. 1977. *Shyness: What it is and what to do about it.* Reading, MA: Addison-Wesley.

Zimmerman, M., Coryell, W., Corenthal, C., and Wilson, S. 1986. A self-report scale to diagnose major depressive disorder. *Archives of General Psychiatry* 43:1076–1081.

Zung, W. W. K. 1969. A cross-cultural survey of symptoms of depression. *American Journal of Psychiatry* 126:116–121.

13

Research and Research Hypotheses about Effectiveness in Intercultural Counseling

NORMAN D. SUNDBERG
DAVID SUE

Ideas about intercultural counseling—abundant and appealing—must be tested systematically. The aim of this chapter is to clarify these views so that research might proceed more readily. In doing so, we have presented an updated research review of the hypotheses discussed in the previous edition.

In their classic book on personality and culture Kluckhohn and Murray (1953) reminded us of a basic principle: Every person in different ways is like all persons, like some persons, and like no other persons. This mixture of similarities and differences underlies the problems of cross-cultural counseling and psychotherapy. The counselor meeting a client for the first time encounters these three aspects in one person— the universal, the group-specific, and the unique. The counselor, too, has these tripartite characteristics. As such, the counseling pair meets in a particular context, and they interact in a social and physical setting with its own history and relationships. Counseling itself is part of Western culture, though it probably has parallels in every society that has ever existed. "Culture is a great storehouse of ready-made solutions to problems which human animals are wont to encounter" (Kluckhohn and Murray 1953, 54). Counseling is a cultural invention for solving personal problems.

This intermixture of universality, group similarity, and uniqueness is not easily untangled and presents many difficulties for research on intercultural counseling and its effectiveness. Almost all research depends on comparisons—condition with condition, person with person. Thus, research concentrates most on group contrast phenomena and ignores both the universal and the unique. Seldom do we think about what we share with others. Like newspaper reporters, social scientists

The authors gratefully acknowledge the help of editor Joe Trimble and his students, who reviewed the literature on the hypotheses, and Crystal Riley, who read the chapter critically and helpfully.

tend to look for the unusual. Even statistical procedures are designed so that they document probable differences rather than commonalities, and the bias of journals seems to be against articles finding no differences, that is, confirming the null hypothesis. Likewise, dealing with uniqueness has never been a strong point in personality research despite Allport's longtime advocacy (1937) and the continuing concern for individuality by prominent psychologists like Tyler (1978, 1983) and Rosenzweig (1986). It is difficult to strike a balance between the two dangers of being overly concerned with group and cultural differences and being not concerned enough—between overdifferentiation and underdifferentiation. We shall return to these problems of similarity and commonality later in this chapter.

Studies on the effectiveness of intercultural counseling and psychotherapy have been relatively few in number, although more have appeared in recent years. This scarcity raises serious questions about the generalization of claimed principles across ethnic or national groups. The general literature does contain several overviews of ideas, examples, and sources for hypotheses on intercultural counseling research. Representative of these are works done by Abel, Métraux, and Roll (1987), Atkinson (1983), Atkinson and Shein (1986), Draguns (1981), Higginbotham (1984), Marsella and White (1982), Pedersen (1985), and Sue and Zane (1987). Draguns (1981) indicates several areas where research is needed: (1) cross-cultural data on the effectiveness of indigenous therapy techniques, (2) comparisons of the effectiveness of indigenous techniques across different cultures, (3) comparisons of the effectiveness of indigenous versus extraneous therapies within the same culture, and (4) determination of the effectiveness of using indigenous mental health workers on therapy outcome. Little research has been directed toward any of these areas, and almost all of it has been with ethnic groups within the United States.

Here the focus will be on those aspects of one-to-one counseling that are most relevant to intercultural and interethnic work. The crucial questions are these: Does the fact that the client and counselor differ in cultural background make for differences in the effectiveness of the counseling? And what special problems may arise or what special opportunities exist in the process of cross-cultural counseling research? It would seem that the greatest value of doing research under intercultural conditions as opposed to the usual unicultural conditions lies in the possibility for studying the effects of similarity-diversity and for determining how universally applicable are our counseling theories and techniques. The variations in expectations, frames of reference, adaptation processes, and communication style offer excellent natural opportunities for experiments if we can record and analyze our observations effectively.

Hypotheses for Research

A principal purpose of this chapter is to propose hypotheses leading toward research in intercultural counseling. Although we call them hypotheses, it might be better to think of some as "protohypotheses," as they are far from having operational definitions. Many will be similar to those found for any kind of counseling. That similarity is to be expected, since, as we will argue in conclusion, counseling cross-culturally must share much with counseling in general. Smith et al. (1978, 159–160) have expressed a similar view through their listing of the necessary minority counselor characteristics: rapport, empathy, interest, appreciation of the minority culture, understanding of special terms and language, knowledge of the person's community, and awareness of problems of living in a bicultural world.

One basic assumption underlying all of these hypotheses is that each person involved in the intercultural counseling dyad has the three components mentioned at the start of this chapter: universal human components shared with all human beings, group-related components shared with certain other human beings, and unique components particular to each individual.

Another assumption is that there is an optimum number of shared components important for the effectiveness of the counseling interaction. The optima for different content areas are yet to be determined. For instance, the counseling pair must share some way of communicating verbally or nonverbally, but beyond a certain level of command of the language it is unlikely that further knowledge adds much to effectiveness in counseling. Knowing 50,000 words of German may add little to a counseling dialogue in German beyond what would be said if one only knew 20,000 words.

A third assumption is that the purposes of counseling or psychotherapy are to be found in systems away from the client-counselor interaction itself. It could be argued that a rewarding experience in the dyadic session is sufficient in itself; the actors would not expect more than what happens at a good party and would leave the session with a sense of enjoyment. One could even argue that society should provide such opportunities for entertainment and encounter, but such an objective is not usually what clients, counselors, or taxpayers expect from a counseling service. The purpose of the artificial counseling setting is to affect either the personal system of the client or the interactional systems of the client outside the counseling session. There should be transsituational effects. In many cases counseling activity by itself must go beyond the office-based dyadic interaction. (For further discussion of assumptions and systems-possibility-developmental theory, see Sundberg, Taplin, and Tyler 1983.)

The following is a series of five areas important for research in intercultural counseling. Each will present some relevant hypotheses—15 in total. Before stating each hypothesis, we will marshal the arguments and evidence for it.

Mutuality of Purposes and Helping Expectations

The process of arriving at expectations for what is to be gained from counseling is particularly important in intercultural work. These intercultural expectations are on a continuum with those in same-culture contacts, but such expectations will be influenced by cultural factors. The first hypothesis has to do with the symbolic and practical meaning of entry into the counseling system itself. In addition to individual motives for contacting the counseling service, the counselor should be aware of the socialization of the person who is seeking help. It is likely that individual members of different cultural and ethnic groups vary in their willingness to come to strangers for help and in their sense of comfort with the bureaucratic aura of services. (Outreach services are designed "to go to the people," but even they must be concerned with the atmosphere of entry.)

Hispanics and Asian Americans prefer family, relatives, or community resources for assistance for emotional problems. Mental illness is considered to be a cultural stigma (Juarez 1985; Root 1985). Webster and Fretz (1978) indicate that American college students of several ethnic backgrounds (Asian, black, and white) all tend to prefer family or relatives as the first source of assistance with both educational-vocational and emotional problems. They go to the university counseling center only as a third choice for educational-vocational problems and as a fifth choice for emotional problems. Ethnic differences were not strong in this study, but other studies (e.g., Andrulis 1977; Sue and Sue 1974; Sue and Kirk 1975) have shown significant differences in usage of counseling by different minority groups; it would seem that research in non-American settings or with non-American populations might show greater divergencies in service usage. Jackson (1976) has argued that there is an African genesis in the attitudes of blacks toward seeking help; the underlying worldview is unlike the dichotomous Western mode of thought and bias toward rationality and quantification. Jackson suggests an authoritative reaching out to bring in blacks with problems. Higginbotham's excellent reviews (1977, 1984) of client expectations also emphasize the need to understand why clients come for services. Degree of acculturation among minority groups affects acceptance of majority American attitudes and practices; for instance, Connor (1975) concluded from a study of third-generation Japanese Americans that they had moved toward general American norms, and Buriel

(1975), Knight and Kagan (1977), and Knight et al. (1978) found that later generations of Mexican Americans approximate American norms more than did earlier generations in regard to competitiveness and field independence. Atkinson's reviews (1985) emphasize that use of mental health services varies within ethnic groups depending on group affiliation and preferences for ethnically similar counselors. Goldstein's work (reviewed by Lorion 1978) emphasizes that therapist expectations are critical at the start of work with lower-income patients. Since the early part of counseling involves the establishment of rapport and trust, the counselor has to be particularly attuned to the client's feelings about meeting with a strange expert and attitudes toward revealing private emotions. One protohypothesis coming from a review of these several reports and research projects can be stated as follows:

1. *Entry into the counseling system will be affected by cultural background, acculturation, and socialization toward seeking help; counselor awareness of such cultural screening—the likely feelings and symbolic meaning of help seeking —will enhance the effectiveness of the counseling program.*

Attitudes toward seeking help are also a factor in whether or not an individual will seek counseling. Vietnamese refugees have less positive attitudes toward seeking professional psychological help, are less likely to recognize the need for help and more concerned with the stigma attached to counseling, and are less confident in being helped by mental health professionals than Anglo-Americans (Atkinson, Ponterotto, and Sanchez 1984). Such attitudes decrease the probability that this group will enter into the counseling system. Idowu (1985) reports that few Nigerian students in the United States seek counseling because they are suspicious of the counseling process and question its usefulness. Entry into the counseling system is also influenced by the degree of acculturation. Less acculturated Mexican Americans make little use of outpatient mental health facilities. The drastic underutulization is hypothesized to be possibly because of factors such as a lack of familiarity of the services, reluctance to enter psychotherapy, or other barriers (Wells et al. 1987). Southeast Asian refugees, who are at very high risk for psychiatric problems, often do not seek mental health services because of their perception that their disorder is physical in nature (Mollica et al. 1987). Some medical agencies have found that it is more useful to start working on the more readily admitted somatic symptoms than to help patients gradually see connections between past events and present feelings. High respect for medical doctors also may be useful with many patients in getting acceptance (C. Riley, personal communication, May 1987).

Minority members coming into counseling may unconsciously see themselves as threatened in a one-down power relationship; for instance, the black client may be ambivalent about the white counselor because whites symbolize oppression. Furthermore, the "helpee role" will be related to how psychological problems or disorders are viewed in the client's culture—how passive one is to be in the presence of the knowledgeable or powerful helper. Understanding parallel or similar roles in the culture—going to a healer, presenting a problem to a member of the family—will help the counselor understand the client from a contrast culture.

A second hypothesis has to do with congruence of purposes, one of the primary concerns of all counseling. Cultural differences in expectations are likely to create incongruence, and the greater the incongruence, the more difficult it will be to establish trust, confidence, and mutual attraction. One of the ideas frequently mentioned in regard to indigenous healing is the manner in which the curer meets the expectations of the "patient" (e.g., Carstairs 1955; Torrey 1986). Among those expectations common acceptance of goals would be particularly important. The second hypothesis is as follows:

2. *The more similar the expectations of the intercultural client and counselor in regard to the goals of counseling, the more effective the counseling will be.*

Not only in regard to goals but also to techniques, process, and relationship, the client and the counselor have expectations that are implicit and explicit before their first meeting and that develop further as the counseling sessions progress. Socialization for dependency, customs of restricting personal communication to the family circle, and attitudes toward social hierarchy are relevant. Another important variable is the symbolic nature of the counselor (as priest, healer, parental figure, scientist, or outcast) in the culture of origin or the culture of residence. Grey (1965) suggested, in discussing his experiences counseling in India, that counselors should be trained to cope with the client's expectations about authority and decision making. Benfari (1969) found that primitive societies that foster a large degree of childhood dependence had person-oriented healers, whereas societies that socialized for low dependence did not. Atkinson, Maruyama, and Matsui (1978) found that directive counselors were rated as more credible and approachable than nondirective ones by Asian Americans. Similar preferences for a directive counseling approach were found in American Indians (Dauphinais, Dauphinais, and Rowe 1981), foreign students (Alexander et al. 1981), and low-income ethnic minorities (De la Cancela 1985). Interestingly enough, however, a study involving white and Asian-American social workers indicated that both groups noted a nondirective style more effective than a directive counseling style in working with Asian clients (Mokuau 1987). In another study involving female black American, Puerto Rican, and Anglo-American analogue clients, Folensbee, Draguns, and Danish (1986) found that all three groups responded more favorably with an affective approach than one involving closed questions. These two studies seem to cast more doubts on the view that minorities respond more positively to a directive rather than a nondirective or affective counseling approach. Aronson and Overall (1966) and Overall and Aronson (1963) found that low-income patients expected stronger, more supportive therapy than comparison groups; these findings are questioned by Lorion (1978), although other studies did find the lowest socioeconomic status level to have less understanding of therapy than others. Low-income people are not necessarily of a different culture, but it is striking how often findings about Americans in poverty approximate the findings of minority and Third World situations, perhaps because the power imbalances are similar. Related to power considerations is the orientation toward locus of control—whether within the person or in the surrounding environment; Sue (1978) presents some interesting hypotheses about differing cultural worldviews regarding internal and external attributions of control and responsibility; oppression occurs when the counselor blindly imposes another view on the client. Expectations are also affected by mass media; the almost universal availability of television may be bringing about a new commonality of expectations about helper-helpee relationships and procedures (Wahl 1976). Tan (1967) found that both American and foreign students tended to be more authoritarian than were graduate students in counseling training in two American universities; foreign students who had been in the United States longer were more similar to American students.

In a study of international students (40 Americans, 39 Chinese from Hong Kong, 35 Africans, and 36 Iranians) it was found that the foreign students expected a counselor to be an authority figure and to offer structure and direction in counseling (Yuen and Tinsley 1981). Szapocznik et al. (1978) indicated that among Cubans in Miami a greater value was placed on hierarchical relations than among Anglos; consequently, therapists were expected to be more effective if they brought the families into the treatment center and in general exerted strong control. Another variable is self-disclosure (e.g., Jourard 1971), a procedure that would seem to be basic to most mainstream American counseling approaches. Because of its seeming importance for counseling, self-disclosure deserves more extensive cross-cultural research attention. It is likely, however, that self-disclosure, much vaunted by the dominant professional subculture, may itself be culturally interactive; there are positive features to such defense mechanisms as denial, as Lazarus (1979) says, and it seems eminently reasonable that revealing one's problems in counseling may not be appropriate for some people in some situations.) In any case, congruence and understanding seem important as stated by the following hypothesis:

3. *Of special importance in intercultural counseling effectiveness is the degree of congruence between counselor and client in their orientations toward dependency, authority, power, openness of communication, and other special relationships inherent in counseling.*

Common understanding of purposes is more important in some instances than in others. A counselor could help someone from another culture with a minor problem more easily than he could help someone from his own culture with a serious problem. Minor problems are more likely to be alleviated by the simple provision of information, or they may just "go away." The clarity of communication is likely to relate to the effectiveness of the contact. The more the "problem" can be identified clearly and targeted, the more likely both parties will be satisfied with the results. This thinking leads to another hypothesis:

4. *The more the aims and desires of the client can be appropriately simplified and formulated as objective behavior or information (such as specific tasks or university course requirements), the more effective the intercultural counseling will be.*

This hypothesis suggests that the intercultural counselor should be prepared to use multiple channels for communication. Brochures, printed explanations, graphic portrayals, and films of procedures for handling problems may be of much more value in intercultural counseling than in ordinary counseling. The counselor may also need to teach the other-culture client specific skills for handling specific situations. It should be noted, however, that the simplification and use of supplementary materials should only be used when relevant to the client's needs and not as an escape from facing crucial emotional issues.

Montijo (1985) emphasizes the importance of a problem-solving approach and indicates that the counselor should first deal with specific and concrete treatment of goals before dealing with more complex issues. The usefulness of formulating specific objectives and tasks was a reason why Asian-American mental health professionals felt that behavioral approaches were useful in working with an immigrant population (Stumphauzer and Davis 1983).

Developing the Counselor's Intercultural Understanding and Communication Skills

In any system, but particularly in the counseling interaction, communication is important. A sensitivity to what the other person is trying to

convey verbally and nonverbally and an ability to respond to that communication are the cornerstones of counseling and psychotherapy. In
the intercultural context we can assume there is always some language
problem. Early language learning seems to be related to expression of
feelings. Achebe (1960, 45) illustrates this in his novel about a young
Nigerian who has just returned from college in London.

> Obi was beginning to feel sleepy and his thoughts turned more and more
> on the erotic. He said words in his mind that he could not say out loud
> even when he was alone. Strangely enough, all the words were in his
> mother tongue. He could say any English word, no matter how dirty, but
> some Ibo words simply would not proceed from his mouth. It was no
> doubt his early training that operated this censorship, English words filter-
> ing through because they were learned later in life.

The book *Cross-Cultural Anxiety* by Spielberger and Diaz-Guerrero
(1976) presents reviews of language learning that corroborate Achebe's
characterization. Saying taboo words in one's mother tongue is more
anxiety provoking than pronouncing them in a second language. Pitta,
Marcos, and Alpert (1978) argue that expression of emotions is more
spontaneous in the first language but more intellectual and less free in
the second language. In any case, the counselor needs to be sensitive to
preferred and natural language qualities and should know something of
the linguistic socialization of the client. Thus, another hypothesis follows:

5. *The more personal and emotion laden the counseling becomes, the more the client
   will rely on words and concepts learned early in life and the more helpful it will
   be for the counselor to be knowledgeable about socialization in the client's culture.*

The counselor's learning could come about before or during the
counseling sessions. Obviously, the counselor needs to be open to learning. Counselors who are open and able to "relate to their client's host
culture" are better equipped to function in an effective manner (Pedersen 1985). Some studies have shown that prejudicial attitudes are associated with ineffective counseling (e.g., Millikan 1965; Millikan and
Patterson 1967). Wampold, Casas, and Atkinson (1981) found that
Anglo-American counselors are more likely to be influenced by stereotypes than ethnic minority counselors. Sometimes prior knowledge is an
impediment; the counselor may think he knows more than he does, and
the result is a less individualized approach.

Sue and Zane (1987) point out that cultural knowledge is often
applied in a stereotypic fashion without considering within-group differ-

ences by mental health professionals. A report of a California survey (Landers 1987) indicated that counselors taking a client's cultural background into account tend to minimize significant problems. Of course, there are many advising and guidance situations in which a large amount of knowledge of cultural background is not necessary; for example, if the focus is on a sharply defined financial or academic information problem, detailed examination may confuse the issue or alienate the client.

In some situations (e.g., with non-English-speaking refugees) an interpreter may be necessary. Anyone who has used an interpreter has questioned the adequacy of translation. A short question by the counselor may be followed by a mystifyingly long interpretation. Kinzie (1972) points out problems with interpreters from his experiences in Malaysia but concluded they have proven their worth. In later work with Southeast Asian refugees he uses a trained counselor of the same ethnic background sitting in on the session (D. Kinzie, personal communication, 1986; Kinzie and Manson 1983). Interpreters in counseling sessions serve not only as translators but also as informants to explain a client's cultural associations and meanings and to provide training.

It must be remembered that interpreters are also influenced by cultural norms and values and may be reluctant to ask about material considered disrespectful, related to sex, or about suicidal or homocidal thoughts (Ishisaka, Nguyen, and Okimoto 1985). Marcos (1979) found that Chinese- and Spanish-speaking interpreters often made distortions of the client's responses through omissions, substitutions, and changes of focus. The counselor should also know the potential effect of differences in the social status or ethnic position between client and interpreter.

In general, learning from the client about his or her background is a necessary part of counseling. In an interview survey of counselors' successes and failures in working with other-culture clients, Bengur (1979) found that the willingness to learn and to request information about practices relevant to the client's problems came up repeatedly as a helpful counselor attribute. If at all possible, the counselor should also become acquainted with the living conditions, customs, and celebrations in the community of the client. Many clients are very pleased that one wishes to learn about their culture.

Counselor sensitivity—the ability to place oneself in the role of the client and to empathize with the client's feelings and environmental context—is crucial. In intercultural work the counselor must be sensitive to the meanings and connotations of language, both in the client's culture and in the contextual culture surrounding the interaction. Words carry different emotional charges and bring different images to persons of different cultures. Likewise, nonverbal aspects of communication enter into the understanding of feedback and reinforcement patterns. Americans often misinterpret as "no" the slight twist of the head that in India signifies "yes" or "agreed"; in bazaars Americans have been known to walk away thinking a haggling proposal has been rejected until the shopkeeper calls them back. Relevant to this illustration, Rubin (1976) cataloged a wide variety of ways to say "no" in different cultures. Hall (1966, 1979) has pointed out that Arabs are much more likely than are northern Europeans to push and touch in public, that is, to invade the "personal bubble" of strangers. Such information is of importance to both client and counselor in interpreting experience in a foreign culture. Within the counseling session itself the study of nonverbal aspects of movement and use of space could prove to be an interesting contribution to basic knowledge as some scientists suggest (Birdwhistell 1970; Boucher 1979; Hall 1966).

Different cultures are also likely to vary in free associations. For instance, one study (Shaffer, Sundberg, and Tyler 1969) found that samples of adolescents in India listed many more words related to food than those of Americans; another study (Bates, Sundberg, and Tyler 1970) showed that Indians reveal much less aggressive and humorous content in drawings than do Americans. Tanaka-Matsumi and Marsella (1976), in their study of associations to words for depression, found that Japanese nationals gave more external and somatic responses, such as "rain" or "headache," whereas Americans, including Japanese Americans, associated more internal mood states, such as "loneliness." The Vietnamese conception of depression included descriptions such as "being angry," "feeling desperate," and "having a feeling of going crazy." Kinzie et al. (1982) state that the lack of correspondence between Western and Vietnamese conceptualization of depression indicates that different constructs may be involved. Johnson (1973) found that foreign students varied widely in the number and kinds of adjectives they used to characterize Americans and other nationalities. The amount of feedback from clients to counselors or among fellow counseling group members in discussion groups is affected by culture. Ogawa and Weldon (1972) reported, for instance, that Japanese Americans respond less to other speakers than do Caucasian Americans, and they attributed the difference to the Japanese norm of *enryo,* shyness or restraint.

Despite the many problems inherent in intercultural communication, one must remember that some immigrants have been highly successful psychotherapists and counselors, for example, many of those psychologists and psychiatrists who fled the Nazis in the 1930s and 1940s. Their success may, however, demonstrate certain commonalities in Western culture as well as a refined sensitivity to other persons. One likely way in which intercultural awareness and empathy in counselors might be increased would be to study the arts of other places (Adinolfi 1971), especially drama, films, and novels, since they often deal with intense emotionality. There are a number of models for multicultural training in counseling (Johnson 1987).

A research project that illustrates well the effective use of culturally sensitive material is the one by Costantino, Malgady, and Rogler (1986). They developed what they called "cuento therapy" by using Puerto Rican folktales as models of adaptive behavior. Working with small groups of high-risk children and their mothers, they found reduced anxiety and aggression and improved intellectual ability as compared with controls.

An obvious hypothesis that arises from these considerations is as follows:

6. *The effectiveness of intercultural counseling will be enhanced by the counselor's general sensitivity to communications, both verbal and nonverbal, and by a knowledge of communication styles in other cultures.*

Reviewing the research, Smith (1966, 177) stated that "most of what we have learned about people we have learned informally. The sensitive people are simply those who have learned the most. The most sensitive person is the most highly motivated, most open to new experiences, most ready to participate in learning about them, and most able to assess the adequacy of what he has learned." Communication sensitivity may be related to language-learning ability (Sundberg 1966), to the sex of the counselor (i.e., women are reputedly more aware of interpersonal nuances), to knowledge and experience in at least one or two cultures other than one's own, to interest and motivation for understanding other cultures, to skill in paraphrasing and reflection of feeling in interviews, and, with specific clients, to some similarity of early experiences, socioeconomic background, and occupational experiences. The likely importance of many of these relationships suggests the use of peers and co-nationals for counseling.

Several reviews of client-counselor differences summarized by Atkinson (1985) present a mixed picture. Atkinson (1983) and Atkinson and Schein (1986) found support for preference among blacks for black counselors. However, little support for an ethnically similar counselor was found among American Indians, Asian Americans, and Hispanic Americans. Most studies indicating a racial preference among blacks did not control for within-group differences involving factors such as level of acculturation and racial identity. Preference for a black counselor has been found to be a function of the stage of cultural identity (Morten and Atkinson 1983; Parham and Helms 1981; Ponterotto, Anderson, and Grieger 1986). In one study, Atkinson, Furlong, and

Williams (1986) found that the five most preferred counselor characteristics were more education; similar attitudes and values; older, similar
personality; and same ethnicity—in this order. Atkinson and his colleagues concluded that preferences for other counselor characteristics
may be more important than for a racially similar counselor and that
more research is needed to examine within-group differences.

Training programs aimed at expanding the awareness and intercultural response repertoire of counselors, such as those of Pedersen (1977,
1978) and Johnson (1987) seem promising. These programs not only
alert the counselor to different assumptions and problems in the contrast culture but they also facilitate sensitivity to the unspoken biases of
the counselor's culture. Analogue studies by Berman (1979) and Woods
and Zimmer (1976) demonstrate how counseling skills and verbal
operant conditioning might be studied in mixed racial interactions. The
latter study, incidentally, found no significant black-white differences in
conditionability, but Berman found that blacks tended to use more
active expression skills, whereas whites used more attending skills.
Selection as well as training should be considered for multicultural
counseling competence. Presumably a person's experience and interest
demonstrated by previous close and favorable cross-cultural contacts
would relate to counseling effectiveness. Lorion (1978) discusses various forms of therapist preparation for work with low-income clients,
many ideas of which would apply to cross-cultural situations. These
considerations lead to the following proposal:

7. *Specific background and training in cross-cultural interactions similar to the
counseling one and an understanding of the day-to-day living problems in other
relevant cultures as compared with their own will enhance the effectiveness of
intercultural counselors.*

Though that hypothesis would seem intuitively to be correct, its
actual testing will likely reveal many subtle problems. The quality of
experience and training and not just the quantity is of importance.

Developing the Client's Intercultural Attitudes and Skills

The other side of the coin in counseling is the preparation and development of the client so that he or she may participate effectively in the
counseling interaction and the counseling program. Expectations and
purposes have already been mentioned. The counselor must also give
consideration to teaching specific skills to clients and to utilizing relevant attitudes and skills already present in the client's repertoire.

Although it is generally advisable "to meet the client where she or he
is" by special outreach programs or by procedures that are congruent
with cultural expectations, sometimes it is not possible to adapt the

activities of a busy counseling service to the style of interaction to which the client is accustomed. The counselor may have to work with the client in developing an understanding of the counselor's point of view and in preparing for participation in the counseling process. With some clients it may be necessary to explain the counseling process carefully, with frequent use of such techniques as paraphrasing and perception checks. For intense counseling the client may need to be taught to speak what is on her or his mind in a relaxed manner, in other words, to develop the skills required to play the counseling role. With lower-class clients Strupp and Bloxom (1973) reported the successful use of a role-induction film for psychotherapy, and Heitler (1973) found that an "anticipatory socialization interview" produced marked improvement in group therapy. These investigators were teaching clients what to expect in counseling and how to participate in the process. Lorion's (1978) review of research found pretreatment preparation for therapy with disadvantaged patients to be consistently favorable; he points out that this pretreatment for clients needs to be paralleled by the preparation of therapists for work with special clienteles.

Lambert and Lambert (1984) also found that immigrants who were given information about the course of psychotherapy, appropriate client and therapist behaviors, and an explanation of typical problems encountered in therapy, attended and completed more sessions than a control group who were not given a role induction. In addition, the experimental group saw the therapist as significantly more interested and accepting and perceived themselves as more satisfied with therapy and changing more significantly. The hypothesis that grows out of these considerations is as follows:

8. *The less familiar the client is with the counseling process, the more the counselor or the counseling program will need to instruct the client in the skills of communication, decision making, and transfer to outside situations.*

In the development of skills for survival in a bicultural or multicultural world, assessment tools have come under considerable recent attack. This extensive field will not be covered in this review, but readers would do well to note that special cautions must be applied in the use of tests (see Lonner and Ibrahim's chapter in this book and discussions in Smith et al. 1978 and Sue and Sue, in press). Probably entirely new procedures need to be developed to improve the understanding of minority and cross-cultural functioning. Of particular importance would be assessment of communication, including the understanding of typical counseling techniques (verbal and nonverbal) and assessment of acculturation to the dominant society. Both of these assessments should help in determining the character of the counseling plan.

Cultural Considerations of the Client's Arenas of Action

So far we have been looking mainly at characteristics of the client and counselor and their interactions. "Off-stage" characteristics—the external environment, daily life as it pertains to intercultural considerations —also deserve attention here. In this regard four factors are salient: cultural assumptions about choice and decision making, the client's reference groups, the process of adapting to intercultural stress, and choice of arenas of action.

Early family influences, religious groups, schools, and mass media inculcate cultural values, many of which are implicit and go unquestioned. Among these is a set of assumptions about choice and possibilities, that is, strategy and openness in searching for possibilities, priority for alternatives, and the responsibility and manner of making life decisions. Cultures vary in the emphasis placed on individual autonomy and on parental responsibility. For instance, in traditional India, as Sundberg et al. (1969) have demonstrated, the father is typically the authority who makes the choices for his adolescent children's future occupation and marriage. Knowledge of the constraints and opportunities in Third World countries is important if one is to assist many clients in career planning. Yeh (1972) demonstrates the family components involved in diagnosing and treating depression and paranoia in Chinese students studying abroad. He notes that paranoia may be treated better after the student returns home. The place of treatment and the cultural meaning of the physical environment may be more important considerations in some cultures than in others; for instance, McShane (1987) demonstrates the importance of geography and rural settings in American Indian mental health. Beliefs about the timing of life's events are critical. For instance, Hindu beliefs emphasize that certain roles should be taken up at various stages in one's life, culminating in a withdrawal from the world—something quite different from Western beliefs. Within the United States there are differences among ethnic groups in the timing expectations about marriage and having children. Timing-related customs have a direct bearing on the immediate counseling interaction as well. This includes the keeping of appointments and the degree of punctuality, as well as the length of acquaintance time before business agreements are reached (Hall and Whyte 1960). A hypothesis (which follows the primary injunction for cross-cultural therapy by Torrey [1972]) may be stated as follows:

9. *The effectiveness of intercultural counseling will be increased by mutual knowledge of the values and assumptive framework of the culture of the client's origin in relation to the cultures of the present and future fields of action.*

The matter of knowledge, however, requires caution. A little information sometimes can be a hindrance if it leads to "typecasting," or stereotyping, or misinterpretations. Greater knowledge may help only in understanding groups and not necessarily individuals. More helpful would be a learning attitude toward the most relevant intercultural phenomena. A learning attitude is closely related to sensitivity, as mentioned in an earlier hypothesis. Several of the books already mentioned could be used in training for knowledge of other cultures, and intercultural learning propensities could be defined operationally by attitudes and problem-solving tests (e.g., Triandis 1976, chap. 2). Of incidental interest here is the research by Matarazzo and Wiens (1977) with police applicants; the researchers found no overlap between blacks and whites on scores for knowledge of black dialect terms. Besides the obvious need to hire black policemen who understand the dialect, these results suggest that white policemen who were relatively familiar with black dialect might be selected for cross-cultural work.

Another significant element in understanding a client is acquaintance with and use of the references groups that the client considers important. With whom does the person identify? Whose judgments about worth and status are accepted? Who will be important to the client in the future? In traditional cultures the family, the neighborhood, and the caste or clan are important. In modern urban settings professional or work groups exert greater influence, and the nuclear family plays a more central role than does the extended family. Being highly select, foreign students on an American campus are more likely to fit into the modern and international setting than the traditional one (see Gordon 1964, 224–232). Some are eager to become a part of the reference group of Americans or of other students rather than to conform to home country norms. As is common knowledge on large campuses, Stecklein et al. (1971) found that foreign students are most likely to seek out other foreign students to help them solve personal problems, and Antler (1970) indicated that commiseration with co-nationals is more important than with Americans. Boyd et al. (1979) describe training for psychological support groups for minority college students. Our experience indicates that three norms or reference groups for foreign students should be taken into account: the host country (e.g., America), the native country, and those who try to relate to both "worlds"; good indexes for deciding which group is strongest for the student seem to be language usage and number of friends in each category. Likewise, with noncollege minority clients in the United States acculturation is probably best evaluated by language usage in the home and extent of interaction at work and leisure with people of the majority culture.

Counselors may find that they can use co-nationals or "co-ethnics" of the client either as consultants, co-counselors, or peer counselors. The counselor should recognize potential pitfalls, however, since co-nationals may have their own disabling biases and may impede the client's adaptation to the host culture and eventual independence. In spite of these cautions, a well-chosen, well-trained co-national is likely to be most helpful. The influence of persons of similar background relates to the strength of identification with the ethnic or cultural group.

Sanchez and Atkinson (1983) found that the degree of commitment to Mexican or Anglo culture influenced preference for counselor ethnicity and willingness to use counseling. Subjects who had strong commitment to Anglo culture were less concerned about seeing an ethnically similar counselor and had more favorable attitudes toward counseling than did those with a strong orientation to Mexican-American culture. Females consistently expressed more favorable attitudes toward counseling than did males. The review by Rogler et al. (1987) also emphasizes the importance of assessing degree of biculturalism in Hispanic Americans. Parham and Helms (1981) hypothesized that there is a relationship between black students' cultural identity and preference for an ethnically similar counselor. At the preencounter stage of racial identity (devaluation of black culture) blacks would prefer a white counselor, but during the encounter and immersion stages (increasing identity with black culture) a black counselor would be preferred. These several foregoing considerations lead to the following hypothesis:

10. *Intercultural counseling is enhanced by the knowledge of the client's degree of identification with the relevant cultures and the use of cultural reference group members who are most important for the client.*

How an individual adapts to another culture has long been of interest to anthropologists and psychologists. The overused term *culture shock* signifies a difficult period of depression and anxiety that follows the initial enthusiasm of the first few weeks in a new and strange country. The newcomer is not yet able to control or predict the new system. In addition, he or she may be physically ill and unable to find familiar food and material comforts. Locke and Feinsod (1982) feel that stress is produced by the inability to perceive cultural cues and norms. Students are often homesick and lack social supports. Traveling professors and business people usually suffer a change of status in moving to a new country. (Sometimes, however, when they are treated with much deference and have servants, they enjoy an increase in status.) Zain (1965), in a survey of foreign students, found a U-shaped adjustment curve, with a high initial adjustment for those who had been in the United States less than six months, a high adjustment again after three years, but poorer adjustment in between. Some groups such as Cambodian refugees, many of whom suffer from post–traumatic stress syndrome, have an extremely difficult time adjusting (Kinzie et al. 1984). The counselor must be sensitive to basic physical needs and must assist the client in getting in touch with others who have successfully gone through the initial adjustment.

During a foreign sojourn, differences between host and home values and mores are likely to become apparent. The counselor must think through the ethical implications of challenging a foreign student's culture-related values. Young male foreign clients in America mention their difficulty in understanding cues about the sexual availability of American girls: they see their revealing clothes, their apparently provocative behavior, and the portrayals of femininity on American television and in films. During youth and young adulthood, identity and values are forming. With the loss of familiar social supports some young people become disoriented. Another aspect for both foreign and minority (and perhaps even most) students is the tension and potential for separation from origins. Rodriguez (1979) poignantly describes the bittersweet pride of poorly educated Mexican-American parents as their child advances in college but grows apart from the family. Older graduate students and sojourners may have their immediate families with them; spouses and children may then be exposed to cultural stress, and the whole family will be a potential concern for counseling.

It is likely that persons who have previously made a successful transition from one environment to another—from a small town to a city or from one country to another—will be better able to deal with other change and culture shock. This problem of adaptation to a new environment applies also to reentry problems to one's own native land. Brislin and Van Buren (1974) have reported a program specifically aimed at training international sojourners to "worry" constructively and to expect problems when they return home. The counselor, in the role of community organizer, can do something about the orientation of students for both entry and return. With all these considerations in mind, the following hypothesis is proposed:

11. *The effectiveness of intercultural counseling is increased by counselor awareness of the process of adaptation to the stress and identity confusion of moving from one culture to another (system boundary crossing) and by consideration of the skills required to gain mastery over the new system.*

A major factor in counseling for the "arena of future action" is whether or not the client intends to stay in the host culture. Sometimes the purpose of counseling is to help a foreign student client make a choice between remaining or returning. There are probably many personality differences between remainers and returners, especially if these persons have come from high-contrast cultures such as those found in

most of the Asian and African countries. (Some of the same considerations pertain to in-country ethnic groups—for instance, for a black
deciding to work in an all-white company or in a black community.)

Most counseling will be oriented toward the short-range problems of
the client. In a college situation the arena of future action will likely center on immediate problems dealing with language, academic work, and
finances (Benson and Miller 1966). Johnson's research (1971) with
international clients led him to conclude that these persons should be
thought of as students first, not foreigners. The study found international students' morale was high during vacations and low during
examinations; the investigators concluded that, contrary to popular
belief, foreign students have greater difficulty in adapting to academic
work, not to American culture. The following hypothesis is proposed:

12. *Effective counseling requires a consideration of both the present living situation
and the future arena of action, its focus determined by the goals and priorities of
the client and an exploration of the bicultural or multicultural nature of these
situations.*

Universality, Group Commonality, and Uniqueness in Intercultural Counseling

Counseling is a social institution in America and Europe. Every culture
probably has some method for handling individual problems that are
not easily solved by the social structure. Frank (1974a) and Torrey
(1986) found common elements between helping procedures in modern
and premodern societies. Torrey's four pancultural commonalities are
most widely noted: (1) shared worldview leading to labeling of the disorder (the "Rumpelstiltskin effect"), (2) benevolent personal qualities in
the therapist or healer, (3) the patient's expectations for being helped,
and (4) an emerging sense of mastery. Certain specific techniques, such
as catharsis and interpretation, are also held in common over wide variations in culture. Draguns (1975) adds another characteristic, that of
therapy as a universally special, intense, and removed experience in
high contrast to daily living. Frank (1974b) points out that the locale, or
setting, usually is clearly designated as a place of healing or help. Counseling and similar processes serve as a refuge from society. In previous
interaction with the surrounding system, the client has lost out in the
judgment of self (regarding sociocultural expectations) or in the judgment of society. He or she is out of step. The counselor typically provides a socially approved antithesis to mainstream society, offering a
confidential, noncritical acceptance in which the client can talk about
weaknesses and dependence and about taboo topics, such as hate, sex,
and egotism.

Dealing with clients' anxiety is a widespread problem. Pedersen (1981) uses a training model that helps the trainees reduce their own defensiveness and to recognize and feel the anxiety of minority clients. In addition, Henderson (1979) and Sue and Sue (1977) indicate the importance of flexibility in choice of approach and techniques in response to clients. Other qualities important in counseling include warmth and acceptance (Rogers 1975), respect (Smith 1977), empathy (Gladstein 1983), and trust (Heppner and Heeacker 1983). Behavior therapists also talk of the importance of positive reinforcement as the client moves toward target behaviors. Well-designed studies by various investigators (e.g., Zeiss, Lewinsohn, and Munoz 1979) have shown that several major kinds of therapy produce improvements over those found with a control group but that the therapies do not differ significantly in effectiveness; so-called nonspecific factors are the effective agents. Bandura (1977, 1982) argues that the essential ingredient in all therapeutic change is the client's increased sense of self-efficacy; this view reflects that of Frank (1974b), who emphasizes demoralization as the root cause of disorder and restoration of a sense of mastery or competence as the key element in change. Feelings and needs of people seem to be the same around the world, though the surface behavior, lifestyles, and communication patterns certainly differ. Butt and Beiser (1987) in a 13-nation survey of well-being over the adult lifespan found high consistency; for instance, those over 50 were more satisfied with life and were more religious than those under 25 in all countries. It may be that an analysis of commonalities in different theories will also lead to the discovery of commonalities across cultures in the helping process. Such potential universality remains to be carefully specified and measured. All of these ongoing considerations of commonality across clients and across theories lead to the following hypothesis:

13. *Despite great differences in cultural contexts, in language, and in the implicit theory of counseling process, a majority of the important elements of intercultural counseling are common across cultures and clients. These elements include such counselor characteristics as a tolerance for anxiety in the client, a manifest positive flexibility in response to the client, a reasonable confidence in one's information and belief system, and an interest in the client as a person.*

Just as there are universal processes that will be shown by research, there are counseling techniques or tactics that may be especially useful within a given culture. Kiev (1969, 1972) and Torrey (1986), while identifying some universals, also question the transcultural generalizability of Western psychiatric practices (Torrey warns of "mental imperialism"). There may be several principles for differentiating between cultures. Prince (1969), for instance, posits that cultures favoring internal controls promote insight-oriented therapy and cultures relying on external controls prefer more directive therapies. The use of charms and magic incantations to cure diseases would seem ridiculous to most Westerners, but their use is very helpful in certain cultures. (We prefer colored pills, comfortable offices, and other trappings.) Western professionals working in non-Western settings differ in the degree to which they believe mental health practice should be bent to meet local belief systems (Draguns 1975). Ho (1985) has found distinct differences between Hong Kong and the West in clinical applications; much of this he attributes to the individualism of the United States with its Calvinistic traditions in comparison with the collectivism and family closeness of the Chinese.

Some have indicated that counseling may have to be altered to be structured and directive for specific ethnic groups and low-income ethnic minorities. Cuento therapy for Puerto Rican children (Costantino, Malgady, and Rogler 1986) was specifically designed to make use of folktales and appears to be effective. This kind of approach may be the next wave in cross-cultural research. However, Sue and Zane (1987) assert that the development of culture-specific techniques may fail to address the problem of within-group differences. The difference between the universal and the culture-specific is likely to parallel the difference between abstract general laws of learning and problem solving and the specific content, tactics, and symbols used in studies of specific languages. The common distinction between etic (transcultural or universal) and emic (in-culture) characteristics is relevant to this issue (Berry 1969; Lonner 1979). This obvious hypothesis may be stated:

14. *Culture-specific modes of counseling will be found that work more effectively with certain cultural and ethnic groups than with others.*

Finally, an overriding caution in counseling is that the counselor should not treat the client as a "foreigner" or as a "stereotype" but as an individual person with his or her own unique background and own personal resources. Roll, Millen, and Martinez (1980, 165) point out "there are some ways in which any particular Chicano is like all other Chicanos and there are some ways in which a particular Chicano is like no other Chicano." Prince (1976) has stated the principle that for the most part people heal themselves spontaneously. On their own they seek special, helpful situations provided by the culture, such as conversations with friends, religious ceremonies, cathartic expression in sports, and in some cultures dissociated trance states. People will often have their own individual therapeutic procedures, for example, their pleasant activities to counteract depression (Lewinsohn 1975). The person chooses a unique way of life from his perceived opportunities and foreseen possibilities (Tyler 1978). The psychologist needs to respect the person's unique history, resources, strengths, and ability to use available cultural resources as well as acts of self-management and self-help. Such attention to the individual, however, should not obscure the fact that cultures vary in the emphasis they place on assertion of individuality. Many American Indian and Mexican groups have norms that stress cooperation and self-effacement. In general, white Americans and other Western-oriented people are more individualistic in their attributions in contrast with Third World peoples, who are more oriented toward societal concerns and traditions. Berman (1979) demonstrated that white Americans, when explaining personal problems, focused almost exclusively on the individual as opposed to the society. Black Americans, on the other hand, were more equally distributed in their attributions. These ideas lead to the final hypothesis about the special character of each person:

15. *Intercultural counseling will be effective to the extent that the counselor views the client as an individual with his or her own competencies and resources for "self-righting" during difficulties.*

Fifteen hypotheses have been mentioned under five headings. As stated earlier, they would be more properly called protohypotheses, since the constructs and propositions must yet be sharpened and assessment methods identified or developed to measure the variables. We hope, however, that they will stimulate research on bringing cultural considerations into counseling theory building and research. It remains to be seen whether some of these hypotheses are in themselves culture-bound.

Research Issues

In developing research from hypothesis, there are many questions. One is the question of how one measures similarities between counselor and client; another is how to incorporate the culture, values, and social environment of the participants. One general hypothesis in psychotherapy and counseling might be stated as follows: As the amount of shared client and counselor expectations, knowledge, and interests increases, the probable success of counseling also increases.

Cross-cultural counseling may also be approached as a multivariate research problem. A number of statistical methods may be used for comparing processes, people, and situations, and the problem of getting sufficiently large samples when there are so many variables is a serious one. Problems of comparison and functional equivalence are also discussed by Lonner (1979).

For highest priority we would choose research on similarities of expectations in counseling, for this topic is close to the very reason for counseling. The research should emphasize not only initial goals and interests but also the process by which people arrive at an agreement to work together. When expectations are clear and congruent, the need for extensive similarity in other ways is less essential. Analogies can be made with other "contact" situations. In cashing a check, it does not matter if the bank teller is foreign-born or local-born, white or black, young or old, male or female, as long as the request is understood and the money handed over. In an inquiry about location of services or where to apply for assistance, the important thing is mutual understanding of the question and ability to deliver the answers. Much of intercultural advising and guidance has this practical aspect, and even personal counseling shares this feature. A training program for intercultural counselors should not ignore the importance of imparting realistic financial, educational, and procedural information, even though many "sophisticated" counselors prefer to become immersed in the more personal and "juicy" aspects of social and sexual relations, emotions, and strange customs.

The degree of salience or importance attached to ethnicity and cultural identity as well as religiosity might be assessed (Bochner and Ohsako 1977) in trying to understand and match for cross-cultural relations. Atkinson and Schein (1986) concluded that most of the research to date on racial similarities and differences in therapy and counseling is poor because many studies only use nonclients and analogue situations. McKitrich (1981) also questions the generalizability of results from analogue research. In addition, Folensbee, Draguns, and Danish (1986) feel that many of the dependent measures used are of questionable validity.

Most of the hypotheses in this chapter refer to the effectiveness of counseling. Thousands of pages have been written about the measurement of outcomes of dyadic or small-group counseling and psychotherapy, and thousands of additional pages have been published about evaluation of programs that are relevant to counseling in the large, or community counseling. (For overviews of evaluation see several chapters in Garfield and Bergin 1986.) It is not necessary to recount here the many kinds of criteria that might be used, such as client reports of satisfaction, counselor ratings, Q sorts, tests, changes in activities, and grade-point averages.

Probably the best kinds of criteria to evaluate the effectiveness of intercultural counseling would employ several judges to check on perceptions of change or benefit. The instruments used in behavioral assessment and the self-anchoring measurements seem promising. Also nonobtrusive measures, such as indexes (for foreign students) of campus participation, grade-average improvement, and observation of dormitory behavior, may be appropriate for certain studies.

Large sample research into the effectiveness of intercultural counseling presents serious obstacles. Even a rather sizable number of international students in America, when classified by sex, country of origin, year in college, and whether or not they sought counseling, would produce extremely small numbers in experimental cell breakdowns. The sheer availability of large numbers of minorities in the United States probably accounts for the fact that the vast majority of the studies have employed such samples; yet as pointed out earlier even the American cross-ethnic studies have seldom been true experiments with variables basic to counseling and therapy.

There seem to be three other directions for realistic cross-cultural research. One is to retain the goal of obtaining a large sample but to broaden the notion of intercultural status to include the category of marginal clients compared with mainstream clients. Marginal clients might include all those with unusual characteristics and backgrounds, such as minority members, handicapped students, and students who speak poor English. In such a sampling foreign students might occupy positions on continua, their position based on such factors as communication ability, knowledge of mainstream social customs, and ability to cope with problem situations. The continua might then be related to the larger problems of counseling effectiveness and process.

The opposite direction would involve the study of individuals—one at a time. Historically, Allport, Skinner, and other psychologists have found conducting intensive studies of personal documents, performances, and reports of experience to be productive. Discussions of single-case designs can be found in Garfield and Bergin (1986). The object of the controlled case study is to demonstrate that changes in behavior and self-report co-vary with changes in counseling. The application need not be limited to the usual behavioral approaches. Similar research programs can be used with free associations and other verbal behavior. Such intensive study, one by one, of the persons involved in intercultural counseling would gradually build up a shared knowledge, the basic objective of all science.

A third direction for intercultural research would be the recruitment of persons with special cultural backgrounds for experiments that mimic the counseling situation. With analogue, or contrived, counseling normal people might be used, and large samples of minorities, refugees, foreign sojourners, and other contrasting cultural groups might be available. Research might usefully be conducted on problems of "at risk" populations at an early point, thereby preventing the need for counseling later.

Centers for the systematic collection of intercultural case data would help a great deal in the development of a knowledge base. What is needed is an organized way by which subjects who represent major problems, major countries with high-contrast cultures (such as India, Hong Kong, Iran, and Nigeria, as compared with Western countries), and major cross-ethnic problems may be sampled, so that over time there might be a comparison across methods and outcomes from intensive individual studies. It would be important to conduct parallel studies testing the same processes within different cultural or ethnic communities. This research would check intracultural utility of principles. Lonner (1975) has asserted that the best research is multimethod, multi-investigator, multicultural, longitudinal, and theory related. Such complex investigations would require close coordination and a high degree of commitment, and these factors might be provided by a center on intercultural human development.

How Widely Applicable Is Counseling?

Another way of looking at the intercultural counseling problem is to raise the question about its utility in different cultures and settings. We already know from many accounts about psychotherapy that there are serious questions about its ethnocentric application to other societies (Draguns 1975). Sanua (1966) pointed out that even our theories and research are ethnocentric. Albee (1977) related psychotherapy to the culture changes accompanying the decline of the Protestant ethic and the glorification of the self in a consumption-oriented capitalistic society. The applicability of counseling also depends on the conceptualization of problems. In Western cultures there is an attempt to seek psychological explanations for emotional and physical problems. In other cultures emotional distress may be interpreted to physical problems. As White (1982, 1520) points out, "it is rather the more psychological and 'psycho-somatic' mode of reasoning found in Western cultures which appears unusual among the world's popular and traditional systems of belief."

For a specific example of problems in the application of Western ideas of helping, let us take India. The Indian psychiatrist Neki (1975) pointed out that Western therapy is applicable only to Westernized Indians. One psychiatrist said that it took him five years in India to unlearn what he had learned in five years abroad. For instance, there are great differences between India and the United States in regard to decision making—an important aspect of counseling young people.

Compared with American teenagers and college students, Indians seem to have fewer choices in making decisions about their lives (Sundberg and Tyler 1968). Sundberg et al. (1969) demonstrated that adolescents' views of decision making in India were much more restricted by family considerations than they are in America. Tyler et al. (1968) concluded that the degree of external structure as it exists in educational arrangements in three countries may be inversely related to internality and individuality in vocational choice making; if the school system splits children into different streams at an early age, the children are less likely to develop cognitively complex structures for life possibilities. Draguns (1975, 284) makes a relevant point: "The nature of psychotherapy practiced would also seem to depend upon the structure of the culture in which it occurs and, especially on the 'degrees of freedom' that are open to most of its members."

One of the important tasks for future research is the study of "folk counseling" and "natural" systems of problem solving and influence for change in various countries (Frank 1974a; Kiev 1969; Torrey 1972). Many cultures do not make the mind-body distinction common in the Western conception of treatment. For instance, in traditional Chinese medicine treatments may involve simultaneous consideration of the psychological and physiological elements (Cheung 1986). The person who would teach or counsel in another country would do well to find out as much as he or she can about the living situations of prospective clients and how they handle personal problems. A visit could help clarify these processes, and the counselor could work within the community to enhance and supplement these processes appropriately rather than superimpose imported counseling concepts and practices. The study of traditional treatments and modern adaptations in the particular culture will be facilitated as researchers in those cultures collaborate. Examples of useful collections of base knowledge in a particular culture are in the recent book by Bond (1986) on Chinese psychology. Articles that review programs and research on particular ethnic groups and make recommendations for treatment such as that by Rogler et al. (1987) are most helpful.

As Kinzie (1978) points out there are many instances in day-to-day psychotherapeutic practice in which one must deal with value systems and social and cultural conditions alien to one's experience. We can conclude that general intercultural sensitivity and professional competence will provide the basis for useful treatment of a wide variety of disorders among a wide variety of people. A counselor needs to become sensitive to his or her own intercultural scope and limitations. Concern for cultural sensitivity in mental health systems is increasing and needs for modifying services and improving methods are arising (Rogler et al. 1987). This sensitivity can be facilitated by training and continuing research as the rest of the non-European, nonwhite world grows steadily more numerous.

Intercultural counseling is an exciting and promising area of study. It not only offers promise for improved services to people but it also brings to psychology and other social sciences opportunities for important learning—how different peoples might understand each other better, how one culture is viewed by another, and new ways of observing our basic human commonalities, similarities, and uniqueness.

References

Abel, T. M., Métraux, R., and Roll, S. 1987. *Psychotherapy and culture.* 2d ed. Albuquerque: University of New Mexico Press.

Achebe, C. 1960. *No longer at ease.* New York: Ivan Obolensky.

Adinolfi, A. A. 1971. Relevance of person perception research to clinical psychology. *Journal of Consulting and Clinical Psychology* 37:167–176.

Albee, G. W. 1977. The Protestant ethic, sex and psychotherapy. *American Psychologist* 32:150–161.

Alexander, A. A., Klein, M. H., Workneh, F., and Miller, M. H. 1981. Psychotherapy and the foreign student. In P. B. Pedersen, J. G. Draguns, W. J. Lonner, and J. E. Trimble (eds.), *Counseling across cultures,* 227–246. Honolulu: University of Hawaii Press.

Allport, G. W. 1937. *Personality: A psychological interpretation.* New York: Holt.

Andrulis, D. P. 1977. Ethnicity as a variable in the utilization and referral patterns of a comprehensive mental health center. *Journal of Community Psychology* 5:231–237.

Antler, L. 1970. Correlates of home and host country acquaintanceship among foreign medical residents in the United States. *Journal of Social Psychology* 80:49–57.

Aronson, H., and Overall, B. 1966. Treatment expectations of patients in two social classes. *Social Work* 11:35–41.

Atkinson, D. R. 1983. Ethnic similarity and counseling psychology. *Counseling Psychologist* 2:79–92.

————. 1985. Research on cross-cultural counseling and psychotherapy: A review and update of reviews. In P. B. Pedersen (ed.), *Handbook of cross-cultural counseling and therapy,* 191–198. Westport, CT: Greenwood Press.

Atkinson, D. R., Furlong, M. J., and Williams, W. C. 1986. Afro-American preferences for counselor characteristics. *Journal of Counseling Psychology* 33:326–330.

Atkinson, D. R., Maruyama, M., and Matsui, S. 1978. Effects of counselor race and counseling approach on Asian Americans' perceptions of counselor credibility and utility. *Journal of Counseling Psychology* 25:76–83.

Atkinson, D. R., Morten, G., and Sue, D. W. 1979. *Counseling American minorities: A cross-cultural perspective.* Dubuque, IA: William C. Brown.

Atkinson, D. R., Ponce, F. Q., and Martinez, F. M. 1984. Effects of ethnic, sex, and attitude similarity on counselor credibility. *Journal of Counseling Psychology* 31:588–590.

Atkinson, D. R., Ponterotto, J. G., and Sanchez, A. R. 1984. Attitudes of Vietnamese and Anglo-American students towards counseling. *Journal of College Student Personnel* 25:448–452.

Atkinson, D. R., and Schein, S. 1986. Similarity in counseling. *Counseling Psychologist* 14:319–353.

Bandura, A. 1977. Self-efficacy: Toward a unifying theory of behavioral change. *Psychological Review* 84:191–215.

———. 1982. Self-efficacy mechanism in human agency. *American Psychologist* 37:122–147.

Bates, B. C., Sundberg, N. D., and Tyler, L. E. 1970. Divergent problem solving: A comparison of adolescents in India and America. *International Journal of Psychology* 5:231–244.

Benfari, R. C. 1969. Relationship between early dependence training and patient-therapist dyad. *Psychological Reports* 24:552–554.

Bengur, B. 1979. Interviews with counselors about effective and ineffective cross-cultural counseling. Typescript. University of Oregon, Eugene.

Benson, A. G., and Miller, R. E. 1966. A preliminary report on users of the Michigan International Student Problem Inventory in research, orientation and counseling, developing a balanced program and evaluating potential for academic success of/for foreign students. Typescript. International Programs Office, Michigan State University.

Berman, J. 1979. Individual versus societal focus in problem diagnosis of black and white male and female counselors. *Journal of Cross-Cultural Psychology* 10 (4):497–507.

Berry, J. W. 1969. On cross-cultural comparability. *International Journal of Psychology* 4:119–128.

Birdwhistell, R. 1970. *Essays in body motion communication.* Philadelphia: University of Pennsylvania Press.

Bloombaum, M., Yamamoto, J., and James, Q. 1968. Cultural stereotyping among psychotherapists. *Journal of Consulting and Clinical Psychology* 32:99.

Bochner, S., and Ohsako, T. 1977. Ethnic role salience in racially homogeneous and heterogeneous societies. *Journal of Cross-Cultural Psychology* 8:477–492.

Bond, M. H. 1986. *The psychology of the Chinese people.* Hong Kong: Oxford University Press.

Boucher, J. D. 1979. Emotion and culture. In A. J. Marsella, R. Tharp, and T. Ciborowski (eds.), *Perspectives on cross-cultural psychology.* New York: Academic Press.

Boyd, V. S., Shueman, S., McMullan, Y. O., and Fretz, B. R. 1979. Transition groups for black freshmen: Integrated service and training. *Professional Psychology* 10:42–48.

Brislin, R. W., and Van Buren, H. 1974. Can they go home again? *Exchange* 9 (4): 19–24.

Buriel, R. 1975. Cognitive styles among three generations of Mexican American children. *Journal of Cross-Cultural Psychology* 6:417–429.

Butt, D. S., and Beiser, M. 1987. Successful aging: A theme for international psychology. *Psychology and Aging* 2:87–94.

Carkhuff, R. R., and Pierce, R. 1967. Differential effects of therapist race and social class upon patient depth of self-exploration in the initial clinical interview. *Journal of Consulting Psychology* 31:632–634.

Carstairs, G. 1955. Medicine and faith in rural Rajasthan. In B. D. Paul (ed.), *Health, culture and community*. New York: Russell Sage Foundation.

Cheung, F. M. C. 1986. Psychopathology among Chinese people. In M. H. Bond (ed.), *The psychology of the Chinese people*, 171–212. Hong Kong: Oxford University Press.

Connor, J. W. 1975. Value changes in third generation Japanese Americans. *Journal of Personality Assessment* 39:597–600.

Costantino, G., Malgady, R. G., and Rogler, L. H. 1986. Cuento therapy: A culturally sensitive modality for Puerto Rican children. *Journal of Consulting and Clinical Psychology* 54:639–645.

Dauphinais, P., Dauphinais, L., and Rowe, W. 1981. Effects of race and communication style on Indian perceptions of counselor effectiveness. *Counselor Education and Supervision* 21:72–80.

De la Cancela, V. 1985. Towards a sociocultural psychotherapy for low-income ethnic minorities. *Psychotherapy* 22:427–435.

Draguns, J. G. 1975. Resocialization into culture: The complexities of taking a worldwide view of psychotherapy. In R. W. Brislin, S. Bochner, and W. J. Lonner (eds.), *Cross-cultural perspectives on learning*, 273–290. New York: John Wiley and Sons.

———. 1981. Counseling across cultures: Common themes and distinct approaches. In P. B. Pedersen, J. G. Draguns, W. J. Lonner, and J. G. Trimble (eds.), *Counseling across cultures*. Honolulu: University of Hawaii Press.

Folensbee, R. W., Draguns, J. G., and Danish, S. J. 1986. Impact of two types of counselor intervention on black American, Puerto Rican, and Anglo-American analogue clients. *Journal of Counseling Psychology* 33:446–453.

Frank, J. D. 1974a. *Persuasion and healing: A comparative study of psychotherapy*. Rev. ed. New York: Schocken Books.

———. 1974b. Psychotherapy: The restoration of morale. *American Journal of Psychiatry* 131:271–274.

Garfield, S. L., and Bergin, A. E., eds. 1986. *Handbook of psychotherapy and behavior change*. 3d ed. New York: John Wiley and Sons.

Gilmore, S. K. 1973. *The counselor-in-training*. New York: Appleton-Century-Crofts.

Gladstein, G. 1983. Understanding empathy: Integrating counseling, development, and social psychology perspectives. *Journal of Counseling Psychology* 30:467–482.

Gordon, M. 1964. *Assimilation in American life*. New York: Oxford University Press.

Gravitz, H. L., and Woods, E. 1976. A multiethnic approach to peer counseling. *Professional Psychology* 7:229–235.

Grey, A. L. 1965. The counseling process and its cultural setting. *Journal of Vocational and Educational Guidance* 11:104–114.

Hall, E. T. 1966. *The hidden dimension.* Garden City, NY: Doubleday.

———. 1979. Learning the Arabs' silent language. *Psychology Today* 12 (8): 45–54.

Hall, E. T., and Whyte, W. F. 1960. Intercultural communication: A guide to men of action. *Human organization* 19:5–12.

Heitler, J. B. 1973. Preparation of lower-class patients for expressive group psychotherapy. *Journal of Consulting and Clinical Psychology* 41:351–560.

Henderson, G. 1979. Overview. In G. Henderson (ed.), *Understanding and counseling ethnic minorities,* 3–27. Springfield, IL: Charles C. Thomas.

Heppner, P., and Heeacker, M. 1983. Perceived counselor characteristics, client expectations and client satisfaction with counseling. *Journal of Counseling Psychology* 30:31–39.

Higginbotham, H. N. 1977. Culture and the role of client expectancy in psychotherapy. In R. W. Brislin and M. P. Hamnett (eds.), *Topics in culture learning.* Vol. 5, 197–224. Honolulu: East-West Center.

———. 1984. The Third World challenge to psychiatry: Culture accommodation and mental health. Honolulu: University of Hawaii Press.

Ho, D. Y. F. 1985. Cultural values and professional issues in clinical psychology: Implications from the Hong Kong experience. *American Psychologist* 40:1212–1218.

Idowu, A. I. 1985. Counseling Nigerian students in United States colleges and universities. *Journal of Counseling and Development* 63:506–509.

Ishisaka, H. A., Nguyen, Q. T., and Okimoto, J. T. 1985. The role of culture in the mental health treatment of Indochinese refugees. In T. C. Owan (ed.), *Southeast Asian mental health: Treatment, prevention, services, training, and research,* 41–64. Washington, DC: U.S. Department of Health and Human Services.

Jackson, G. G. 1976. The African genesis of the black perspective in helping. *Professional Psychology* 7:292–308.

Jackson, G. G., and Kirschner, S. A. 1973. Racial self-designation and preferences for a counselor. *Journal of Counseling Psychology* 20:560–564.

Johnson, D. C. 1971. Problems of foreign students. *International Educational and Cultural Exchange* 7:61–68.

———. 1973. Ourselves and others: Comparative stereotypes. *International Educational and Cultural Exchange* 9 (2–3): 24–28.

Johnson, S. D. 1987. Knowing that versus knowing how: Toward achieving expertise through multicultural training for counseling. *Counseling Psychologist* 15:320–331.

Jones, A., and Seagull, A. A. 1977. Dimensions of the relationship between the black client and the white therapist: A theoretical overview. *American Psychologist* 32:850–855.

Jourard, S. M. 1971. *Self-disclosure.* New York: John Wiley and Sons.

Juarez, R. 1985. Core issues in psychotherapy with the Hispanic child. *Psychotherapy* 22:441–448.

Kiev, A. 1969. Transcultural psychiatry: Research, problems and perspectives.

In S. C. Plog and R. B. Edgerton (eds.), *Changing perspectives in mental illness*. New York: Holt, Rinehart and Winston.

―――. 1972. *Transcultural psychiatry*. New York: Macmillan, Free Press.

King, L. M. 1978. Social and cultural influences on psychopathology. *Annual Review of Psychology* 29:405–434.

Kinzie, J. D. 1972. Cross-cultural psychotherapy: The Malaysian experience. *American Journal of Psychotherapy* 26:220–231.

―――. 1978. Lessons from cross-cultural psychotherapy. *American Journal of Psychotherapy* 32:510–520.

Kinzie, J. D., Frederickson, R. H., Ben, R., Fleck, J., and Karls, W. 1984. Posttraumatic stress disorder among survivors of Cambodian concentration camps. *American Journal of Psychiatry* 141:645–650.

Kinzie, J. D., and Manson, S. 1983. Five years' experience with Indochinese refugee psychiatric patients. *Journal of Operational Psychiatry* 14:105–111.

Kinzie, J. D., Manson, S. M., Vinh, D. T., Tolan, N. T., Anh, B., and Pho, T. N. 1982. Development and validation of a Vietnamese-language depression rating scale. *American Journal of Psychiatry* 139:1276–1281.

Kluckhohn, C., and Murray, H. A. 1953. Personality formation: The determinants. In C. Kluckhohn, H. A. Murray, and D. M. Schneider (eds.), *Personality in nature, society and culture*. New York: Random House, Alfred A. Knopf.

Knight, G. P., and Kagan, S. 1977. Acculturation of prosocial and competitive behaviors among second and third generation Mexican-American children. *Journal of Cross-Cultural Psychology* 8:273–284.

Knight, G. P., Kagan, S., Nelson, W., and Gumbiner, J. 1978. Acculturation of second and third generation Mexican-American children: Field independence, locus of control, self-esteem and school achievement. *Journal of Cross-Cultural Psychology* 9:87–97.

Lambert, R. G., and Lambert, M. J. 1984. The effects of role preparation for psychotherapy on immigrant clients seeking mental health services in Hawaii. *Journal of Community Psychology* 12:263–275.

Landers, S. 1987. Sensitivity backfires. *APA Monitor* 18 (5): 26.

Lazarus, R. S. 1979. Positive denial: The case for not facing reality. *Psychology Today* 18 (6): 44–60.

Leff, J. 1973. Culture and the differentiation of emotional states. *British Journal of Psychiatry* 123:229–306.

Lewinsohn, P. M. 1975. The use of activity schedules in the treatment of depressed individuals. In J. D. Krumboltz and C. E. Thoresen (eds.), *Counseling methods*. New York: Holt, Rinehart and Winston.

Locke, S., and Feinsod, F. 1982. Psychological preparation for young adults traveling abroad. *Adolescence* 17:815–819.

Lonner, W. J. 1975. An analysis of the prepublication evaluation of cross-cultural manuscripts: Implications for future research. In R. W. Brislin, S. Bochner, and W. J. Lonner (eds.), *Cross-cultural perspectives on learning*. New York: John Wiley and Sons, Halsted.

―――. 1979. Issues in cross-cultural psychology. In A. J. Marsella,

R. Tharp, and T. Ciborowski (eds.), *Perspectives on cross-cultural psychology.* New York: Academic Press.

Lorion, R. P. 1978. Research on psychotherapy and behavior change in the disadvantaged. In S. L. Garfield and A. E. Bergin (eds.), *Handbook of psychotherapy and behavior change: An empirical analysis,* 2d ed., 903–938. New York: John Wiley and Sons.

McKitrich, D. 1981. Generalizing from counseling analogue research on subjects perception of counselors. *Journal of Counseling Psychology* 28:357–360.

McShane, D. 1987. Mental health and North American Indian/Native communities: Cultural transactions, education and regulation. *American Journal of Community Psychology* 15:95–116.

Manson, S. M. 1979. Personal communication.

Marcos, L. R. 1979. Effects of interpreters on the evaluation of psychopathology in non-English-speaking patients. *American Journal of Psychiatry* 136:171–174.

Marsella, A. J. 1979. Cross-cultural studies of mental disorders. In A. J. Marsella, R. Tharp, and T. Ciborowski (eds.), *Perspectives on cross-cultural psychology.* New York: Academic Press.

Marsella, A. J., and Pedersen, P. B., eds. 1981. *Cross-cultural counseling and psychotherapy: Foundations, evaluation, and cultural considerations.* Elmsford, NY: Pergamon Press.

Marsella, A. J., Tharp, R., and Ciborowski, T., eds. 1979. *Perspectives on cross-cultural psychology.* New York: Academic Press.

Marsella, A. J., and White, G. M. 1982. Cultural conceptions of mental health and therapy. Dordrecht, Holland: D. Reidel Publishing.

Matarazzo, J. D., and Wiens, A. N. 1977. Black Intelligence Test of Cultural Homogeneity and Wechsler Adult Intelligence Scale scores of black and white police applicants. *Journal of Applied Psychology* 62:157–163.

Merluzzi, T. V., and Merluzzi, B. H. 1977. Counselor race and power base: Effects on attitudes and behavior. *Journal of Counseling Psychology* 24:430–436.

Millikan, R. L. 1965. Prejudice and counseling effectiveness. *Personnel and Guidance Journal* 43:710–712.

Millikan, R. L., and Patterson, J. J. 1967. Relationship of dogmatism and prejudice to counseling effectiveness. *Counselor Education and Supervision* 6:125–129.

Minuchin, S., Montalvo, B., Guerney, B., Rosman, B. L., and Schumer, F. 1967. *Families of the slums.* New York: Basic Books.

Mokuau, N. 1987. Social workers' perceptions of counseling effectiveness for Asian American clients. *Social Work* 32:331–335.

Mollica, R. F., Wyshak, G., de Marneffe, D., Khuon, F., and LaVelle, J. 1987. Indochinese versions of the Hopkins Symptom Checklist–25: A screening instrument for the psychiatric care of refugees. *American Journal of Psychiatry* 144:497–500.

Montijo, J. A. 1985. Therapeutic relationships with the poor: A Puerto Rican perspective. *Psychotherapy* 22:436–440.

Morten, G., and Atkinson, D. R. 1983. Minority identity development and preference for counselor race. *Journal of Negro Education* 52:156–161.

Naditch, M. P., and Morrissey, R. F. 1976. Role stress, personality, and psychopathology in a group of immigrant adolescents. *Journal of Abnormal Psychology* 85:113–118.

Neki, J. S. 1975. Psychotherapy in India: Past, present and future. *American Journal of Psychotherapy* 29:92–100.

Ogawa, D. M., and Weldon, T. A. 1972. Cross-cultural analysis of feedback behavior within Japanese American and Caucasian American small groups. *Journal of Communication* 22:189–195.

Overall, B., and Aronson, H. 1963. Expectations of psychotherapy in patients of lower socioeconomic class. *American Journal of Orthopsychiatry* 33:421–430.

Parham, T. A., and Helms, J. E. 1981. The influence of black students' racial identity attitudes on preference for counselor's race. *Journal of Counseling Psychology* 28:250–257.

Parloff, M. B., Waskow, I. E., and Wolfe, B. B. 1978. Research on therapist variables in relation to process and outcome. In S. L. Garfield and A. E. Bergin (eds.), *Handbook of psychotherapy and behavioral change: An empirical analysis,* 233–282. 2d ed. New York: John Wiley and Sons.

Pedersen, P. B. 1977. The triad model of cross-cultural counselor training. *Personnel and Guidance Journal* 55:94–100.

———. 1978. Four dimensions of cross-cultural skill in counselor training. *Personnel and Guidance Journal* 56:480–484.

———. 1981. Triad counseling. In R. Corsini (ed.), *Innovative psychotherapies.* New York: John Wiley and Sons.

———. 1985. Intercultural criteria for mental-health training. In P. B. Pedersen (ed.), *Handbook of cross-cultural counseling and therapy.* Westport, CT: Greenwood Press.

Pedersen, P. B., Lonner, W. J., and Draguns, J. G., eds. 1976. *Counseling across cultures.* Honolulu: University of Hawaii Press.

Pitta, P., Marcos, L., and Alpert, M. 1978. Language switching as a treatment strategy with bilingual patients. *American Journal of Psychoanalysis* 38:255–258.

Ponterotto, J. G., Anderson, W. H., and Grieger, I. Z. 1986. Black students' attitudes toward counseling as a function of racial identity. *Journal of Multicultural Counseling and Development* 14:50–59.

Prince, R. H. 1969. Psychotherapy and the chronically poor. In J. C. Finney (ed.), *Culture change, mental health and poverty.* Lexington: University of Kentucky Press.

———. 1976. Psychotherapy as the manipulation of endogenous healing mechanisms: A transcultural survey. *Transcultural Psychiatric Research Review* 13:115–133.

———. 1979. Variations in psychotherapeutic procedures. In A. J. Marsella, R. Tharp, and T. Ciborowski (eds.), *Perspectives on cross-cultural psychology.* New York: Academic Press.

Raskin, A., Crook, T. H., and Herman, K. D. 1975. Psychiatric history and symptom differences in black and white depressed inpatients. *Journal of Counseling and Clinical Psychology* 43:73–80.

Rodriguez, R. 1979. Going home again: The new American scholarship boy.

In D. Atkinson, G. Morten, and D. W. Sue (eds.), *Counseling American minorities: A cross-cultural perspective,* 149–158. Dubuque, IA: William C. Brown.

Rogers, C. 1975. Empathic: An unappreciated way of being. *The Counseling Psychologist* 5:2–10.

Rogler, L. H., Malgady, R. G., Costantino, G., and Blumenthal, R. 1987. What do culturally sensitive mental health services mean? The case of Hispanics. *American Psychologist* 42:565–570.

Roll, S., Millen, L., and Martinez, R. 1980. Common errors in psychotherapy with Chicanos: Extrapolations from research and clinical experience. *Psychotherapy: Theory, Research and Practice* 17:158–168.

Root, M. P. P. 1985. Guidelines for facilitating therapy with Asian American clients. *Psychotherapy* 22:349–356.

Rosenzweig, S. 1986. Idiodynamics vis-à-vis psychology. *American Psychologist* 41:241–245.

Rubin, J. 1976. How to tell when someone is saying "no." In R. W. Brislin (ed.), *Topics in culture learning.* Vol. 4, 61–65. Honolulu: East-West Center.

Ruiz, R. A., Padilla, A. M., and Alvarez, R. 1978. Issues in the counseling of Spanish-speaking surnamed clients: Recommendations for therapeutic services. In G. Walz and L. Benjamin (eds.), *Transcultural counseling,* 13–56. New York: Human Sciences Press.

Sanchez, A. R., and Atkinson, D. R. 1983. Mexican-American cultural commitment, preference for counselor ethnicity, and willingness to use counseling. *Journal of Counseling Psychology* 30:215–220.

Sanua, V. D. 1966. Sociocultural aspects of psychotherapy and treatment: A review of the literature. *Progress in Clinical Psychology* 7:151–190.

Sattler, J. M. 1970. Racial "experimenter effects" in experimentation, testing, interviewing and psychotherapy. *Psychological Bulletin* 73:137–160.

Shaffer, M., Sundberg, N. D., and Tyler, L. E. 1969. Content differences on word listing by American, Dutch and Indian adolescents. *Journal of Social Psychology* 79:139–140.

Smith, E. 1977. Counseling black individuals: Some stereotypes. *Personnel and Guidance Journal* 55:390–396.

Smith, H. G. 1966. *Sensitivity to people.* New York: McGraw-Hill.

Smith, W. D., Berlew, A. K., Mosley, M. H., and Whitney, W. M. 1978. *Minority issues in mental health.* Reading, MA: Addison-Wesley.

Spielberger, C. D., and Diaz-Guerrero, R., eds. 1976. *Cross-cultural anxiety.* New York: John Wiley and Sons.

Stecklein, J. K., Liu, H. C., Anderson, J. F., and Gunararatne, S. A. 1971. *Attitudes of foreign students toward educational experiences at the University of Minnesota.* Minneapolis: University of Minnesota, Bureau of Institutional Research.

Strauss, J. S. 1979. Social and cultural influences on psychopathology. *Annual Review of Psychology* 30:397–416.

Strupp, H. H., and Bloxom, A. L. 1973. Preparing lower-class patients for group psychotherapy: Development and evaluation of a role-induction film. *Journal of Consulting and Clinical Psychology* 41:373–384.

Stumphauzer, J. S., and Davis, L. C. 1983. Training community-based Asian-American mental health personnel in behavior modification. *Journal of Community Psychology* 11:253–258.

Sue, D. W. 1978. Eliminating cultural oppression in counseling: Toward a general theory. *Journal of Counseling Psychology* 25:419–428.

Sue, D. W., and Kirk, B. 1975. Asian-Americans: Use of counseling and psychiatric services on a college campus. *Journal of Counseling Psychology* 22:84–86.

Sue, D. W., and Sue, D. 1977. Barriers to effective cross-cultural counseling. *Journal of Counseling Psychology* 24:420–429.

Sue, D. W., and Sue, S. In press. Cultural factors in the clinical assessment of Asian Americans. *Journal of Consulting and Clinical Psychology.*

Sue, S., and Sue, D. W. 1974. MMPI comparisons between Asian-American and non-American students utilizing a student psychiatric clinic. *Journal of Counseling* 21:423–427.

Sue, S., and Zane, N. 1987. The role of culture and cultural techniques in psychotherapy. *American Psychologist* 42:37–45.

Sundberg, N. D. 1966. A method for studying sensitivy to implied meanings. *Gawein* 16:1–8.

Sundberg, N. D., Sharma, V., Wodtli, T., and Rohila, P. 1969. Family cohesiveness and autonomy of adolescents in India and the United States. *Journal of Marriage and the Family* 31:403–407.

Sundberg, N. D., Taplin, J. R., and Tyler, L. E. 1983. *Introduction to clinical psychology: Perspectives, issues and contributions to human service.* Englewood Cliffs, NJ: Prentice-Hall.

Sundberg, N. D., and Tyler, L. E. 1968. Adolescent views of life possibilities in India, the Netherlands and the United States. *Student Services Review* 3 (1): 8–13.

Sundland, D. M. 1977. Theoretical orientations of psychotherapists. In A. S. Gurman and A. M. Razin (eds.), *Effective psychotherapy: A handbook of research.* New York: Pergamon Press.

Szapocznik, J., Scopetta, M. A., Aranalde, M. A., and Kurtines, W. 1978. Cuban value structure: Treatment implications. *Journal of Consulting and Clinical Psychology* 46:961–970.

Tan, H. 1967. Intercultural study of counseling expectancies. *Journal of Consulting Psychology* 14:122–130.

Tanaka-Matsumi, J., and Marsella, A. J. 1976. Cross-cultural variations in the phenomenological experience of depression: Pt. 1, Word association studies. *Journal of Cross-Cultural Psychology* 7:379–396.

Thompson, R. A., and Cimbolic, P. 1978. Black students' counselor preference and attitudes toward counseling center use. *Journal of Counseling Psychology* 25:570–575.

Torrey, E. F. 1972. *The mind game: Witchdoctors and psychiatrists.* New York: Emerson Hall Publishers.

———. 1986. *Witchdoctors and psychiatrists: The common roots of psychotherapy and its future.* New York: Harper and Row.

Triandis, H. C., ed. 1976. *Variations in black and white perceptions of the social environment.* Champaign/Urbana: University of Illinois Press.

Triandis, H. C., and Draguns, J. G., eds. 1980. *Handbook of cross-cultural psychology.* Vol. 6, *Psychopathology.* Boston: Allyn and Bacon.

Trimble, J. E. 1981. Value differentials and their importance in counseling American Indians. In P. B. Pedersen, J. G. Draguns, W. J. Lonner, and J. E. Trimble (eds.), *Counseling across cultures.* Honolulu: University of Hawaii Press.

Tyler, L. E. 1978. *Individuality: Human possibilities and personal choice in the psychological development of men and women.* San Francisco: Jossey-Bass.

————. 1983. *Thinking creatively: A new approach to psychology and individual lives.* San Francisco: Jossey-Bass.

Tyler, L. E., Sundberg, N. D., Rohila, P. H., and Greene, M. M. 1968. Patterns of choices in Dutch, American and Indian adolescents. *Journal of Counseling Psychology* 15:522–529.

Wahl, O. 1976. Six TV myths about mental illness. *T. V. Guide* (March 13): 4–8.

Walz, G. R., and Benjamin, L. 1978. *Transcultural counseling: Needs, programs and techniques.* New York: Human Sciences Press.

Wampold, B. E., Casas, J. M., and Atkinson, D. R. 1981. Ethnic bias in counseling: An information processing approach. *Journal of Counseling Psychology* 28:498–503.

Webster, D. W., and Fretz, B. R. 1978. Asian American, black and white college students' preferences for help-giving sources. *Journal of Counseling Psychology* 25:124–130.

Wells, K. B., Hough, R. L., Golding, J. M., Burnam, M. A., and Karno, M. 1987. Which Mexican-Americans underutilize health services. *American Journal of Psychiatry* 144:918–922.

Westbrook, F. D., Miyares, J., and Roberts, J. H. 1978. Perceived problem areas by black and white students and hints about comparative counseling needs. *Journal of Counseling Psychology* 25:119–123.

White, G. M. 1982. The role of cultural explanations in "somatization" and "psychologization." *Social Science Medicine* 16:1519–1530.

Woods, E., and Zimmer, J. M. 1976. Racial effects in counseling-like interviews: An experimental analogue. *Journal of Counseling Psychology* 23:527–531.

Yeh, E. K. 1972. Paranoid manifestations among Chinese students studying abroad: Some preliminary findings. In W. Lebra (ed.), *Transcultural research in mental health,* vol. 2 of *Mental health research in Asia and the Pacific,* 326–340. Honolulu: University Press of Hawaii.

Yuen, R. K., and Tinsley, H. E. A. 1981. International and American students' expectancies about counseling. *Journal of Counseling Psychology* 28:66–69.

Zain, E. K. 1965. A study of the academic and personal-social difficulties encountered by a select group of foreign students at the University of Oregon. Ph.D. diss., University of Oregon.

Zeiss, A. M., Lewinsohn, P. M., and Munoz, R. F. 1979. Nonspecific improvement effects in depression using interpersonal skills training, pleasant activity schedules of cognitive functioning. *Journal of Consulting and Clinical Psychology* 47:427–439.

Contributors

Gary Althen is assistant director of the Foreign Students and Scholars Program in the Office of International Education and Services at the University of Iowa. He has worked with international students for over 16 years. He has written *The Handbook of Foreign Student Advising* and *American Ways: A Guide for Foreigners in the United States* and is the author, co-author, or editor of more than 30 other publications on intercultural communication or foreign student affairs. He is the recipient of the National Association for Foreign Student Affairs' Marita Houlihan Award for innovative contributions to his field. His interests are in cross-cultural communication and training.

J. Manuel Casas is an associate professor in the Counseling Psychology Program at the University of California, Santa Barbara. He has worked extensively with ethnic minorities and as co-founder of JMC & Associates serves as a consultant to various organizations and corporations that are interested in working more effectively with ethnic minorities. A major area of interest includes the identification of sociocultural variables that affect cross-cultural communication. He has published widely in this area and is presently devoting much of his time to identifying the sociocultural variables and institutional interventions that contribute significantly to the success of ethnic minorities in educational and corporate settings.

Juris G. Draguns was born and completed his primary schooling in Riga, Latvia. He graduated from high school while a refugee in Germany and completed his undergraduate and graduate studies in the United States. His Ph.D. in clinical psychology is from the University of Rochester. He held a number of clinical, research, and academic positions before accepting a faculty appointment at The Pennsylvania State University, where he is now professor of psychology. He has traveled extensively in Europe, Latin America, Asia, and Australia and has occupied visiting appointments at the Johannes Gutenberg University in Mainz, West Germany; the East-West Center in Honolulu, Hawaii; Flinders University in Bedford Park, South Australia; and Florida Institute of Technology in Melbourne, Florida. His interests in cross-cultural psychology are focused on abnormal behavior, personality, psychotherapy, and counseling. He co-edited the *Handbook of Cross-Cultural Psychology,* Volume 6: *Psychopathology* and *Counseling across Cultures.* In addition to these publications, he has written numerous articles and chapters that have appeared in psychological, psychiatric, and anthropological journals.

Candace M. Fleming, who received her Ph.D. from the University of North Carolina, Chapel Hill, is an assistant professor in the Department of Psychiatry at the University of Colorado Health Sciences Center in Denver and an Alcohol Research Scholar in the National Center for American Indian and Alaska Native Mental Health Research. Before joining the Faculty at the University of Colorado, she worked as a clinical psychologist for the Indian Health Service directing American Indian mental health programs. Her research interests include an investigation of family issues as they relate to the prevention of substance abuse among American Indians and the interrelationship between addiction and mental health problems.

Sandra L. Foster is a counselor and consultant in Mountain View, California. A graduate of Stanford's Counseling Psychology Program, she has conducted research on social skills training for shy men. Her consulting interests include assisting managers and supervisors from Silicon Valley companies in the development of cross-cultural awareness and competencies.

Mary Fukuyama, a counseling psychologist at the University of Florida Counseling Center, received her Ph.D. from Washington State University. She has taught cross-cultural counseling in the University of Florida Department of Counselor Education and supervised psychology doctoral interns in training in multicultural counseling issues. She has co-authored research articles on the Cultural Attitudes Repertory Technique (CART), an instrument designed to measure personal constructs of cultural perceptions.

Anne Heath is a graduate student in the Counseling Psychology Program at the University of Florida, Gainesville. She recently completed a Delphi Study on the future of multicultural counseling and is currently examining the effects of multicultural training on attitudes and perceptions of counselors.

H. Nick Higginbotham received his Ph.D. in clinical-community psychology from the University of Hawaii in 1979. He directed New Zealand's first community psychology graduate program at Waikato University and has held appointments at the East-West Center and the University of Hawaii-Hilo. Currently he teaches health psychology at the Hunter Institute in New South Wales, Australia, and coordinates the social science component of the Centre for Clinical Epidemiology and Biostatistics at the University of Newcastle. This program trains Third World physicians as part of the Rockefeller Foundation's International Clinical Epidemiology Network. He has written *Third World Challenge to Psychiatry: Culture and Mental Health Care,* based on work in Southeast Asia, and co-authored *Psychotherapy and Behavior Change.* He continues studies of cultural accommodation of clinical services among Native Hawaiians and Australian Aboriginals.

Farah A. Ibrahim, an immigrant to the United States from South Asia, is a licensed psychologist and an associate professor of educational psychology (counseling psychology) at the University of Connecticut, Storrs. She is a consulting editor for *Psychotherapy,* a past member of the editorial board of the *Journal for Counseling and Development,* and past co-editor of *Counsellor,* a journal published in Pakistan. A past chair of the Human Rights Committee of the American Association for Counseling and Development (AACD) and the Human Rights Task Force of the Association for Counselor Education and Supervision, she is now serving on the AACD International Relations Committee. She is the author and co-author of two AACD Position Papers on Human Rights. Her research interests include cross-cultural/multicultural counseling, psychotherapy, assessment, evaluation, training, and ethics.

Harry H. L. Kitano is professor of social welfare and sociology at the University of California, Los Angeles. His major books include *Asian Americans,* 1988, co-authored with Roger Daniels; *Race Relations,* 1985; and *Japanese Americans: The Evolution of a Subculture,* 1976.

Teresa D. LaFromboise, an assistant professor in the Counseling Psychology Program at Stanford University, Stanford, California, is one of the few psychologists conducting empirical research on American Indian student adjustment, especially women. She has conducted a number of studies on the efficacy of culturally adapted counseling and educational interventions with American Indian adolescents. She has acted as a consultant to university programs, tribal organizations, and other community agencies on problems related to American Indian mental health.

Harriet P. Lefley is professor of social and cultural psychiatry, University of Miami School of Medicine, and director of the Collaborative Family Training Project supported by the National Institute of Mental Health. Formerly director of the Cross-Cultural Training Institute for Mental Health Professionals and author of multiple publications, she has been involved in cross-cultural research and community mental health services for multiethnic and refugee groups for more than 15 years.

Walter J. Lonner is a professor in the Department of Psychology at Western Washington University, Bellingham. He is the founding editor (and currently senior editor) of the *Journal of Cross-Cultural Psychology* and the co-author or co-editor of several books on cross-cultural psychology. During 1986–1988 he served as the ninth president of the International Association for Cross-Cultural Psychology.

Paul B. Pedersen taught in Asia for six years, counseled foreign students at the University of Minnesota for seven years as a faculty member of Psychoeducational Studies, and for four years directed a National Institute of Mental Health training grant for developing interculturally skilled counselors through the Department of Psychology and Social Work of the University of Hawaii and the East-West Center. At present he is chairman of counselor education and professor of education at Syracuse University.

Charles R. Ridley received his Ph.D. from the University of Minnesota. He is currently an associate professor at the Graduate School of Psychology, Fuller Theological Seminary, Pasadena, California. Previously he was a consulting psychologist in private industry and taught at the University of Maryland and Indiana University. The focus of much of his research has been directed toward explicating the effects of ethnicity and culture on psychotherapy process and outcome.

David Sue is professor of psychology and serves as the chairperson of the Clinical/Counseling Program at Western Washington University. For 10 years, he was on the psychology faculty at the University of Michigan, Dearborn. He has co-authored *Understanding Abnormal Psychology* (3d edition) and *Counseling the Culturally Different: Theory and Practice* (2d edition) with his brothers, Derald and Stan Sue. He has research and writing interests in Asian Americans and cross-cultural counseling.

Norman D. Sundberg is a professor in the Department of Psychology at the University of Oregon. He received his Ph.D. in clinical psychology from the University of Minnesota and is the former director of the

Oregon Clinical/Community Psychology Program. He is a Fellow of the APA divisions of Clinical, Counseling, and Community Psychology and a Diplomate of the American Board of Professional Psychology. He has taught and conducted research in India, Hong Kong, Germany, Spain, France, and Australia, and has published many articles on cross-cultural topics, including family decision making, values, and time perspectives. He has written and lectured on multicultural issues in assessment, therapy, and counseling.

Junko Tanaka-Matsumi is an associate professor of psychology at Hofstra University, Hempstead, New York. She received her Ph.D. in clinical psychology from the University of Hawaii and was an East-West Center degree scholar as well as a research intern from Japan. Her current research interests include investigations of dyadic interactions of depressed people, behavior influence processes in psychotherapy, and cross-cultural research methods to facilitate these investigations.

Kay Thomas is associate director and psychologist with the Office of International Education at the University of Minnesota, where she directs the Counseling and Advising Division. She received her Ph.D. in counseling and student personnel psychology at the University of Minnesota, where she has taught cross-cultural counseling and other counseling process courses. Through the National Association of Foreign Student Affairs she has been active in promoting training in cross-cultural counseling for advisers of international students and scholars. She has given numerous workshops and presentations throughout the country on cross-cultural counseling and cultural adjustment. In addition, she has interests in the impact of cultural values on the counseling process and in intercultural groups.

Joseph E. Trimble, who received his Ph.D. from the University of Oklahoma, is professor of psychology at Western Washington University, Bellingham, where he is the coordinator for the cross-cultural counseling program and a research associate in the Center for Cross-Cultural Research and the Western Institute for Social and Organizational Research. He is also a research associate for the National Center for American Indian and Alaska Native Mental Health Research at the University of Colorado Health Sciences Center in Denver. He has written extensively on mental health and substance abuse topics on American Indians. Currently, his research interests focus on the prevention of substance abuse among American Indian youth and an investigation of problematic life events among American Indian adolescents.

Melba J. T. Vasquez is a staff psychologist at the Counseling and Mental Health Center at the University of Texas at Austin and is also in part-time private practice. She has written and published in the areas of Hispanic women's psychology, training and supervision, and professional ethics. She received her Ph.D. in counseling psychology from the University of Texas in 1978. She serves on several editorial boards and is active in several professional organizations, including the Society for the Study of Ethnic Minority Psychology, a division of the American Psychological Association.

Julian Wohl is professor of psychology at the University of Toledo, where he has served at different times as chairman of the Department of Psychology and director of the Clinical Psychology Program and has taught and supervised graduate students in psychotherapy for many years. He is a Diplomate in Clinical Psychology of the American Board of Professional Psychology. His cross-cultural experience includes Fulbright lectureships at Rangoon University in Burma and Chiang Mai University in Thailand. He has taught summer courses in Hong Kong and participated in the founding of the Association of Psychological and Educational Counselors in Asia.

Author Index

Subject Index

Abnormal behavior, medical model of, 270–272

Academic: difficulty for foreign students, 214, 226–227, 353; setting for foreign students, 210–212

Acceptance: passive, 34; of situations, 14–15

Accommodation, 14–15; for foreign students, 214, 222

Acculturation: as aid to therapy, 101–102; of Asian Americans, 142–149; and counseling usage, 338–339; as counseling variable, 186; for foreign students, 214, 222; and Hispanic diversity, 164–166, 168; in refugee counseling, 247–250

Acculturative: status, 200; styles, 195–200

Acquiescence: as response set, 308

Activity: and cultural values, 207–208, 302

Adaptation: as counseling goal, 160

Adaptive behavior models, use of folktales for, 346

Adaptive Behavior Scale. See Tests and scales

Adjective checklist. See Tests and scales

Adjustment, 225; to foreign cultures, 221, 223; problems, 214–217, 233–235; reactions, 246, 250–251; stress, 220–226

Affective: approach, 341; awareness, 40

African(s), 233, 317; psychology, 34, 89

Afro-American values, 34. See also Blacks

Aging, 171

Agism: and cultural bias, 161

Ajase complex, 148–149

Alcoholism: among American Indians, 178, 182, 194

Altered states: of consciousness, 36, 92

Alternative modes: of counseling, 23

Amaeru: and emic strategy in research, 12

Amerasian children: problems as refugees, 254–255

American Association for Counseling and Development (AACD), 120

American Indians, 98; behavioral therapy for, 284; counseling expectations of, 341, 346; and counselor credibility studies, 32; indigenous healing rituals of, 13; lack of service providers for, 122; legal definition of, 179; locus of control studies, 315; providing counseling for, 177–200; traditional healing systems of, 88

American Psychological Association: Accreditation Criterion II, 124–126; Committee on International Relations, 120–121; committee on professional standards, 127; Counseling Psychology Division, 123; Education and Training Committee, 39; Ethical Principles, 115–121, 124, 126, 128; program time, 26; Subcommittee on Culturally Sensitive Models, 38–39

American School Counselor Association, 120

Amok, 272

Analogue Procedures. See Tests and scales

Anthropological perspective, 23–24

Anxiety: assessment of, 316–317, 321; and lack of social skills, 274, 285; of minority clients, 70–71

Arts: and counselor training, 346

Asian Americans: behavioral therapy for, 284; and counselor credibility studies, 32; expectations of, as clients, 104; a model for counseling, 139–149; use of counseling services by, 338, 346

Assertiveness: as cultural dimension, 209–210

Assessment, 17, 299–324; diagnostic, 251–252

Assimilation: as acculturation stage, 248; in counseling approaches, 14–15; in counseling Asian-Americans, 142–149

391

Production Notes

This book was designed by Roger Eggers.
Composition and paging were done on the
Quadex Composing System and typesetting
on the Compugraphic 8400 by the design and
production staff of University of Hawaii
Press.

The text typeface is Baskerville and the display typeface is Compugraphic Optima.

Offset presswork and binding were done by
Vail-Ballou Press, Inc. Text paper is Writers
RR Offset, basis 50.